Multimodality Therapy
for Head and Neck Cancer

Multimodality Therapy for Head and Neck Cancer

Edited by

Gordon B. Snow, M.D., Ph.D.

Professor, Department of Otorhinolaryngology
Free University Hospital
Amsterdam, The Netherlands

and

John R. Clark, M.D.

Division of Clinical Oncology
Harvard Medical School
Dana-Farber Cancer Institute
Boston, Massachusetts, USA

with contributions by

Janet W. Andersen, M.S., Boston
S. B. Bader, M.D., Boston
H. Bartelink, M.D., Ph.D., Amsterdam
D. A. Bowdler, FRCS, London
P. M. Busse, M.D., Ph.D., Boston
J. R. Clark, M.D., Boston
L. Dewit, M.D., Ph.D., Amsterdam
F. Eschwège, M.D., Villejuif, France
H. T. Hoffman, M.D., Ph.D., Iowa City
W. K. Hong, M.D., Houston
J. Jassem, M.D., Gdansk

L. A. Kalish, D. Sc., Boston
R. B. Keus, M.D., Amsterdam
C. J. Krause, M.D., Ann Arbor
S. M. Lippman, M.D., Houston
B. W. Morrison, M.D., Boston
D. R. Parkinson, M.D., Bethesda
S. P. Schantz, M.D., New York
G. B. Snow, M.D., Ph.D., Amsterdam
P. M. Stell, Ch.M., FRCS, Liverpool
J. B. Vermorken, M.D., Ph.D., Amsterdam

17 illustrations, 41 tables

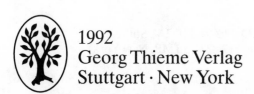

1992
Georg Thieme Verlag
Stuttgart · New York

Thieme Medical Publishers, Inc.
New York

Library of Congress Cataloging-in-Publication Data

Multimodality therapy for head and neck cancer /
  edited by Gordon Snow and John Clark ; with
  contributions by Janet W. Andersen . . . [et al.].
        p.   cm.
    Includes bibliographical references and index.
    1. Head--Cancer--Treatment.
    2. Neck--Cancer--Treatment.
    3. Squamous cell carcinoma--Treatment.
    4. Cancer--Adjuvant treatment.
  I. Snow, Gordon Brian.   II. Clark, John, 1953
  III. Andersen, Janet.
      [DNLM: 1. Combined Modality Therapy.
    2. Head and Neck Neoplasms--Therapy.
    WE 707 M9602]
    RC280.H4M83   1992
    616.99'49108--dc20
    DNLM/DLC
    for Library of Congress   92-3210
                                                  CIP

Important Note:

Medicine is an ever-changing science undergoing continual development. Research and clinical experience are continually expanding our knowledge, in particular our knowledge of proper treatment and drug therapy. Insofar as this book mentions any dosage or application, readers may rest assured that the authors, editors and publishers have made every effort to ensure that such references are in accordance with the state of knowledge at the time of production of the book.

Nevertheless this does not involve, imply, or express any guarantee or responsibility on the part of the publishers in respect of any dosage instructions and forms of application stated in the book. Every user is requested to examine carefully the manufacturers' leaflets accompanying each drug and to check, if necessary in consultation with a physician or specialist, whether the dosage schedules mentioned therein or the contraindications stated by the manufacturers differ from the statements made in the present book. Such examination is particularly important with drugs that are either rarely used or have been newly released on the market. Every dosage schedule or every form of application used is entirely at the user's own risk and responsibility. The authors and publishers request every user to report to the publishers any discrepancies or inaccuracies noticed.

Cover drawing by Renate Stockinger

© 1992 Georg Thieme Verlag, Rüdigerstrasse 14,
D-7000 Stuttgart 30, Germany
Thieme Medical Publishers, Inc.,
381 Park Avenue South, New York, NY 10016
Typesetting by Druckhaus Götz GmbH,
D-7140 Ludwigsburg
Printed in Germany by
Druckerei K. Grammlich GmbH
D-7401 Pliezhausen

ISBN 3-13-778801-3 (GTV, Stuttgart)
ISBN 0-86577-433-1 (TMP, New York)

1 2 3 4 5 6

Preface

It has long been recognized that patients with early stage squamous cell carcinoma of the head and neck (SCCHN) can in many instances be treated effectively by single modality surgery or radiotherapy, but that these modalities when used alone fail in the majority of patients with advanced disease. In an attempt to increase the effectiveness of therapy, planned combined radiation therapy and surgery gained popularity in the 1960s and today is considered standard local–regional treatment for patients with advanced staged squamous cell carcinoma at most sites within the head and neck. Local–regional control of disease has been further improved by developments in reconstructive surgery which allow wide surgical margins without excessive cosmetic or functional morbidities, and by recent refinement in radiation planning and dose delivery. However, this decrease in local–regional failure is not reflected in a proportionate increase in survival. As fewer patients die from uncontrolled disease of the head and neck, more are exposed to the risk of disseminated disease below the clavicles and the risk of second primary cancers in the respiratory and upper digestive tracts.

Since the 1970s chemotherapy has been used widely in the multidisciplinary treatment of patients with advanced SCCHN in an attempt to improve the survival of these patients by enhancing local–regional control as well as eliminating micrometastatic disease at distant sites. Unfortunately, despite progress in the development of increasing active regimens of chemotherapy, an improvement in survival after multidisciplinary treatment that includes chemotherapy has not been documented. A specific role for chemotherapy in the routine management of patients with advanced SCCHN remains uncertain. However, the great majority of studies evaluating multimodality treatment with chemotherapy suffer from serious methodologic shortcomings. SCCHN is not a single disease. Rather each site within the head and neck has its own natural history. In most studies carried out to date the various sites and stages of SCCHN are grouped together. This, as well as the insufficient sample sizes in many trials has precluded definite evaluation of chemotherapy.

In the first part of this book a state of the art overview of SCCHN is given. The natural history, prognostic factors, evaluation, and staging are reviewed. The principles of single modality treatment, surgery, and radiotherapy, are discussed, emphasizing their limitations and indicating areas in which advances of each of these modalities might be expected. Much attention is given to the biostatistical issues in the design and interpretation of clinical trials in SCCHN.

In the second and greater part of this book the principles and applications of the various multimodality treatments for patients with SCCHN are reviewed. The rationale and treatment strategies of combined surgery and radiotherapy are considered and controversial areas are identified. Multimodality therapy with chemotherapy in its various settings —neoadjuvant, adjuvant, or synchronous with radiotherapy—is critically assessed and strategies including chemotherapy which are most likely to benefit patients are indicated. Finally, therapies which are in development, such as immunobiological therapy and differentiation therapy, are reviewed.

The limiting factor in the development of multidisciplinary therapies of patients with SCCHN is not a deficiency in creative ideas or potentially effective treatment, but rather the availability of patients for clinical studies. New combinations and novel modalities are first evaluated in small phase I–II studies, but can only be assessed definitively in large well designed cooperative trials. The failure to consider patients for investigative treatment due to inappropriate pessimism, or false optimism with the injudicious use of "off-protocol" therapy must be discouraged. The probability that properly administered multimodality treatment can improve the natural history of SCCHN remains high.

We hope that *Multimodality Therapy for Head and Neck Cancer* will assist all oncologists towards a better understanding of the management of patients with advanced head and neck cancer, and will provide a stimulus and guide for the essential interdisciplinary approach required of all, surgical and nonsurgical specialists, involved in this complex field of oncology.

Amsterdam and Boston,   *Gordon B. Snow, M.D.*
January 1992   *John R. Clark, M.D.*

Addresses of Contributors

Janet W. Andersen, M.S., Biostatistician, Division of Biostatistics, Dana-Farber Cancer Institute, 44 Binney Street, Boston, MA 02115, USA

Stephen B. Bader, M.D., Radiation Oncologist, Joint Center for Radiation Therapy, Harvard Medical School, Boston, MA 02115, USA

Harry Bartelink, M.D., Ph.D., Professor, and Chairman, Department of Radiotherapy, The Netherlands Cancer Institute, Plesmanlaan 121, 1066 CX Amsterdam, The Netherlands

D. A. Bowdler, FRCS, Department of Otolaryngology/Head and Neck Surgery, Lewisham Hospital, High Street, Lewisham, London SE13 6LH, U.K.

Paul M. Busse, M.D., Ph.D., Assistant Professor of Radiation Oncology, Chief, Department of Radiation Oncology, Joint Center for Radiation Therapy, Harvard Medical School, 50 Binney Street, Boston, MA 02115, USA

John R. Clark, M.D., Instructor in Medicine, Medical Coordinator of the Head and Neck Tumor Clinic, Harvard Medical School, Dana-Farber Cancer Institute, 44 Binney Street, Boston, MA 02115, USA

Luc Dewit, M.D., Ph.D., Department of Radiotherapy, The Netherlands Cancer Institute, Plesmanlaan 121, 1066 CX Amsterdam, The Netherlands

François Eschwège, M.D., Professor and Chairman, Department of Radiotherapy, Institut Gustave Roussy, 39 Rue Camille Desmoulins, 94805 Villejuif Cedex, France

Henry T. Hoffman, M.D., Ph.D., Department of Otolaryngology/Head and Neck Surgery, The University of Iowa Hospitals and Clinics, Iowa City, IA 52242, USA

Waun K. Hong, M.D., Professor and Chief, Section of Head and Neck, Thoracic Medical Oncology, The University of Texas M.D. Anderson Cancer Center, 1515 Holcombe Blvd, Houston, TX 77030, USA

Jacek Jassem, M.D., Head, Radiotherapy Dept., Klinika Radioterapii, ul. Dębinki 7, 80.211 Gdansk, Poland

Leslie A. Kalish, D. Sc., Assistant Professor of Biostatistics, Harvard School of Public Health, Dana-Farber Cancer Institute, 44 Binney Street, Boston, MA 02115, USA

Ronald B. Keus, M.D., Department of Radiotherapy, The Netherlands Cancer Institute, Plesmanlaan 121, 1066 CX Amsterdam, The Netherlands

Charles J. Krause, M.D., Professor and Chairman, Department of Otolaryngology/Head and Neck Surgery, University of Michigan Hospitals, Ann Arbor, MI 48109, USA

Scott M. Lippman, M.D., Assistant Professor of Medicine, Department of Medical Oncology, The University of Texas M.D. Anderson Cancer Center, 1515 Holcombe Blvd, Houston, TX 77030, USA

Briggs W. Morrison, M.D., Clinical Fellow in Medical Oncology, Division of Clinical Oncology, Harvard Medical School, Dana-Farber Cancer Institute, 44 Binney Street, Boston, MA 02115, USA

David R. Parkinson, M.D., Head, Biologics Evaluation Section, Investigation Drug Branch, Cancer Therapy Evaluation Program, and Senior Staff Immunotherapy Service Surgical Branch, Division of Cancer Treatment, National Cancer Institute, Bethesda, MD, 28092, USA

Stimson P. Schantz, M.D., Associate Professor of Surgery, Head and Neck Surgery Service, Department of Surgery, Memorial Sloan-Kettering Cancer Center, 1275 York Avenue, New York, NY 10021, USA

Gordon B. Snow, M.D., Ph.D., Professor and Chairman, Department of Oto-Rhino-Laryngology, Free University Hospital, De Boelelaan 1117, 1081 HV Amsterdam, The Netherlands

Philip M. Stell, Ch.M., FRCS, Professor and Chairman, Department of Otolaryngology/Head and Neck Surgery, The Royal Liverpool Hospital, Prescot Street, P.O. Box 147, Liverpool L69 3BX, U.K.

Jan B. Vermorken, M.D., Ph.D., Department of Medical Oncology, Free University Hospital, De Boelelaan 1117, 1081 HV Amsterdam, The Netherlands

Contents

Introduction

1 Evaluation and Staging

G. B. Snow

Introduction

Thorough history taking and careful physical examination are the cornerstones of the evaluation of the patient with head and neck cancer. Special studies including high-technology imaging techniques, such as computed tomographic scanning, magnetic resonance imaging and echography, and endoscopy may provide important additional information on the extent of local and regional disease. It is debatable how far examinations aimed at detecting distant metastases are to be extended. In connection with the high overall incidence of second primary tumors in head and neck cancer patients, thorough inspection of the mucous membranes of the respiratory and upper digestive tracts through panendoscopy is commonly included in the initial work-up. Its benefits, however, are being questioned because the incidence of synchronous tumors is low. In contrast, surprisingly little attention is generally paid during follow-up to screening for second primary tumors, although the incidence of metachronous tumors is high.

To establish the true nature of the disease, in most instances a biopsy specimen is taken and sent for histopathologic examination. In certain situations for example, in patients presenting with a neck mass, aspiration cytology is an effective technique for establishing a tentative diagnosis.

The two most commonly applied systems for staging are those of the American Joint Committee on Cancer (AJCC) and of the International Union against Cancer (UICC). Until recently, these two systems displayed considerable differences, particularly regarding the staging of neck nodes. Their use of the same symbols T, N, and M for, respectively, the primary tumor, neck nodes, and distant metastases, consequently has led to much confusion. Therefore, it is gratifying to notice that the revised 1987 edition of the UICC classification is much closer to that of the AJCC than it has been in the past. Remember that both classification systems are primarily based almost exclusively on the anatomic extent of disease as determined clinically. As yet, biologic tumor markers and, more importantly, characteristics of the host are not included in these two systems.

When the diagnosis has been made and the patient's disease has been staged, treatment is planned. The choice of treatment is based primarily on the stage of the disease, but may have to be modified or altered if the general medical status or the psychosocial status of the patient necessitate so. As the majority of patients with squamous cell carcinoma of the head and neck are heavy cigarette smokers, cardiovascular and chronic respiratory diseases are common in this group. Many also suffer from alcohol abuse.

The various aspects of evaluation and staging are discussed in this chapter. As knowledge of the epidemiology and the natural history of head and neck cancer is considered important, these topics are briefly reviewed first. Much attention is paid to prognostic factors, as knowledge of prognostic factors is considered essential for evaluation and staging, as well as for the management of head and neck cancer patients. Unless otherwise stated, the following relates to squamous cell carcinoma only.

Epidemiology

Squamous cell carcinoma can occur anywhere in the mucous membranes of the head and neck. Generally the peak incidence is in the sixth and seventh decades of life. Oral (pharyngeal) cancer is one of the ten most common cancers in the world (1). Almost three-quarters of these cases occur in developing countries and in such countries it is the third most common cancer behind only cancers of the cervix and the stomach. In developed countries oral cancer ranks as the eighth most common cancer. Within this figure, however, there is a great deal of heterogeneity. In some areas of France, for example, oral cancer is the most common form of cancer. The disease is more common in males than in females. The sex ratio, however, varies considerably. In the United Kingdom, where incidence and mortality data are available over long periods of time, the incidence and mortality rates of tongue cancer have been declining steadily in this century. This fall is attributed almost entirely to a fall in the incidence in males (2). It is remarkable that in most developed countries in recent years both the incidence and the mortality in males are apparently rising (3). The increase in mortality is particularly observed among younger age-groups. A similar general pattern of increasing incidence is observed for cancers at other sites within the mouth as well as for cancers in the oro- and hypopharynx. The trends in females are difficult to interpret, since the disease is so much rarer.

The larynx is a site of cancer of rather low incidence in many countries. However, incidence rates are high among males in Brazil and in a number of European countries like France, Spain, Italy and Poland. The incidence is much lower among females. The higher male preponderance may be expected to relatively diminish as a direct consequence of increased smoking in the female population as already seen in carcinoma of the bronchus (4). In some areas there are quite substantial increases taking place in laryngeal cancer incidence (3). Between 1970 and 1980 the average annual age adjusted incidence rates per 100000 in males in Quebec rose from 6,5 to 10,4 in Sao Paulo from 14,1 to 17,8 and in Warsaw from 7,6 to 11,4. Again, the incidence rates among females appear to change less, but this may reflect difficulty in interpretation because of the low incidence rates in women.

It is very likely that the pathogenesis of head and neck cancer is multifactorial (5). In the developed countries both tobacco and alcohol are important risk factors for oral, oropharyngeal, hypopharyngeal, and laryngeal cancer. In southeast Asia the wide spread habit of chewing betel quid and areca nut are important in regard to oral and pharyngeal cancer. For both tobacco and alcohol consumption there is a strong dose−risk relationship, heavy smokers and drinkers carrying an increased risk as compared, respectively, to light smokers and drinkers (6−8). Among consumers of both products, the risk of oral and pharyngeal cancer tends to combine in a multiplicative, rather than in an additive fashion, the risk increasing 35-fold among those who consumed two or more packs of cigarettes and more than four alcoholic drinks per day, as compared to nonsmokers and nondrinkers (6). The relationship between cigarette smoking and cancer of the larynx has been demonstrated consistently (9). However, it has been noted that the incidence and mortality patterns for laryngeal cancer do not reflect trends in cigarette consumption in the manner that has been demonstrated for lung cancer. There is increasing evidence that alcohol consumption is also an important etiologic factor in cancer of the larynx (10, 11). The considerable variation in geographic distribution of laryngeal cancer within Europe—high incidence in the south versus low rates in the north-west—may be correlated to some extent with patterns of alcohol consumption, particularly wine. In this regard it appears important to note that in southern Europe, supraglottic cancer of the larynx is more common than glottic cancer, whereas the reverse is true for north-western Europe. The fact that laryngeal cancer rates are higher in Latin countries while lung cancer rates are higher in the United Kingdom and Benelux countries may also be related to the kinds of tobacco—black versus blond and nonfilter versus filter cigarettes—used (12, 13).

Recent epidemiologic and laboratory evidence has suggested that vitamins A and C and caretenoids may be protective against epithelial cancer (14−16). In a large population-based study of oral and pharyngeal cancer, the major finding was an inverse relationship with fruit intake (17). In another study a significant increased pharyngeal cancer risk associated with low intake of vitamin C from food was found (18). Occupational factors have long been suspected of playing a role, particularly in the etiology of laryngeal cancer. The evaluation of possible associations between occupation and laryngeal cancer requires separation of the confounding effects of tobacco and alcohol in view of their strong association with the disease. Evidence for an occupational association with laryngeal cancer among various workers is comprehensively reviewed by Maier et al. (19). Finally, it seems very likely that individual genetic susceptibility to the forementioned external carcinogens is important, if only because so many individuals have been and are being exposed, for instance, to tobacco and alcohol, whereas only relatively few actually develop cancer in the upper air and food passages. Advances in molecular biology and genetics provide the opportunity to explore the concept of genetic susceptibility to environmental carcinogenesis in this population (20−22).

Cancer of the nasopharynx has completely different epidemiologic characteristics. It is among the most common cancers in the Chinese, with the highest incidence rates for both sexes in Hong Kong and in areas of China bordering Hong Kong (23). The Epstein−Barr virus (EBV) has been implicated as a factor in its etiology (24). Substantial increases in risk have emerged in association with childhood consumption of salted fish and its use in weaning (25, 26).

Natural History

At the Primary Site

Spread at the primary site is dictated by local anatomy, and each anatomic site has its own peculiar spread patterns. Squamous cell carcinoma may extend superficially widely beneath intact mucosa. Invasion of muscle is a common feature, and tumor may spread along muscle and fascial planes for a surprising distance from the visible and palpable lesion. In particular, carcinoma of the mobile tongue is notorius for such spread.

It is not uncommon for squamous cell carcinomas of the head and neck and particularly those in the oral cavity to spread along perineural spaces (27). The site of the primary tumor is of major importance in determining the pattern of perineural spread. Once within perineural spaces, tumor cells can invade axially in either direction. This may have important surgical implications. However, clinical features suggesting perineural infiltration are by no means always found. It has been reported that patients with a carcinoma of the mobile tongue demonstrating perineural spread are at high risk of harboring occult nodal metastases in the neck (28).

A feature that has not received much attention is invasion of the microcirculation, although this is probably not uncommon in head and neck squamous cell carcinoma. It has been demonstrated that microvascular invasion by carcinoma cells correlates with an increased incidence of lymph node metastases (29). If discovered in the initial biopsy, this may be a reason to plan for more extensive treatment than would be indicated by the clinical stage alone.

A squamous cell carcinoma invades underlying bone or cartilage by a biphasic process (30). At first the tumor plays an indirect role, acting mainly by stimulating local osteoclasts. It is only after the osteoclastic response wanes that carcinoma cells themselves invade the bone. Bone and cartilage invasion are usually a late event.

Lymph Node Metastasis

Squamous cell carcinomas of the head and neck have a proclivity to metastasize to regional lymph nodes rather than to spread hematogenously. It is rare to observe distant metastases in patients who never suffered from nodal metastasis in the neck. However, it is not uncommon for patients with nodal metastasis to develop distant metastases, usually at a later stage.

The incidence of lymph node metastasis depends mainly on the site and size of the primary tumor. Depth of infiltration at the primary site is more important than surface area of the primary tumor for predicting the probability of cervical nodal metastasis (31). There is conflicting evidence on the role of the degree of histologic differentiation in this regard. The great majority of metastases to regional lymph nodes occur within 2 years following treatment of the primary tumor.

It is evident from clinical practice that lymph nodes quite often appear to be a very fertile soil for tumor growth. Everyone involved in head and neck oncology is only too familiar with patients presenting with a very small or even unknown primary tumor and a huge neck node metastasis. Also, tumor deposits in lymph nodes may have a surprisingly high growth rate. This is well demonstrated by patients with an initially clinically negative neck who, after treatment of the primary tumor only, may develop nodal metastases of substantial size between two follow-up visits that lie only a few weeks apart. This

is the main reason that patients with head and neck squamous cell carcinoma should have frequent follow-ups in the first 2 years after initial diagnosis.

The presence or absence of extranodal spread is of particular importance (see Prognostic Factors, below). The incidence of extranodal spread is about 55% (32, 33). Histologic judgement in this regard, however, may at times be difficult. In general, it has been thought that extranodal spread is limited to large nodes with clinical fixation. Although indeed nodal size correlates strongly with extranodal spread, it has been shown that extranodal spread does occur in a substantial percentage of small nodes as well (33–35). This appears to be in agreement with the demonstration that primary arrest of tumor emboli within the nodal capsule or juxtacapsular tissues rather than in the subcapsular sinus may lead to extranodal spread at a comparatively early phase in the progress of the disease (36).

The distribution of lymphatic metastasis is for the most part explicable in mechanical and anatomic terms (37). The filter and barrier function of lymph nodes usually appears to be effective in the initial stage as lymphatic spread initially is generally limited to the first echelon of lymph nodes. As a node is increasingly replaced by metastatic tumor, the local lymphatic flow will be distorted, reflected, and perhaps reversed, directing new lymph-borne tumor cells to fresh nodes. The cancerous node will itself act as a focus for further "tertiary" spread (38). This can occur via lymphatic vessels and via the bloodstream, not only through the large communications between the lymphatic and blood systems at the base of the neck, but also through small lymphaticovenous shunts or through full thickness invasion and penetration of the internal jugular vein by direct spread from adjacent nodal metastases (39).

Distant Metastases

It is not surprising that the rate of distant metastases correlates more with the appearance of cervical node metastasis than with the T-stage (40, 41). Eighty percent of distant metastases become manifest within 2 years after the appearance of nodal metastasis. The lungs are the most frequent site of distant metastases (45%) followed by the skeletel system (25%) (42).

Prognostic Factors

The prognosis of any patient with cancer is determined by three types of factor: those determined by the host, those by the tumor and those by the treatment. The effect of these three types of factor on death from head and neck cancer will be reviewed. Such a review has certain limitations. Firstly, it has been recognized for a long time that the prognosis of squamous cell carcinoma is different for the various sites within the head and neck. Ideally therefore, prognostic factors should be discussed for each of the head and neck sites separately. Such a discussion, however, would be too detailed for the scope of this chapter. This review will thus necessarily be limited to a discussion of prognostic factors common to all head and neck sites and only occasionally site-specific factors will be mentioned. Secondly, there is the problem that many of the prognostic factors are associated with each other, while few true multivariate analyses of prognostic factors for recurrence and survival have been carried out. Accurate information on the significance of each individual prognostic factor is therefore often lacking.

Host Factors

Age

There are at least five ways that age can affect survival (43). Firstly, the proportion of patients who can be treated falls with increasing age. Secondly, the death rate from second tumors rises with increasing age. Thirdly, the death rate from intercurrent disease rises with increasing age. Fourthly, the stage of presentation might change with age, and fifthly, there might be some fundamental biologic effect dependent on age which would influence the rate of growth of the tumor itself. Although the literature on this topic is conflicting, it appears that survival rates fall with increasing age (2, 44). It has been stated that prognosis is poor in the very young patients, particularly in children and young adults with carcinoma of the tongue (45, 46). However, it appears that it is the intrinsic characteristics of the tumor, its site and extent rather than the chronologic age of its host which determine the outcome of therapeutic efforts (47).

Sex

Survival in females with oral cancer is very much better than in males (2, 48). This is intriguing. It could not be demonstrated that this is so because females present with smaller lesions, at an earlier age, with an excess of tumor at favorable sites, or with more highly differentiated tumors (48). It has been suggested that hormonal, genetic, or immunologic differences could account for a better prognosis in females. Similarly, it has been recognized that females with laryngeal cancer carry a better prognosis compared to their male counterparts to such a degree that primary irradiation for all female patients irrespective of TNM staging has been advocated (49).

Likewise, in a large series of patients with carcinoma of the tonsil, sex could be identified as an important prognostic factor, females doing considerably better than males regardless of tumor stage or treatment modality (50).

Immunologic Competence

The immunoreactivity of head and neck cancer patients has been studied extensively in the past 15 years (51, 52). From the data it appears that cell-mediated immunity is seriously affected in these patients. Although many investigators have found correlations between deficiencies in cellular immunity and prognosis, assays of cellular immunity have found extremely limited clinical application.

It has been questioned whether the impairments in host defense mechanisms are direct reflections of tumor–host interaction. It has been demonstrated that cell-mediated immune functions are severely impaired in individuals who abuse alcohol (53). Similarly, a highly significant correlation has been found between nutritional status and defective cellular immunity (54). It is well known that many head and neck cancer patients are alcohol abusers. Also, malnutrition is a very common accompanying condition in head and neck cancer patients. This suggests that nutrition deficiency is of major prognostic value and that defects in immunocompetence are secondary phenomena. Also, it is a general clinical experience that patients who have lost considerable weight over a relatively short period of time carry a bad prognosis.

Attempts have also been made to assess the immunologic response of the host to head and neck cancer. Lymphocytic or inflammatory infiltrate in or around a tumor has been found to correlate with a favorable prognosis (55, 56). However, such parameters are difficult if not impossible to quantify. The occurrence of sinus histiocytosis and the presence or absence of reactive lymphocyte proliferation in regional lymph nodes have also been studied. Some investigators have found that lymphocytic stimulation correlates well with survival (57), others (58) could show no correlation between lymph node morphology and survival or metastasis.

Tumor Factors

T-factors

The site of the primary tumor within the head and neck and even within the same organ is of importance. This is well illustrated for patients with cancer of the larynx: patients with supraglottic carcinoma in general have a worse prognosis than patients with glottic carcinoma.

It is generally assumed that the size of the primary tumor influences prognosis. It may well be, however, that size in itself is not all that important. It has been found, for instance, in patients with oral cancer that the size of the primary tumor did not seem to affect 5-year survival except inasmuch as the larger tumors resulted in a higher rate of cervical metastasis and in this way affected prognosis (59).

N-factors

It is generally recognized that the status of the cervical lymph nodes is the single most important prognostic factor in squamous cell carcinoma of the head and neck (34, 42, 60, 61). When nodal metastases are present on admission or develop subsequently during follow-up, cure rates drop roughly by half. The following clinical parameters of nodal metastasis are of importance: size, number, fixation, and level. Laterality, that is, contralateral or bilateral metastases, appears to be of prognostic importance only in patients with strictly unilateral primary tumors, but does not seem to bear on prognosis in patients with tumors that are close to or cross the midline (33, 62). As clinical assessment of the status of the neck is far from accurate, it is not surprising that retrospective clinicopathologic analyses of large series of patients who underwent a radical neck dissection have demonstrated that histologic parameters are of much more prognostic reliability than clinical parameters (33–35, 60, 63–67). Extranodal spread (capsular rupture) and number of histologically positive nodes are of most prognostic significance in regard to failure in the neck and failure at distant sites. Patients who were found pathologically to have four or more positive nodes and extranodal spread had a greater than 60% likelihood of developing distant metastases (42). Likewise, it has been shown that the pathologic extent of nodal metastasis at neck dissection in terms of levels in the neck involved is a very sensitive prognostic indicator for distant metastases (68).

Histologic Pattern

It is traditionally held that the more differentiated the squamous cell cancer, the less likely it is to recur locally after treatment and to metastasize. An overall impression of the degree of differentiation is the method commonly used by pathologists (69). The assessment is based on the least differentiated parts of the tumor and three categories are distinguished: well differentiated, moderately differentiated, and poorly differentiated squamous cell carcinoma. For carcinoma of the larynx, support for the validity of this method has been provided by some pathologists (69). However, the method has serious shortcomings: it carries a large subjective element and it lacks quantitation. The well known Broders system (70) based on counting of differentiated cells meets part of this criticism, but is impracticable. More refined modifications—taking into account not only tumor

differentiation but also mitotic index and tumor host relationship in terms of mode of invasion—have been introduced (71), but have not found wide acceptance by pathologists. Regardless of the grading system used, one should realize that there may be differences in degree of differentiation from place to place in the same tumor and that therefore the biopsy may not be representative for the whole tumor. The value of histological grading for predicting prognosis and planning treatment has remained limited.

Ploidy

The first milestone in the study of ploidy in human malignancy was a paper by Atkin and Kay (72), based on 1465 tumors, in which they showed that patients with diploid tumors at all tumor sites except the uterine cervix had a better survival prospects than those with nondiploid tumors. At that time ploidy studies were done by static photometry. Flow cytometry was the next major step forward (73). The third milestone was the development of a method allowing the cellular DNA content of already fixed specimens to be assessed (74). The ploidy could thus be measured on previously treated patients and its relation to survival assessed. Reports on the relation of ploidy to head and neck squamous cell carcinoma have been controversial (75). Stell (76) recently has reviewed and meta-analysed the twenty-six series published to date, which address the relationship of ploidy to squamous cell carcinoma of the head and neck. Stells' analysis shows that about two-thirds of squamous cell carcinomas of the head and neck are nondiploid. There is no relation between host factors and ploidy. Tumors with a poorer degree of differentiation are more likely to be nondiploid, but there is no relation with stage group. Oral cancer patients with diploid tumors show improved survival when compared to patients with nondiploid tumors (77). The outcome in laryngeal cancer patients is not affected by ploidy and there were too few tumors at other sites to draw any conclusions. A surprising outcome of Stell's meta-analysis is that ploidy affected response neither to chemotherapy nor to radiotherapy. On the basis of this meta-analysis it appears that the prognostic significance of ploidy in head and neck cancer patients is limited.

Tumor Markers

During the course of the tumor development, quantitative changes occur in the level of a variety of substances in serum. Such substances are collectively referred to as tumor markers or biochemical serum markers. The origin of these markers could be from the tumor itself, as is the case with ectopic hormone secretion, oncofetal antigens, or excess of some metabolic products of these neoplastic cells. Alternatively, markers may be produced by the host in response to developing tumor. Potential uses of tumor markers include monitoring reduction in tumor mass, detecting recurrence of metastases after therapy, and predicting patient prognosis based on initial levels of marker or changes in serum levels after therapy (78). A perfect tumor marker should ideally have certain characteristics. Firstly, the marker used should have a high degree of sensitivity, as well as a high degree of specificity. Secondly, the level of the marker should correlate with tumor burden. Thirdly, the level of a marker should correlate with tumor biologic behavior and provide an additional prognostic index. To date, unfortunately, no such ideal marker has been found. The current status of serum markers of head and neck cancer has recently been reviewed extensively by Hanna et al. (79). In this section only the two most tested of the currently available markers will be discussed briefly: SCC-Ag and CEA. Both are tumor products secreted by the neoplastic cells. SCC is a tumor associated antigen. CEA is an oncofetal antigen.

Squamous cell carcinoma antigen (SCC-Ag) was first described in the sera of patients with squamous cell carcinoma of the uterine cervix (80). Elevated pretreatment levels of SCC-Ag are found in 38−53% of head and neck cancer patients (81, 82, 83). Pretreatment levels appear to correlate with tumor burden. The potential clinical value of SCC-Ag therefore lies in monitoring the course of the disease in patients with elevated pretreatment levels. However, Clasen et al. (82) point to the fact that pretreatment levels of SCC-Ag may vary considerably in the same individual when measured several times. Carcinoembryonic antigen (CEA) has been known since 1965 (84). Its clinical value for establishing prognosis and monitoring therapy has been demonstrated for carcinoma of the colon (85). Elevated pretherapeutic levels of CEA are reported in 28%−58% of head and neck cancer patients (86−87) depending on the chosen upper normal limit of serum CEA concentration. There appears to be a positive correlation between serum CEA levels and tumor size, but the evidence on monitoring treatment is conflicting. Importantly, the serum level of CEA is most probably mainly determined by the smoking habits of the patients (89).

From these two examples it is clear, as it is for all other tumor markers tested in head and neck cancer patients, that they have a low sensitivity. This means that a substantial number of patients with head and neck cancer fails to show any change in the level of these markers. Also most markers, like CEA, show a low degree of specificity, being elevated also in non-cancer bearing patients. Other disadvantages include the inconstant correlation with tumor burden for some markers. Taking into account that the great

majority of currently tested markers have been around for quite some time and still have not found routine acceptance, the role of these markers appears very limited, if useful at all. It has been suggested, however, that serial determination of a combination of markers may be of some value in monitoring head and neck cancer (79).

Treatment Factors

There is a voluminous literature on the conflicting methods of treatment for the various stages of cancer at the various sites within the head and neck. There is surprisingly little literature on the quality of the treatment administered, whereas it is generally recognized that treatment quality is an important factor for the final outcome of success or failure for the patient. The issue of treatment quality has recently been addressed in both the surgical and the radiotherapeutic literature, albeit from different points of view.

Loré (90) in a commentary in the *Archives of Otolaryngology−Head and Neck Surgery,* focused on the problem of the dabbler in head and neck oncology, defined as one who manages only a few patients with head and neck cancers a year. The major cause of this problem in the USA, according to Loré, is the practice of training excess numbers of physicians, including surgeons, radiotherapists, and medical oncologists in the field of head and neck surgery and oncology. To maintain one's expertise, one must have reasonable continuing experience. It is difficult to set exact numbers of patients, but it appears that to meet this criterion, any facility with a number of physicians in the various disciplines involved, should manage a minimum of 75−100 patients with head and neck cancer per year.

In the radiotherapeutic literature, the issue of quality control has received considerable interest in the last decade as a corollary of the increased use of multi-institutional controlled clinical trials. It was realized that what should be the strength of a collaborative study, namely its multicentricity, could also be its fundamental weakness, unless the intrinsic quality of the data presented by the participating centers could be guaranteed. Within the EORTC (European Organization on Research and Treatment of Cancer) the cooperative group of radiotherapy has carried out a quality control study including site visits among participating institutions in controlled clinical studies (91−93). It was found that there were substantial differences between institutions in equipment, treatment techniques, and dosimetry, which could seriously interfere with the reliability of the data and thus the results of controlled clinical trials. Recommendations for improvements were made and it was concluded that a quality insurance program must be included in controlled clinical trials. It is clear that this also emphasizes once more the importance of the quality of individual patient care.

One of the treatment associated prognostic factors which has received considerable interest in the last decade is the effect of blood transfusion on the recurrence and survival rates of cancer patients undergoing surgical resection. Burrows and Tartter (94) first reported in 1982 that intraoperative transfusion was associated with adverse effects on both the recurrence and the survival rates of patients with adenocarcinoma of the colon. However, some question exists as to whether this effect is seen in all types of cancer, whereas even in colorectal cancer conflicting results have been published. The mechanism of how blood transfusion affects tumor viability is still unclear, although the weight of evidence suggests that some type of immune suppression is involved. For head and neck cancer patients the issue has recently been addressed by Johnson et al. (95) and Jones and Weissler (96) through retrospective analyses. Johnson et al. found that blood transfusion is associated with reduced survivorship in patients undergoing surgery followed by postoperative radiotherapy. Such a correlation, however, was not demonstrable in patients treated by surgery alone. Jones and Weissler (96) carried out a multivariate analysis of sixteen risk factors for recurrence of head and neck cancer and found that the presence or absence of a blood transfusion is a statistically highly significant predictor of recurrence. Methodologically it is very difficult, if not impossible, to study the prognostic importance of blood transfusion prospectively and thus its precise role will remain unclear. However, the findings of Johnson et al. (95) and Jones and Weissler (96) should be taken seriously by all head and neck surgeons and emphasize the importance of keeping the amount of blood loss during surgery as low as possible, thus avoiding the need for blood transfusions.

Obviously there are many other treatment-related prognostic factors, such as the surgical margins in surgical treatment and the dose and fields of radiation therapy, but these factors will be discussed in another section of this chapter or in other chapters of this book.

Initial Evaluation

History

Evaluation starts with a thorough history taking. It is important that the physician is a good listener, that he takes ample time and makes the patient feel as comfortable as is possible under the circumstances. After the patient has presented the problem, the examiner directs more specific questions to the patient, depending on the (likely) site of the primary tumor. One should try to get an impression of the growth rate of the tumor, although unfortunately in many cases the patient will provide insufficient clues on this point. Questions pertaining to the patient's use of tobacco and alcohol with respect to both amount and duration are important. It is mandatory to ask the patient about any medical or surgical problems in the past and about any medications.

It is essential to seek information concerning the patients' psychosocial status. It is an inherent quality of man, particularly under these circumstances, to be in want of human attention. Patients will therefore in general appreciate questions about their work record and marital history. If the questions are put forward in a subtle and gentle way, the patient will usually loosen up. The way patients respond to these questions gives important information on how motivated they are to overcome their disease as well as on the support that they can expect from their families during and after treatment. A more thorough assessment of the patient's psychological status, if necessary, can best be carried out at the time of the patient's hospitalization.

Physical Examination and Special Studies of the Head and Neck

It is not within the scope of this chapter to describe in detail the specific techniques associated with the examination of the head and neck. It rather focuses on a number of aspects of both primary tumors at the various sites within the head and neck and nodal metastases in the neck, which need particular attention. In association with these aspects, those features of the examination and of the special investigations that have been found useful for their assessment are discussed. Furthermore, the accuracy and the reliability of some of the clinical and investigational findings are reviewed.

A division is to be made between patients presenting with a primary tumor and patients presenting with cervical nodal metastases of unknown origin. The latter situation is rare and demands a specific approach; this will be discussed separately. For the rest, the following relates to patients presenting with a primary tumor. Assessment of cancer at the two most commonly involved sites, the larynx and the oral cavity, will be reviewed in more detail than that of cancers at other sites.

Assessment of the Status of Neck Lymph Nodes

Clinical Assessment

The detection of nodal metastases is based on clinical assessment of deviation from expected normal size and a firmer-than-normal consistency (and/or reduced mobility) of regional lymph nodes at risk, and this is still based on palpation. The palpability of a lymph node depends on its location, size, and consistency, the type of neck, and the experience of the examiner. In a neck of average size and in the hands of an experienced examiner, the lower limit of palpability is approximately 0.5 cm in a superficial area, such as the submental or submandibular area, and 1 cm in a deeper area (97). Therefore, nodes containing small deposits of carcinoma may not be clinically palpable. A palpable node in the neck of a patient with a primary lesion in the head and neck region generally is considered to contain metastatic deposits. However, a normal-sized lymph node in an adult may vary from 2 mm to 2 cm. The latter could be readily palpable in any part of the neck, especially in the submental and submandibular area. Therefore, not all palpable nodes will be enlarged, and not all enlarged nodes contain metastatic deposits. Furthermore, large interobserver variations have been reported. It is not surprising therefore that the overall error in assessing the presence or absence of cervical lymph node metastasis is reported in the range of 20–30% (61, 97, 98). Nevertheless, in most institutions around the world, nodal disease in the neck is still staged on the basis of clinical examination only.

Also, it is useful to have a look at the accuracy of palpation regarding the various clinical prognostic parameters of nodal metastasis, such as size, number, and fixation. It is often surprising, judging from day-to-day practice in a large head and neck tumor clinic run by a group of head and neck surgeons, how subjective clinical assessment is in regards to size determination, particularly for nodal metastases in deeper areas, such as the subdigastric area. Regarding the number of clinically involved nodes, palpation is unreliable (33). This holds particularly true for the situation of a clinically solitary enlarged node: in nearly 20% of patients the node is tumor negative on histologic examination, whereas in about 30% of patients more than one positive node is found; in other words, the diagnosis is correct in only approximately 50% of the cases. When it appears that more than one node is involved clinically, the situation is not as bad: there is a 75% chance of a correct diagnosis. The term "fixation" or "fixed" is by no means clearly defined. Some reserve this term for lymph nodes that are immobile and fixed to the underlying muscles; others include nodes that demonstrate reduced mobility. Because of this dilemma and the subjective nature of this parameter, it has been dropped from the latest UICC classification. Nevertheless, it has been shown to have a statistically significant relation with extranodal spread and as such to be of prognostic significance (33).

Other Methods

The question arises whether modern imaging techniques like CT scanning, MR imaging, or ultrasonog-raphy can do better than palpation for the assessment of neck nodes. The majority of reports derive from clincan's experience using CT scanning. In most studies, the use of CT compares favorably to palpation in assessing the status of the lymph nodes; the overall error rates ranges from 7.5 to 19% (99–102). Only one publication cites an overall error rate of 28% with use of CT (103). Furthermore, CT is certainly more accurate than palpation in determination of size and number of involved nodes, which are important parameters in the UICC and AJCC staging classifications. Moreover, CT scans provide a permanent document of the status of the neck.

A problem is, that many different radiologic criteria are being used to assess the presence or absence of metastasis in cervical lymph nodes (99–105). The criteria include the maximal axial diameter, the irregular enhancement due to tumor necrosis, and the shape and the grouping of nodes. The difference in criteria used account in part for the difference in reported overall error rates. Most authors define their criteria by retrospective radiologic–histopathologic correlation. Such retrospective comparison obviously has many disadvantages. Recently, van den Brekel et al. (106) reported on a careful prospective study assessing the radiologic criteria. These authors reemphasize that irregular contrast enhancement in the nodes, which can be caused by tumor necrosis, cystic tumor growth, or keratinization, is the most specific criterion for metastatic growth, although occasionally it can be mimicked by centrally located adipose metaplasia. It is to be realized, however, that contrast-enhanced CT or MR imaging with a section thickness of 3–6 mm can only detect central necrosis measuring 3 mm or larger. Furthermore, these authors found that the minimal diameter in the axial plane is the most accurate size criterion for predicting lymph node metastasis. A minimal axial diameter of 10 mm was determined the most effective size criterion. The size criterion for lymph nodes in the subdigastric region was 1 mm larger (11 mm). Groups of three or more "borderline" nodes were proved to increase the sensitivity. It is hoped that the radiologic criteria as defined by van den Brekel et al. (106) will find general acceptance.

Much less experience assessing neck nodes has been gained with MR imaging. The freedom of parameter choice with this technique allows the same tissue to be depicted in various ways and the contrast to surrounding tissues to be manipulated. In a search for ways better to localize lymph nodes, a recently obtained MR technique, gradient–echo imaging, is very promising. Furthermore, administration of gadolinium in conjunction with the use of gradient-echo technique constitutes a very sensitive tool for demonstrating metastatic tumor in lymph nodes (107). Using these MR techniques and applying the forementioned radiologic criteria (106) van den Brekel et al. (108) compared prospectively MR findings and clinical staging (palpation) with the histopathologic findings in a series of 100 patients undergoing 136 neck dissections. The overall error of palpation and MR imaging was respectively 32% and 16%. MR reliably upstaged 60% of the clinically negative necks. MR was thus found to improve the preoperative staging of the neck.

The introduction of hig-resolution real-time equipment has increased the role of ultrasonography in the exploration of small body parts. Continuous advances in ultrasonography have made the technique more sensitive in the detection of lymph nodes (105, 109, 110). Several ultrasonographic size criteria have been developed for detection of neck nodes (5−8 mm). However, differentiation between benign and metastatic nodes is not possible. Ultrasonographically guided fine-needle aspiration cytology is an effective technique and has a high diagnostic significance in the assessment of the neck, with a low rate of complications (111).

From the foregoing it can be concluded that CT, MRI, and ultrasound-guided aspiration cytology can all three improve the preoperative staging of the lymph nodes in the neck in head and neck cancer patients. Studies comparing these three methods are ongoing. It is hoped that the best and most cost-effective method for the assessment of the neck nodes will emerge from these studies shortly.

A different approach to the problem of small cancer deposits in cervical lymph nodes is radioimmunolocalization using monoclonal antibodies against cell surface antigens of squamous cell carcinoma. When tagged with isotopes, these antibodies may be used for diagnosis. However, production of monoclonal antibodies against cell surface antigens of squamous cell carcinoma in general and in head and neck patients in particular has been found to be extremely difficult (112). Only recently Quak et al. (113) have been able to develop a monoclonal antibody, E48, that has strong and selective reactivities to squamous cell carcinoma and thus appears very promising for radioimmunoscintigraphy in humans.

Assessment of Oral Cancer

In the assessment of the extent of primary cancers in the oral cavity, three aspects are of particular importance: depth of infiltration, relationship to the mandible, and the status of the oral mucosa. To begin with the last, oral cavity carcinoma is quite often associated with leukoplakic and erythroplakic changes of the mucosa in the vicinity of the tumor. To determine the extent of such changes, the use of the operating microscope can at times be helpful.

Depth of Infiltration

Most important is the assessment of the depth of infiltration. This can be done best by digital palpation and, for a carcinoma of the tongue, by careful evaluation of the mobility of the tongue. Whenever doubt exists about the true extent of the tumor in this regard, local examination under general anesthesia should be performed. This is particularly helpful when the lesion is painful or posteriorly situated in the oral cavity.

Relationship to Mandible

In tumors of the inferior complex of the oral cavity, consisting of the tongue, the floor of the mouth, and the lower gum, a potential problem is that of management of the mandible. From the point of view of mandible, patients fall into three categories: those with gross invasion, in whom resection is inevitable, those with a degree of involvement, and those in whom there is still a measurable distance of a few millimeters of normal mucosa between the gross edge of the lesion and the mandible. In most patients in the last two categories mentioned above, a more conservative management of the mandible, marginal mandibulectomy, is to be considered.

Whether marginal mandibulectomy can be carried out safely depends on the relationship between the tumor and the mandible. In this regard, it is significant whether the patient is edentulous or not. First, the edentulous mandible looses considerable height after resorption of the alveolar element of the mandible, and this by itself makes marginal mandibulectomy hazardous from the technical point of view. Second, the edentulous occlusal ridge that forms fails to develop a complete covering of cortical bone and it is through this ridge that tumors easily enter the bone (114). Moreover, the inferior dental canal is no longer sited deeply in the body of the mandible but lies close to the alveolar mucosa. Consequently, a tumor involving bone may readily spread along the inferior dental nerve. The presence or absence of bone involvement is traditionally assessed by radiology. However, conventional imaging techniques including panoramic radiography, bone scans, and computed tomography can be unreliable in defining the extent of neoplastic marrow invasion. Magnetic resonance imaging appears to be superior to these methods for the evaluation of tumor invasion of the mandible (115). The relationship between a tumor and the mandible is best assessed by bimanual palpation, preferably under general anesthesia.

The appraisal of the defect likely to result after excision is important in terms of its several components, mucosa, soft tissue, and bone, so that a general outline of the ensuing reconstructive procedure can be made if necessary. Whenever a segmental resection of the mandible or maxillectomy is envisaged, this appraisal should be carried out with a dentist to allow for preparation of necessary appliances. The dentist should also be utilized heavily to evaluate the remaining dentition as well as the oral soft tissues. Frequently, dental restorations and extractions must be carried out prior to, or in concert with, the treatment program.

Assessment of Laryngeal Cancer

Indirect and direct laryngoscopy and conventional radiologic techniques are traditionally the cornerstones in the examination of the larynx. However, these methods each have their limitations. The introduction of CT in the 1970s and of MRI in the 1980s has greatly enhanced our diagnostic potential for the assessment of the extent of laryngeal cancer in that both methods are capable of visualizing tumor extension in the horizontal or axial plane deep to the laryngeal mucosal surface.

Indirect Laryngoscopy

Indirect laryngoscopy offers an excellent preliminary overall survey of the larynx. However, its limitation is the inaccessibility of certain recesses of the larynx, such as the undersurface of the ventricular bands, the lateral extent of the ventricles, the undersurface of the vocal cords, the postcricoid region and the apex and medial wall of the piriform sinuses. In addition, there are variations in patients' response to the procedure of mirror examination, and in some patients anatomic factors, such as an overhanging infantile epiglottis, interfere with mirror examination. For these patients the recent introduction of the small flexible fiberoptic laryngoscope is a breakthrough in our diagnostic armamentarium. After topical anesthesia of the mucous membranes of the nose, oropharynx, and larynx, this scope can be introduced readily through the nose, permitting an adequate view of the intralaryngeal structures.

Radiologic Examinations

Radiographic studies should be done before direct laryngoscopy and biopsy, because these procedures may cause anatomic changes. The following radiologic techniques are most commonly used: conventional frontal tomography, CT, and MRI. In early glottic cancers, T1 and "small" T2, conventional frontal tomography is usually still sufficient. In larger glottic tumors, frontal tomography provides a good demonstration of tumor size. However, cartilage destruction and extralaryngeal extension cannot be visualized by this technique. Because of these limitations, frontal tomography has been superseded by CT or MRI in the evaluation of large tumors.

CT is of particular value in the visualization of the preepiglottic space, the thyroid cartilage, and the extralaryngeal soft tissues and of tumor infiltration into these structures (116). However, CT too has its limitations. It often fails in detecting minor cartilage invasion owing to extreme variations in calcifications. Calcified cartilage invaded by cancer is frequently seen by CT as having an intact contour (117, 118). On the other hand, tumor approaching nonossified cartilage may simulate cartilage invasion (119, 120).

An advantage of MRI over CT is its ability to provide multiplanar images: the laryngeal structures can be visualized in transverse, sagittal, and frontal planes. Moreover, MRI appears superior to CT in detecting minor invasion of laryngeal cartilages (121, 122). MRI therefore will play an increasingly important role in the diagnostic work-up of laryngeal cancer patients. MRI images, however, are much more difficult to read than CT images, particularly for the clinician, and this will probably somewhat delay widespread acceptance of MRI as an important tool for the assessment of the extent of laryngeal cancer.

Direct Laryngoscopy

Direct laryngoscopy with rigid tubes is usually performed under general anesthesia. It is important that the anesthetic technique provides an unobstructed view of the lesion. For small glottic cancers, it may be helpful for accurate delineation of the lesion to use the operating microscope through the suspension laryngoscope, which can be fixed to the anterior chest wall. In most instances, and particularly in the more advanced tumors, a more versatile endoscope is advantageous. With the tip of the scope placed intraluminally and a hand placed externally on the thyroid cartilage, all recesses of the larynx can be inspected. By palpating the tumor mass with the tip of the suction tube, one can estimate the degree of infiltration in depth. After the extent of the tumor is assessed, the tumor is then biopsied. In supraglottic cancers spreading to the vallecula, digital palpation of the base of the tongue is important in order to detect submucosal tumor extension in this area; this is best done after the completion of the direct laryngoscopy when the patient is still under general anesthesia.

Assessment of Pharyngeal Cancer

Cancer of the Nasopharynx

Fiberoptic endoscopy is a great improvement in the examination of the nasopharynx and is rapidly replacing mirror examination. The nasopharynx has a very close relationship to the base of the skull. Direct infiltration of the skull base with cranial nerve involvement is common. Cranial nerve examination and CT scanning of the base of the skull are routinely performed.

Cancer of the Oropharynx

The oropharynx includes the base of the tongue, the tonsillar area, the soft palate, and the posterior pharyngeal wall. Except for the rare early lesions, examination under general anesthesia is usually carried out permitting careful palpation of the tumor area. This is particularly important for the assessment of the extent of involvement of the base of the tongue. CT and MRI have proven extremely valuable for the determination of soft tissue extension and for the detection of nodal metastases in the parapharyngeal and retropharyngeal spaces, which are not accessible to palpation (123).

Although the mandible and the maxilla are usually not invaded by cancer, the relationship of the tumor to one or both of these structures is often so close that portions of these structures must be encompassed within the resection specimen. When this is envisaged, a dentist should be involved to prepare appropriate appliances, if these are found necessary.

Cancer of the Hypopharynx

The hypopharynx consists of the piriform sinuses, the postcricoid area, and the posterior pharyngeal wall. On presentation, carcinoma of the hypopharynx is usually well advanced and it is easily recognized by indirect laryngoscopy. However, accurate assessment of the extent of the lesion is often difficult because cancer of the hypopharynx has a tendency to spread submucosally. Also, it may have "skip areas". A barium swallow esophagogram is essential to evaluate involvement of the cervical esophagus. CT or MRI are very useful in demonstrating extension into the larynx, the neck, and posteriorly into prevertebral fascia. Direct laryngoscopy and hypopharyngoscopy are performed routinely, most importantly for determination of the distal extent of the tumor as well as depth of penetration in cases of cancer of the posterior wall.

Assessment of Paranasal Sinus Cancer

The complex anatomy of this region accounts for easy spread between the nose and other sinuses via innumerable foramina and fissures. The assessment of these tumors relies almost exclusively on imaging techniques, that is, CT (124) and MRI (125). Particularly, destruction of small bony structures is well seen on CT (126). However, CT does not differentiate between tumor and nontumor soft tissues. MRI is superior to CT in that regard, as it is particularly capable of differentiating tumor from inflammatory changes on T2 weigthed images (127, 128). However, small bony structures are not well seen on MRI (129). Therefore, MRI does not replace CT, but it is a valuable complementary procedure for the diagnostic work-up of paranasal sinus tumors.

Assessment of Cervical Nodal Metastasis of Unknown Origin

It is important to distinguish between patients who present with nodal metastases in the upper neck and those with cervical nodal metastases in the lower neck. In the first group, the primary tumor is very likely to be found within the head and neck, whereas metastases in the supraclavicular fossa more likely originate from a primary tumor below the clavicles. The following relates to the first group.

A complete history and physical examination is performed with emphasis on a thorough otolaryngologic examination. If this work-up is negative, aspiration cytology of the neck mass is carried out (130). If metastatic squamous cell carcinoma is found, endoscopy of the upper air and food passages is performed. The nasopharynx, tonsil, base of the tongue, supraglottic larynx, and piriform fossa are common sites of primary tumors. In this situation, special attention is paid to these areas. Palpation under general anesthesia of the oropharynx is important. All suspicious areas should undergo biopsy. Selected random biopsies (so-called "blind" biopsies) can be taken from areas of high probability based on the predictibility of lymphatic drainage. Homolateral tonsillectomy has also been advised as a routine procedure in this situation (131).

Open (excisional) biopsy of the neck mass is rarely needed. The most common situation in which this is indicated is when the cytology findings reveal malignancy but the pathologist is not sure about its nature. The node should be sent immediately to the laboratory. Special tests can then be carried out which can differentiate between, for instance, carcinoma or lymphoma.

Screening for Second Primary Cancers

Definition and Incidence

There is a growing interest in multiple primary tumors in head and neck cancer patients (132). This reflects the increased incidence of second cancers, which probably results from the fact that as fewer patients die from uncontrolled cancer in the head and neck today as compared with 30 years ago, more patients are exposed to the risk of developing a second primary cancer. For analysis of the occurrence of multiple primary tumors, it is common practice to use the criteria proposed by Warren and Gates (133). Furthermore, it has been proposed to regard solitary lung tumors appearing in patients treated successfully for laryngeal cancer as being primary lung malignancies if the index larynx tumor was T1 or T2 without lymph node metastases and without signs of local or regional recurrence (134). Skin tumors, carcinoma in situ lesions or carcinomas found at autopsy as second primary tumors are usually not included for analysis.

The incidence of multiple primary tumors varies from 10–35% (135–138). The great majority of these second primary tumors in head and neck cancer patients occur in the respiratory tract and in the upper digestive tract, including the esophagus. In index tumors of the upper digestive tract, for instance, in the oral cavity or oropharynx, the second primary tumor is relatively frequently also in the digestive tract, whereas in laryngeal cancer patients, the second primary frequently appears in the respiratory tract. This might be explained by common etiologic factors, such as smoking and alcohol consumption. The great majority of second primary tumors occur metachronously, that is more than 6 months after the diagnosis of the index tumor. Surprisingly, the interest in practical terms of early detection of the second primary tumor through panendoscopy has almost exclusively focused on initial evaluation. Also, little attention has been given to high-risk groups.

High-Risk Groups

First, remember that findings in one patient population, in view of geographic differences in exposure to carcinogens, do not necessarily apply to other patient populations. Nevertheless, in our material more second primary tumors occur in patients with oral cancer than in patients with laryngeal cancer (138). Probably the incidence is highest for patients with cancer of the hypopharynx. In laryngeal cancer patients the incidence is 14% in all sites and 10% in the lung (139). The following subgroups of laryngeal cancer patients carry an even higher risk of developing lung cancer: patients with supraglottic cancer as compared to those with glottic cancer (139–141), males versus females (139), and those continuing smoking versus those stopping (142). In oral cancer, more second primary tumors appear to occur in patients with an index tumor in the lower part of the oral cavity (lower part: floor of mouth, inferior alveolar process, and retromolar trigone) than in the rest of the oral cavity (tongue, buccal mucosa, and palate) and in males than in females (138).

Recently, it has also been demonstrated that the occurrence of second primary tumors in head and neck cancer patients is also related to certain immunoglobulin allotypes; patients who lack immunoglobulin light-chain marker Km(1) are higher at risk than Km(1)-positive patients (143). Furthermore, there is a relationship to certain HLA antigens; head and neck cancer patients with HLA-B8, HLA-DR3, and HLA-DQw2 are especially at risk (144).

Panendoscopy

The incidence of simultaneous primary tumors as reported in the literature varies considerably: from 2.5% up to as high as 25% (145–148). The panendoscopy is the only way to detect these tumors in roughly half the cases. Accordingly, panendoscopy at initial work-up is advocated by some and questioned by others. The reported differences in incidence might be related to endoscopic techniques. The group from Switzerland reporting the above quoted incidence of 25% routinely uses supravital staining with toluidine-blue for screening of early second primary cancer in the pharynx and the esophagus and indeed find the majority of second primary tumors at these sites, regardless of the localization of the index tumor. It is not unlikely, however, that the role of the upper digestive tract as the site of second primary tumors is more important in some of the more Southern European countries such as Switzerland and France than it is in Northwestern Europe and North America, where the lung is more important as the site of second primary tumors, particularly when the index tumor is in the larynx. For instance, in a series of 748 patients with a laryngeal carcinoma, we did not encounter a single case of second primary cancer in the esophagus (139). Accordingly, we do not routinely perform esophagoscopy in laryngeal cancer patients. However, a barium swallow is done in all patients, and in those in whom the esophagograph shows abnormalities, esophagoscopy will then be carried out.

A thorough examination of the mucous membranes of the head and neck for detection of second primary tumors should be performed routinely in all patients at initial work-up. In general, panendoscopy is advocated for all heavy smokers and drinkers, regardless of the site of the primary tumor. For the rest, risk factors are to be taken into account when screening for secondary tumors is considered at initial work-up. For instance, in laryngeal cancer patients bronchoscopy should always be carried out. In oral cancer patients we take sex and site of the index tumor into account. Aged women with no history of smoking and drinking and with a primary tumor in the buccal mucosa, for instance, will have neither esophagoscopy nor bronchoscopy.

Pathological Evaluation

It is essential that the pathologist and the head and neck physician, whether surgeon, radiation therapist, or medical oncologist, develop a cooperative relationship. This is especially so for the head and neck where the anatomy is difficult and tumors are among the most complex found anywhere in the human body. The latter holds particularly true for the rarer types of tumor, occurring in the head and neck, such as salivary gland tumors, sarcomas, etc. This section will be limited to a brief discussion of the histopathologic aspects of squamous cell carcinoma. For more extensive reviews, including the rarer tumor types, the reader is referred to the excellent textbooks on head and neck pathology by Batsakis (149) and Barnes (150).

The tissue diagnosis of invasive squamous cell carcinoma arising from the mucous membranes of the head and neck is generally straight forward. However, it is the surgeon's responsibility that the tissue biopsy obtained is representative. Ideally, the biopsy specimen should include both normal and abnormal tissue. The biopsy therefore is preferably taken from the margin rather than from the necrotic center of the tumor. In general, the biopsy material can be placed in a regular fixative. However, if the differential diagnosis includes malignant lymphoma, it is important that the biopsy material is delivered immediately to the pathologist in an unfixed state to allow testing for T- and B-cell markers. When tumors appear anaplastic or undifferentiated on routine histologic sections, newer techniques based primarily on immunohistochemistry are being used to study the tumor specimens. These methods rely on the binding of specific antibodies to cellular antigens in order better to define the tumor according to cell type (151, 152).

The pathologic evaluation of a surgical specimen should contain information on the extent of disease, on the status of the surgical margins, and on any other histologic features that are of prognostic importance, such as perineural spread and microvascular invasion at the primary site and extranodal spread in the neck. As the status of the lymph nodes in the neck is the single most important prognostic factor in squamous cell carcinoma of the head and neck, it is mandatory that the pathology report provides accurate data on number and size of metastatic nodes, levels of involved nodes (153), presence —gross or microscopic— or absence of extranodal spread (33, 35, 42), as well as the total number of lymph nodes examined. The last item gives an indication of the thoroughness of the investigation. In head and neck cancer, little attention has so far been paid to the method of sampling of the lymph nodes from the specimen by the pathologist: conventional versus serial sectioning. Saska and McDonald (154) in a recent study concluded that the small additional yield from examination of multiple blocks of each node does not justify the extra work involved.

The aim of surgical treatment of cancer is complete excision with adequate surgical margins if cure is to be expected. Although negative surgical margins do not guarantee a favorable outcome, positive surgical margins are associated with significantly increased local (regional) recurrence and mortality rates (155, 156). What constitutes positive or negative surgical margins lacks standardization (157). Irrefutable microscopic evidence is the presence or absence of invasive carcinoma at the margins. In a study from the Memorial Hospital in New York it has been shown that carcinoma in situ, or severe dysplasia at the margin or invasive carcinoma close to the margin (within 0,5 cm), also carry a high risk of recurrence and mortality (155). Frozen section evaluation can be helpful to obtain free margins of excision (158), but is has been observed that patients who had positive margins on initial frozen section examination and who were subsequently rendered negative at the completion of the procedure, still had a significantly increased local recurrence rate and decreased survival when compared with patients similarly treated with surgery alone, who had initially negative margins (159). It will be clear that in all the forementioned instances of positive or doubtful margins, additional therapy if possible is needed.

General Evaluation

Other Serious Diseases

Many patients with head and neck cancer are of advanced age and have a variety of other serious diseases. In particular, the incidence of chronic obstructive pulmonary disease and of cardiovascular disease is high. A majority of patients are heavy smokers and many use alcohol excessively. Some have associated liver disease. Operations for cancer of the head and neck may be limited, but often they are major procedures. Irradiation is often referred to as a type of conservative treatment when compared to surgery, but in fact irradiation of large fields in the head and neck is far from easily tolerated by the patients. It is of paramount importance therefore to identify other serious diseases and to bring the general condition of the patients to its most favorable state before instituting treatment. Total evaluation of the patient requires a multidisciplinary approach and the liberal use of consultants is recommended.

Psychosocial Status

Evaluating the patient's psychosocial status may be more difficult than evaluating the physical status. Many head and neck cancer patients are alcoholics. It is important to identify these patients, so that appropriate measures can be taken to prevent serious postoperative problems. However, they are often by no means easy to identify, as they usually minimize and deny their problem. It is highly recommended to involve a psychiatrist at an early stage when such difficulties are anticipated.

Nutritional Status

Awareness of the necessity of proper nutritional support is critical in the management of patients with head and neck cancer. These patients often have a history of poor dietary habits, which may be associated with alcoholism, resulting in protein, vitamin, and mineral deficiencies. Head and neck cancer itself can cause an insufficient dietary intake because of pain on swallowing and inability to chew properly. As a result, patients with head an neck cancer are often protein–calorie malnourished at the time the tumor is diagnosed and they are admitted to undergo surgical treatment. Major operative therapy puts a metabolic stress on the patient at the time when food intake is absent, and surgical therapy for head and neck cancer in particular often results in diminished oral intake for a prolonged period. In addition, subsequent irradiation is often required, which produces oral mucositis and diminished salivary secretions and may thus further decrease oral intake. A vicious catabolic cycle may readily result, which greatly enhances the risk of complications of treatment. The same holds true when primary irradiation is considered. Every effort, therefore, should be taken to restore the patient's nutritional condition and maintain it at an optimal level.

Metastatic Work-up

It is common practice to omit a diligent search for distant tumor deposits, probably because head and neck cancer poses predominantly a locoregional problem. Usually only a chest radiograph and liver function studies are done, which will be performed anyway within the framework of the preoperative work-up. Patients with extensive nodal disease in the neck, that is multiple nodes at multiple levels or huge tumor masses with extranodal spread, carry a high risk of distant metastases (42). In such patients, a metastatic work-up should be done. Taking into account that the lungs, the skeletal system, and the liver are the sites of predilection of distant metastases in head and neck cancer patients, such work-up includes CT scanning of the lungs, bone scanning, and liver scanning.

Classification and Staging

They are called wise who put things in their order.
—Thomas Aquinas

Purpose

The practice of dividing cancer patients into groups according to so-called stages arose from the fact that survival rates were higher for patients in whom the disease was localized than for those in whom the disease had extended beyond the organ of origin. These groups were often referred to as early cases and late cases, implying some regular progression with time. Actually, the stage of disease at the time of diagnosis may be a reflection not only of the rate of growth and extension of the neoplasm but also of the type of tumor and of the tumor–host relationship.

Staging of cancer is a method of gathering groups of classified patients for the purpose of analysis. Recording accurate information on the extent of disease for each site serves a number of related objectives: to aid the clinician in the planning of treatment, to give some indication of prognosis, to assist in evaluation of the results of treatment, to facilitate the exchange of information between treatment centers, and to contribute to the continuing investigation of human cancer. The principal purpose to be served by international agreement on the classification of cancer patients by extent of disease is to provide a method of conveying clinical experience to others without ambiguity (160).

History

The TNM system for the classification of malignant tumors was developed by Pierre Denoix of France in 1943. In 1953, agreement was reached between the International Union against Cancer (Union Internationale Contre le Cancer, UICC) and the International Congress of Radiology on a general technique for classification by *anatomic extent of disease*, using the TNM system. In 1954, the UICC set up a special committee on clinical stage classification and applied statistics to extend this general technique for classification to cancer at all sites. This committee became later known as the TNM committee. Between 1958 and 1967, the committee published nine brochures describing proposals for the classification of twenty-three sites. The committee recommended that for each site an initial 5-year trial period be undertaken. In 1968, these brochures were combined in a pocket book, which was translated into eleven languages. In 1974 and 1978, second and third edition were published, containing new site classifications and amendments to previously published classifications. The third edition was enlarged and revised in 1982. Over the years, some users introduced variations in the rules of classification of certain sites. To correct this development, the national TNM committees in 1982 agreed to formulate a single TNM system. A series of meetings was held to unify and update classifications as well as to develop new ones. The result is the 1987 fourth edition of the UICC TNM booklet (160).

The American Joint Committee on Cancer (AJCC) was first organized in 1959 as the American Joint Committee for cancer staging and end results reporting (AJC), for the purpose of developing a system of clinical staging of cancer by site that was acceptable to the American medical profession. The AJC decided to use the TNM system, where applicable, to describe the anatomic extent of the cancer at the time of diagnosis and from this information to develop a classification into stages, which would be useful as a guide to treatment and prognosis and in comparing the end results of treatment. Retrospective studies have resulted in recommendations for stage classifications for cancer at various sites, which have been published in separate fascicles. These were brought together to form a *Manual for Staging of Cancer*, published in 1977. This was revised and reprinted in 1978 and reprinted again in 1980. A second edition appeared in 1983 and a third edition in 1988 (161).

The TNM committee of the UICC and AJCC have been working along similar lines and with similar objectives, although points of view and methods sometimes have differed. The TNM committee and the AJCC have attempted to come to agreement on staging of cancer at all anatomic sites. The recommendations of AJCC and UICC are now identical and thus, an international system of staging cancer is available.

General Rules

The rules of classification and stage grouping according to UICC correspond exactly with those appearing in the third edition of the AJCC *Manual for Staging of Cancer* (1988). The TNM system for describing the anatomic extent of disease is based on the assessment of three components:

T – extent of primary tumor
N – status of regional lymph nodes
M – presence or absence of distant metastases.

The addition of numbers to these three components (e. g. T1, T2, N0, N1, etc.) indicates the extent of the malignant disease.

All cases should be confirmed microscopically. All cases are identified by T, N, and M categories, which must be determined and recorded *before any therapy is started*. This *clinical* classification is based on evidence acquired from physical examination, imaging, endoscopy, biopsy, surgical exploration, or other relevant examinations. Apart from this widely used pretreatment clinical classification, pathologic classification can be carried out postsurgically, designated as pTNM. This is based on the evidence acquired before treatment, supplemented or modified by the additional evidence acquired from surgery and from pathologic examination. The pathologic assessment of the primary tumor (pT) entails a resection of the primary tumor or biopsy adequate to evaluate the highest pT category. The pathologic assessment of the regional lymph nodes (pN) entails removal of nodes adequate to validate the absence of regional lymph node metastasis (pN0) and sufficient to evaluate the highest pN category. The pathologic assessment of distant metastasis (pM) entails microscopic examination.

After T, N, and M or pT, pN and pM categories are assigned, they may be grouped into stages. The TNM classification and stage grouping, once established, must remain unchanged in the medical records. The clinical stage is essential to select and evaluate therapy, whereas the pathologic stage provides the most precise data to estimate prognosis and calculate end results.

If there is doubt concerning the correct T, N, or M category to which a particular case should be allotted, then the lower, that is, less advanced, category should be chosen. This will also be reflected in the stage grouping.

Head and Neck Cancer

Definitions

In the UICC TNM booklet and the AJCC *Manual for Staging of Cancer,* the following head and neck sites are included: lip and oral cavity, pharynx (nasopharynx, oropharynx, hypopharynx), larynx, and maxillary sinus. (There are separate classifications on tumors of the salivary glands and tumors of the thyroid gland.) For the various T classifications pertaining to these sites, the reader is referred to the UICC booklet and the AJCC manual. In this section, a few comments on these two classification systems will be made.

The anatomic definitions of the various primary sites within the head and neck are almost identical in the UICC and AJCC classifications. However, some of the subdivisions in regards to the larynx are not sufficiently precise, particularly in the UICC classification. The boundaries of the glottis and subglottis, for example, are not clearly defined. In the AJCC classification, the lower boundary of the glottis is a horizontal plane 1 cm below the apex of the ventricle. However, many consider 5 mm below the free margin of the vocal cord, that is, approximately the line of junction between squamous and respiratory epithelium, as the border (162). In the past, there has been controversy as to the superior border of the supraglottis. This has been settled now, within the UICC and the AJCC including the lingual surface of the epiglottis within the supraglottis.

The definitions of the N-categories, which have been so different in the past, are now identical (Table 1.1). It is unfortunate that the level of involvement of cervical lymph nodes is not incorporated in the UICC and AJCC staging systems, as it has been shown that the level of nodal involvement has prognostic importance (61, 153). UICC has even abandoned in its latest 1987 classification its former recommendation to use four levels of involvement of cervical lymph nodes. AJCC recommends to indicate only regional lymph nodes involved on diagrams. The author highly recommends applying to this end the diagrams which have been in use at the Memorial Hospital in New York for some decades and which distinguish five levels or regions of involvement

Table 1.1 N-Classification regional lymph nodes according to UICC and AJCC

NX	Regional lymph nodes can not be assessed
N0	No regional lymph node metastasis
N1	Metastasis in a single ipsilateral lymph node, 3 cm or less in greatest dimension
N2	Metastasis in a single ipsilateral lymph node, more than 3 cm, but not more than 6 cm in greatest dimension or in multiple ipsilateral lymph nodes, none more than 6 cm in greatest dimension, or in bilateral or contralateral lymph nodes, none more than 6 cm in greatest dimension
N2a	Metastasis in a single ipsilateral lymph node, more than 3 cm, but not more than 6 cm in greatest dimension
N2b	Metastasis in multiple ipsilateral lymph nodes, none more than 6 cm in greatest dimension
N2c	Metastasis in bilateral or contralateral lymph nodes, none more than 6 cm in greatest dimension
N3	Metastasis in a lymph node more than 6 cm in greatest dimension

Table 1.2 Stage grouping for all head and neck sites according to UICC and AJCC

Stage I	T1, N0, M0
Stage II	T2, N0, M0
Stage III	T3, N0, M0
	T1 or T2 or T3, N1, M0
Stage IV	T4, N0 or N1, M0
	any T, N2 or N3, M0
	any T, any N, M1

(Fig. 1.1). Region I includes the contents of the submental and the submandibular triangles. Regions II, III, and IV include the lymph nodes adjacent to the internal jugular vein and the lymph nodes contained within the fibroadipose tissue located medial to the sternocleidomastoid muscle. These are arbitrarily divided into equal thirds. Region V includes the contents of the posterior triangle of the neck. Such a diagrammatical division of the lymph nodes of the neck into regions may also serve a rational classification of neck dissections.

Stage grouping is identical in the UICC and AJCC classifications and is similar for all sites (Table 1.2).

For all head and neck sites except salivary glands and the thyroid gland, only squamous cell carcinomas are to be included in the TNM system. Although the grade of the tumor does not enter into staging of the tumor, it should be recorded. The definitions of the tumor grade (G) categories are as follows:

GX – grade of differentiation cannot be assessed
G1 – well differentiated
G2 – moderately differentiated
G3 – poorly differentiated
G4 – undifferentiated.

Staging Procedures

A variety of procedures and special studies may be used in the process of staging a given tumor. Both UICC and AJCC recommend specific methods of investigation for assessment of the T (N and M) categories for each primary site within the head and neck. The UICC is less precise in this regard than AJCC. For instance, for the assessment of T categories in carcinoma of the larynx, UICC recommends physical examination, laryngoscopy, and imaging, without further indication as to the type of imaging, for example, conventional radiographic techniques, CT, or MRI. However, UICC recognizes an optional additional descriptor, the so-called C-factor, reflecting the validity of classification according to the diagnostic methods used. The C-factor definitions are: C1, evidence from standard diagnostic means (e. g. physical examination, standard radiography, intraluminal endoscopy); and C2, evidence obtained by special diagnostic means (e. g. CT, MRI, etc.).

Problems in Staging

Problems in staging can be divided basically into two categories. First, a given tumor may not fit into a specific site definition, although this definition per se

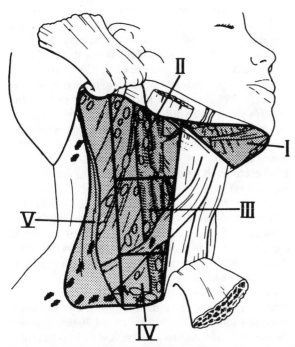

Fig. 1.1 **Lymph node regions of the neck**

is precise. For instance, in advanced carcinomas extending into both the oropharynx and the posterior part of the oral cavity, it may be extremely difficult if not impossible to define the tumor as primarily oropharyngeal or primarily orginating from the oral cavity. Second, the definition of a particular T category may be interpreted differently by different examiners. An example of this situation is a glottic carcinoma with fixation, in which there is radiographic but not endoscopic evidence of involvement of the medial wall of the piriform sinus without evidence of thyroid cartilage destruction on CT or MRI. Such a tumor most likely will be staged T3 by most clinicians, although some would prefer T4.

It appears that in general there is a tendency to upstage rather than downstage. However, whenever there is doubt concerning the correct T, N, or M category, the lower (i. e. less advanced) category should be chosen, according to one of the general rules of the TNM system.

Comments

The TNM system takes into account only the anatomic extent of local invasion of the primary tumor, along with the presence of clinically detectable regional metastases or distant metastases. Other factors of the disease, such as the growth rate of the tumor, are not reflected in the TNM system. Host factors of proved or suggested prognostic significance, such as the patients's age, sex, and resistance to the spread of cancer, are not taken into account.

The biologic aggressiveness of the tumor is reflected to a certain extent by its structural differentiation as assessed on biopsy material and expressed as grade of differentiation by the pathologist. Other prognostic histologic characteristics such as perineural spread and microvascular invasion usually become apparent only in the surgical specimen and therefore are of no help in pretreatment staging.

It is hoped that in the not too far future useful tumor markers predictive for the biologic behavior of the cancer will be identified in head and neck cancer

patients not only in the serum but also at the local tumor level (i. e. in biopsy material). Such biologic markers could then be added to those of anatomic extent in classifying head and neck cancer.

Host Performance Scale

The host performance status or the condition of the patient does not enter into determination of stage of the tumor but may be a factor in deciding type and time of treatment. Several scales are in use. The AJCC scale is presented in Table 1.**3**.

Evaluation during Follow-up

The main objective of the follow-up of cancer patients is to detect and treat early recurrences and thereby to improve the chance of survival. It is important in this regard to realize that the great majority of recurrence in head and neck cancer patients, about 85%, occur within 2 years and only 5% occur later than 3 years (163). It is common practice, therefore, to have patients come back to the outpatient clinic frequently during the first 2 years. In our department, patients are seen at from 1- to 1½-month intervals in the first year, at 2-month intervals in the second year, at 3-month intervals in the third year, and at from 4- to 6-month intervals in the fourth year. After the fifth year, patients will be seen once a year.

It is important to pay particular attention, also in terms of frequency of follow-up visits, to those patients for whom the benefit of early detection of recurrent disease in terms of survival gain will be high. First, this concerns all patients who initially, for one or another reason, had only their primary tumor treated and who run a substantial risk of developing nodal metastases in the neck. Second, there is a category of patients in whom early detection of local recurrence is not only of importance for survival but also for the quality of life. An example of this group are patients with T1 glottic carcinomas who have been treated initially by irradiation. If recurrent tumor is found early in these patients, vertical partial laryngectomy as a salvage procedure has very gratifying results (164).

In general, salvage treatment (i. e. surgery) is relatively frequently successful in patients whom irradiation failed to help (particularly in laryngeal cancer), whereas few patients will survive when cancer recurs after primary major surgery or primary combined irradiation−surgery.

The evaluation during follow-up consists of a complete physical examination of the head and neck. Special studies are only performed if the situation demands. Unfortunately, there are still no available imaging methods that can distinguish between radia-

---

Table 1.3   **Host performance scale** (AJCC)

H	The physical state (performance scale) of the patient, considering all cofactors determined at the time of stage classification and subsequent follow-up examinations
H0	Normal activity
H1	Symptomatic and ambulatory; cares for self
H2	Ambulatory more than 50%; occasionally needs assistance
H3	Ambulatory 50% or less of time; nursing care needed
H4	Bedridden; may need hospitalization

tion fibrosis or edema and carcinoma. However, aspiration cytology can be helpful in this situation, if feasible.

All through the follow-up period, there is a high risk of second primary tumors. In our patients, these occur particularly in the head and neck and in the lung. After 2 years, the detection of second primary tumors is indeed the main reason of the follow-up. Although bronchoscopy, often as part of panendoscopy, is an established procedure at the initial workup of head and neck cancer patients, it is rarely done routinely during follow-up. The usual follow-up policy in this regard consists of biannual chest radiographs only, and not surprisingly it is often inadequate. The bronchial carcinomas usually are found beyond the curative stage, and the survival rate of these patients is as poor as that of lung cancer patients in general.

With the availability of the flexible fiberoptic bronchoscope, regular bonchoscopy during follow-up of high-risk patient has become feasible. Regular bronchoscopy is rational, because the slight majority of second primary lung cancers in laryngeal cancer patients occur centrally in the lung—centrally defined as visible by bronchoscopy (165). Preliminary experiences with fiberoptic bronchoscopy with sputum cytology every 6 months in patients previously treated for laryngeal cancer demonstrate that a significantly higher number of cases of lung cancer are diagnosed at a stage at which curative treatment is possible as compared with historical controls (166). However, in our own experiences routine biannual bronchoscopy in laryngeal cancer patients demands a lot of extra work with little gain and for that reason is hardly, if at all, feasible.

Next to early detection, prevention of second primary tumors, if possible, is an attractive approach. Since it is well known that patients who continue smoking are more at risk of developing a second primary than patients who stop smoking (142), an intensive effort is necessary to get the head and neck cancer patient to stop smoking. It has to be realized, however, that the chance of developing a second primary tumor after stopping smoking only gradually decreases in the course of years. Furthermore, antismoking campaigns in these patients are at most only partially successful. It may be more effective to add to the average diet specific micronutrients, such as vitamin A, which have been suggested as possible inhibitors of cancer at various stages of carcinogenesis (167, 168). Studies testing the concept of chemoprevention are to be encouraged, particularly in high-risk groups (169, 170).

Conclusions

Careful evaluation and accurate staging of the disease as well as total evaluation of the patient are mandatory for the planning of treatment and assist in evaluation of the results of treatment. Furthermore, they facilitate the exchange of information between treatment centers and contribute to the continuing investigation of head and neck cancer.

References

1. Parkin DM, Laara E, Muir CS. Estimates of the worldwide frequency of sixteen major cancers in 1980. Int J Cancer 1988; 41: 184–97.
2. Easson EC, Palmer MK. Prognostic factors in oral cancer. J Clin Oncol 2: 1976; 2: 191–202.
3. Boyle P, Macfarlane GJ, McGinn R, et al. International epidemiology of head and neck cancer. In: de Vries N, Gluckman JL, eds. Multiple primary tumors in the head and neck. Stuttgart, New York: Georg Thieme, 1990; 80–139.
4. Boyle P, Robertson P. Statistical modelling of lung cancer and laryngeal cancer incidence in Scottland, 1960–1979. Am J Epidemiol 1987; 125: 731–44.
5. Boyle P, Zheng T, Macfarlane GJ, et al. Recent advances in the etiology and epidemiology of head and neck cancer. Curr Opinion Oncol 1990; 2: 539–45.
6. Blot WJ, McLaughlin JK, Winn DM. Smoking and drinking in relation to oral pharyngeal cancer. Cancer Res 1989; 48: 3282–7.
7. Brugère J, Guenel P, Leclerc A, et al. Differential effects of tobacco and alcohol in cancer of the larynx, pharynx and mouth. Cancer 1986; 57: 391–5.
8. Merletti F, Boffeta P, Ciccone G. Role of tobacco and alcoholic beverages in the etiology of cancer of the oral cavity/oropharynx in Torino, Italy. Cancer Res 1989; 49: 4919–24.
9. International Agency for Research on Cancer. Tobacco smoking (IARC monographs on the evaluation of the carcinogenic risk of chemicals to humans, 38). Lyons: International Agency for Research on Cancer, 1986.
10. Ramadan MF, Morton RP, Stell PM, et al. Epidemiology of laryngeal cancer. Clin Otolaryngol 1982; 7: 417–28.
11. Tuyns AJ. Incidence trends of laryngeal cancer in relation to national alcohol and tobacco consumption. In: Magnus K ed. Trends in cancer incidence. Washington: Hemisphere, 1982: 199–214.
12. Tuyns AJ, Esteve J, Raymond L, et al. Cancer of the larynx/hypopharynx; tobacco and alcohol. Int J Cancer 1988; 41: 481–3.
13. Esteve J, Tuyns AJ, Raymond L, et al. Tobacco and the risk of cancer: importance of kinds of tobacco. In: O'Neill IK, von Borstel RC, Miller CT, et al., eds. N-nitroso compounds: occurrence, biological effects, and relevance to human cancer, vol. 57. Lyons: IARC Scientific Publications, 1984: 867–76.
14. Colditz GA, Branch LG, Lipnick RJ, et al. Increased green and yellow vegetable intake and lowered cancer deaths in an elderly population. Am J Clin Nutr 1985; 41: 32–6.
15. Schwartz J, Scklar G. Regression of experimental oral carcinomas by local injection of beta-carotene and canthaxantine. Nutr. Cancer 1988; 11: 35–40.
16. Graham S, Mettlin C, Marshall J, et al. Dietary factors in the epidemiology of cancer of the larynx. Am J Epidemiol 1981; 113: 675–80.
17. McLaughlin JK, Gridley G, Block G. Dietary factors in oral and pharyngeal cancer. J Natl Cancer Inst 1988; 15: 1237–43.
18. Rossing MA, Vaughan TL, McKnight B. Diet and pharyngeal cancer. Int J Cancer 1989; 44: 593–7.
19. Maier H, de Vries N, Weidauer H. Beruf und Krebs im Bereich von Mundhöhle, Pharynx und Larynx. HNO 1990; 38: 271–278.
20. Hsu TC, Johnston DA, Cherry LM, et al. Sensitivity to

genotoxic effects of bleomycin in humans: possible relationship to environmental carcinogenesis. Int J Cancer 1989; 43: 403–9.

21. Schantz SP, Hsu TC. Mutagen-induced chromosome fragility within peripheral blood lymphocytes of head and neck cancer patients. Head Neck Surg 1989; 11: 337–42.

22. Spitz MR, Fueger JJ, Beddingfield NA, et al. Chromosome sensitivity to bleomycin-induced mutagenesis, an independent risk factor for upper aerodigestive tract cancers. Cancer Res 1989; 49: 4626–8.

23. Muir C, et. al. Cancer incidence in five continents. vol. V. Lyons: IARC Scientific Publications, 1988.

24. Pearson GR, Weiland LH, Neel HB, et al. Application of Epstein–Barr virus (EBV) serology to the diagnosis of North American nasopharyngeal carcinoma. Cancer 1983; 51: 260–268.

25. Yu MC, Mo CC, Chong WX, et al. Preserved foods and nasopharyngeal carcinoma: a case-control study in Guangxi, China. Cancer Res 1988; 48: 1954–9.

26. Yu MC, Huang TB, Henderson BE. Diet and nasopharyngeal carcinoma: a case-control study in Guangzhou, China. Int J Cancer 1989; 43: 1077–82.

27. Carter RL, Tanner NSB, Clifford P, et al. Perineural spread in squamous cell carcinomas of the head and neck: a clinicopathological study. Clin Otolaryngol 1979; 4: 271–81.

28. Maddox WA. Vicissitudes of head and neck cancer. Am J Surg 1984; 148: 428–32.

29. Poleksic S, Kalwaic HJ. Prognostic value of vascular invasion in squamous cell carcinoma of the head and neck. Plast Reconstr Surg 1978; 61: 234–40.

30. Pitam MR, Carter RL. Framework invasion by laryngeal carcinomas. Head Neck Surg 1982; 4: 200–8.

31. Mohit-Tabatabai MA, Sobel HJ, Rush BF, et al. Relation of thickness of floor of mouth stage I and II cancers to regional metastasis. Am J Surg 1986; 152: 351–3.

32. Micheau C, Sancho H, Gerard-Marchant R. Prognostic des adenopathies cervicales metastatiques en fonction des facterus anatomo-pathologique. Nuovo Arch Ital Otol VI 1978; 1: 5–9.

33. Snow GB, Annyas AA, van Slooten EA, et al. Prognostic factors of neck node metastasis. Clin Otolaryngol 1982; 7: 185–92.

34. Cachin Y, Sancho-Garnier H, Micheau Ch, et al. Nodal metastasis from carcinoma of the oropharynx. Otolaryngol Clin North Amer 1979; 12: 145–54.

35. Johnson JT, Barns EL, Myers EN, et al. The extracapsular spread of tumors in cervical node metastasis. Arch Otolaryngol 1981; 107: 725–9.

36. Toker, C. Some observations on the deposition of metastatic carcinoma within cervical lymph nodes. Cancer 1963; 16: 364–74.

37. Lindberg RD. Distribution of cervical lymph node metastasis for squamous cell carcinoma of the upper respiratory tract. Cancer 1972; 29: 1446–9.

38. Carter RL. Metastasis. In: Symington T, Carter RL, eds. Scientific foundations of oncology. London: William Heinemann Medical, 1976.

39. Djalilian M, Weiland LH, Devine KD, et al. Significance of jugular vein invasion by metastatic carcinoma in radical neck dissection. Am J Surg 1973; 126: 566–9.

40. Berger DS, Fletcher GH. Distant metastasis following local control of squamous cell carcinoma of the nasopharynx, tonsillar fossa and base of tongue. Radiology 1971; 100: 141–3.

41. Merino OR, Lindberg RD, Fletcher GJ. An analysis of distant metastases from squamous cell carcinoma of the upper respiratory and digestive tracts. Cancer 1977; 40: 145–51.

42. Snow GB, Balm AJM, Arendse JW, et al. In: Larson DL, Guillamondequi OM, Ballantyne AJ, eds. Cancer in the Neck. New York: Macmillan, 1986.

43. Stell PM. Prognostic factors in laryngeal carcinoma. Clin Otolaryngol 1988; 13: 399–409.

44. Huygen PLM, van den Broek P, Kazem I. Age and mortality in laryngeal cancer. Clin Otolaryngol 1980; 5: 129–37.

45. Amsterdam JT, Strawitz JG. Squamous cell carcinoma of the oral cavity in young adults. J Surg Oncol 1982; 19: 65–8.

46. Usenius T, Kärjä J, Collan Y. Squamous cell carcinoma of the tongue in children. Cancer 1987; 60: 236–9.

47. Lund VJ, Howard DJ. Head and neck cancer in the young: a prognostic conundrum? J Laryngol Otol 1990; 104: 544–8.

48. Langdon JD. Epidemiology and aetiology. In: Henk JM, Langdon JD, eds. Malignant oral cavity. London: Edward Arnold, 1985: 1.

49. Lederman M. Cancer of the larynx, part I: natural history in relation to treatment. Br J Radiat 1971; 44: 569–78.

50. Rudert H, Neumann FW, Gremmel H. Die Behandlungsergebnisse von 197 platten epithel Karzinomen des oropharynx. HNO 1986; 34: 357–64.

51. Katz AE. Immunobiologic staging of patients with carcinoma of the head and neck. Laryngoscope 1983; 93: 445–63.

52. Wolf GT, Tumor immunology, immune surveillance and immunotherapy of head and neck squamous carcinoma. In: Wolf GT, ed.: Head and neck oncology. Boston: Martinus Nijhoff, 1984; 375–410.

53. Lundy J, Raaf JH, Deakins S, et al.: The acute and chronic effects of alcohol on the human immune system. Surg Gynaecol Obstet 1975; 141: 212–18.

54. Brookes GB, Clifford P. Nutritional status and general immune competence in patients with head and neck cancer. J R Soc Med 1981; 74: 132–9.

55. Bennett SH, Futrell JW, Roth JA, et al. Prognostic significance of histologic host response in cancer of the larynx or hypopharynx. Cancer 1971; 28: 1255–65.

56. Guo M, Rabin BS, Johnson JT, et al. Lymphocyte phenotypes at tumor margins in patients with head and neck cancer. Head Neck Surg 1987; 9: 265–71.

57. Ortega IS, Nieto CS, Fresno ME, et al. Lymph node response and its relationship to prognosis in carcinomas of the head and neck. Clin Otolaryngol 1987; 12: 241–7.

58. Gilmore BB, Repola DA, Batsakis JG. Carcinoma of the larynx: lymph node reaction patterns. Laryngoscope 1978; 88: 1333–8.

59. Hibbert J, Marks NJ, Winter PH, et al. Prognostic factors in oral squamous carcinoma and their relation to clinical staging. Clin Otolaryngol 1983; 8: 197–203.

60. Kalnins IK, Leonard AG, Sako K, et al. Correlation between prognosis and degree of lymph node involvement in carcinoma of the oral cavity. Am J Surg 1977; 134: 450–4.

61. Spiro RH, Alfonso AE, Farr HW, et al. Cervical node metastasis from epidermoid carcinoma of the oral cavity and oropharynx. A critical assessment of current staging. Am J Surg 1974; 128: 562–7.

62. Cachin Y. Cancers of the head and neck: prognostic factors and criteria of response to treatment. In: Staquet MJ, ed. Cancer therapy: prognostic factors and criteria of response. New York: Raven Press, 1975: 353–66.

63. Grandi C, Alloisio M, Moglia D, et al. Prognostic significance of lymphatic spread in head and neck carcinomas: therapeutic implications. Head Neck Surg 1985; 8: 67–73.

64. Noone RB, Bonner H, Raymond S, et al. Lymph node metastases in oral carcinoma. A correlation of histopathology with survival. Cancer 1974; 53: 158–66.

65. Sessions DG. Surgical pathology of cancer of the larynx and hypopharynx. Laryngoscope 1976; 86: 814–39.

66. Shah JP, Cendon RA, Farr HE, et al. Carcinoma of the oral cavity. Factors affecting treatment failure at the primary site and neck. Am J Surg 1976; 132: 504–7.

67. Zoller M, Goodman ML, Cummings CW. Guidelines for prognosis in head and neck cancer with nodal metastasis. Laryngoscope 1978; 88: 135–40.

68. Vikram B, Strong EW, Shah JP, et al. Failure at distant sites following multimodality treatment for advanced head and neck cancer. Head Neck Surg 1984; 6: 730–3.

69. Michaels L. Pathology of the larynx. Berlin, Heidelberg, New York: Springer, 1984.

70. Broders AC. Squamous cell epithelioma of the lip. JAMA 1920; 74: 656–64.

71. Jakobsson PA, Eneroth CM, Killander D. Histological classification and grading of malignancy in carcinoma of the larynx. Acta Radiol. Ther 1973; 12: 1–8.

72. Atkin NB, Kay R. Prognostic significance of modal DNA value and other factors in malignant tumours, based on 1465 cases. Br J Cancer 1979; 40: 210–21.

73. Barlogie B, Raber MN, Schuman J, et al. Flow cytometry in clinical research. Cancer Res 1983; 43: 3982−97.
74. Hedley DW, Friedlander ML, Taylor IW. Method for analysis of cellular DNA content of paraffin-embedded pathological material using flow cytometry. J Histochem Cytochem 1983; 31: 1333−35.
75. Head and Neck Oncology Research Conference, September 26−28, 1990, Las Vegas. Book of abstracts.
76. Stell PM. Ploidy in head and neck cancer: a review and meta-analysis. Clin Otolaryngol 1991; 16: 510−516.
77. Tytor M, Franzen G, Olofsson J. DNA ploidy in oral cavity carcinomas with special reference to prognosis. Head Neck Surg. 1989; 11: 257−63.
78. Veltri RW, Maxim PE. Tumor immunity and tumor markers in head and neck cancer. In: Wolf GT, ed. Head and neck oncology. Boston: Martinus Nijhoff, 1984.
79. Hanna EYN, Papay FA, Gupta MK, et al. Serum tumor markers of head and neck cancer: Current status. Head Neck Surg. 1990; 12: 50−9.
80. Kato H, Torigoe T. Radioimmunoassay for tumor antigen of human cervical squamous cell carcinoma. Cancer 1977; 40: 1621−28.
81. Eibling CE, Johnson T, Wagner R, et al. SCC−RIA in the diagnosis of squamous cell carcinoma of the head and neck. Laryngoscope 1989; 99: 117−24.
82. Clasen B, Péré P, Senekowitsch R, et al. Das plattenepithel-karzinom assoziierte Antigen (SCC) als Tumormarker bei der Initialdiagnostik von Karzinomen des Kopf−Hals−Gebietes. Ergebnisse einer prospektiven Studie nach 24 Monaten. Laryngol Rhinol Otol (Stuttg) 1990; 69: 275−80.
83. Fischbach W, Meyer Th, Barthel K. Squamous cell carcinoma antigen in the diagnosis and treatment follow-up of oral and facial squamous cell carcinoma. Cancer 1990; 65: 1321−24.
84. Gold P, Freeman SO. Demonstration of tumor-specific antigens in human colonic carcinomata by immunological tolerance and absorption techniques. J Exp Med 1965; 121: 439−62.
85. Wanebo H, Rao B, Pinsky CM, et al. Preoperative carcinoembryonic antigen level as a prognostic indicator in colorectal cancer. N Engl J Med 1978; 299: 448−51.
86. Silverman NA, Alexander JC, Chretien PB. CEA levels in head and neck cancer. Cancer 1976; 36: 2204−11.
87. Demard F, Chauvel P, Vallicioni J, et al. Le dosage de l'antigène carcino-embryonnaire dans les cancers des voies aérodigestives supérieures. Ann Otolaryngol (Paris) 1982; 99: 367−74.
88. Schröder M, Meyer T. CEA−Verlaufsbeobachtungen bei Plattenepithelcarcinomen im Kopf−Hals−Bereich. HNO 1986; 34: 334−42.
89. Laarman DAW, van Kamp GJ, Balm AJM, et al. Carcinoembryonic antigen and head and neck cancer. Clin Otolaryngol 1991; 16: 152−156.
90. Lore JM. Dabbling in head and neck oncology (A plea for added qualifications). Arch Otolaryngol Head Neck Surg 1987; 113: 1165−8.
91. Horiot JC, Johansson KA, Gonzalez DG, et al. Quality assurance control in the EORTC cooperative group of radiotherapy. 1. Assessment of radiotherapy staff and equipment. Radiother Oncol 1986; 6: 275−84.
92. Johansson KA, Horiot JC, Van Dam J. Quality assurance control in the EORTC cooperative group of radiotherapy. 2. Dosimetric intercomparison. Radiother Oncol 1986; 7: 269−279.
93. Johansson KA, Horiot JC, van der Schueren E. Quality assurance control in the EORTC cooperative group of radiotherapy. 3. Intercomparison in an anatomical phantom. Radiother Oncol. 1987; 9: 289−98.
94. Burrows L, Tartter P. Effect of blood transfusions on colonic malignancy recurrence rate. Lancet 1982; 2: 662−4.
95. Johnson JT, Taylor FH, Thearle PB. Blood transfusion and outcome in stage III head and neck carcinoma. Arch Otolaryngol Head Neck Surg 1987; 113: 307−10.
96. Jones KR, Weissler MC. Blood transfusion and other risk factors for recurrence of cancer of the head and neck. Arch Otolaryngol Head Neck Surg 1990; 116: 304−9.
97. Sako K, Pradier RN, Marchetta FC, et al. Fallibility of palpation in the diagnosis of metastases to cervical nodes. Surg Gynecol Obstet 1964; 118: 989−90.
98. Ali S, Tiwari RM, Snow GB. False-positive and false-negative neck nodes. Head Neck Surg 1985; 8: 78−82.
99. Friedman M, Shelton VK, Mafee M, et al. Metastatic neck disease: evaluation by computed tomography. Arch Otolaryngol Head Neck Surg 1984; 110: 443−7.
100. Stevens MH, Harnsberger R, Mancuso AA, et al.: Computed tomography of cervical lymph nodes: staging and management of head and neck cancer. Arch Otolaryngol Head Neck Surg 1985; 735−9.
101. Close LG, Merkel M, Vuitch MF, et al. Computed tomographic evaluation of regional lymph node involvement in cancer of the oral cavity and oropharynx. Head Neck Surg. 1989; 11: 309−17.
102. Mancuso AA, Maceri D, Rice D, et al. CT of cervical lymph node cancer. AM. J. Roentgenol. 1981; 136: 381−5.
103. Feinmesser R, Freeman JL, Nojek AM, et al. Metastatic neck disease: a clinical/radiographic/pathologic correlative study. Arch Otolaryngol Head Neck Surg 1987; 113: 1307−10.
104. Som PM. Lymph nodes of the neck. Radiology 1987; 165: 593−600.
105. Bruneton JN, Roux G, Caramella MLEE, et al. Ear, nose and throat cancer: ultrasound diagnosis of metastasis to cervical lymph nodes. Radiology 1984; 152: 771−3.
106. Brekel MWM van den, Stel HV, Castelijns JA, et al. Cervical lymph node metastases: assessment of radiologic criteria. Radiology 1990; 177: 379−84.
107. Brekel MWM van den, Castelijns JA, Stel HV, et al. Detection and characterization of metastatic cervical adenopathy by MR Imaging: comparison of different MR techniques. J Comput Assist Tomogr 1990; 14: 581−9.
108. Brekel MWM van den, Castelijns JA, Croll GA, et al. MRI versus palpation of cervical lymph node metastasis. Arch Otolaryngol Head Neck Surg. 1991; 117: 666−673
109. Hajek PC, Salomonowitz E, Turk R, et al. Lymph nodes of the neck: evaluation with US. Radiology 1986; 158: 739−42.
110. Grasl MCh, Neuwirth-Riedl K, Gritzmann N, et al. Wertigkeit sonomorphologischer Kriterien bei der Identifikation regionärer Metastasen von Plattenepithelkarzinomen des HNO-Bereiches. HNO 1989; 37: 333−7.
111. Baatenburg de Jong RJ, Rongen RJ, Lameris JS. Metastatic neck disease. Arch Otolaryngol Head Neck Surg 1989; 115: 689−90.
112. Watkinson JC, Maisey MN. Imaging of the head and neck cancer using radioisotopes. J R Soc Med. 1988; 81: 657−63.
113. Quak JJ, Balm AJM, Brakkee JGP, et al. Localization and imaging of radiolabeled monoclonal antibody against squamous cell carcinoma of the head and neck in tumor bearing nude mice. Int J of Cancer 1989; 44: 534−8.
114. McGregor IA, McGregor FM. Cancer of the face and mouth: pathology and management for surgeons. Edinburgh: Churchill Livingstone, 1986.
115. Ator GA, Abemayor E, Lufkin RB. Evaluation of mandibular tumor invasion with magnetic resonance imaging. Arch Otolaryngol Head Neck Surg. 1990; 116: 454−9.
116. Gerritsen GJ, Valk J, van Velzen DJ, et al. Computed tomography: a mandatory investigational procedure for the T-staging of advanced laryngeal cancer. Clin Otolaryngol 1986; 11: 307−16.
117. Archer CR, Yeager VL. Computed tomography of laryngeal cancer with histopathological correlation. Laryngoscope 1982; 92: 1173−80.
118. Silverman PM, Bossen EH, Fisher SR, et al. Carcinoma of the larynx and hypopharynx: computed tomographic−histopathologic correlations. Radiology 1984; 151: 697−702.
119. Hoover LA, Calcaterra TC, Walter GA, et al. Preoperative CT-scan evaluation for laryngeal carcinoma: correlation with pathological findings. Laryngoscope 1984; 94: 310−15.
120. Yeager VL, Lawson C, Ancher CR. Ossification of the laryngeal cartilages as it relates to computed tomography. Invest Radiol 1982; 17: 11−29.
121. Castelijns JA, Gerritsen GJ, Kaiser MC, et al. MRI of normal or cancerous laryngeal cartilages: histopathologic correlation. Laryngoscope 1987; 97: 1085−93.

122. Castelijns JA, Gerritsen GJ, Kaiser MJ, et al. Invasion of laryngeal cartilage by cancer: comparison of CT and MR imaging. Radiology 1988; 167: 199–206.

123. Lufkin RB, Wortham DG, Dietrich RB, et al. Tongue and oropharynx: findings on MR imaging. Radiology 1986; 161: 69–75.

124. Hasso AN. CT of tumours and tumour-like conditions of the paranasal sinuses. Radiol Clin North Am 1984; 22: 119–30.

125. Mancuso AA, Hanafee WN. Malignant sinus, benign sinus. In: CT and MRI of the head and neck. 2nd ed. Baltimore: Williams & Wilkins 1985: chaps 1 and 2.

126. Tiwari RM, Gerritsen GJ, Balm AJM, Snow GB. A critical evaluation of the role of CT scanning in ethmoidal cancer. J Laryngol Otol 1986; 100: 421–8.

127. Ziedsés des Plantes BG, de Slegte RGM, et al. Magnetic resonance imaging in malignant lesions of the paranasal sinuses. In: Partain CL, ed. Magnetic resonance imaging. Philadelphia: WB Saunders, 1987.

128. Som PM, Shapiro MD, Biller HF, et al. Sinonasal tumors and inflammatory tissues: Differentiation with MR imaging. Radiology 1988; 167: 803–8.

129. Virapongse C, Mancuso A, Fitzsimmons J, et al. Value of magnetic resonance imaging in assessing bone destruction in head and neck lesions. Laryngoscope 1986; 96: 284–91.

130. Frable WJ, Frable MA. Thin-needle aspiration biopsy: the diagnosis of head and neck tumors revisited. Cancer 1979; 43: 1541–48.

131. Tytor M, Olofsson J. Cervical lymph node metastases with occult primary. Clin Otolaryngol 1986; 11: 463–7.

132. de Vries N. Magnitude of the problem. In: de Vries N, Gluckman JL, eds. Multiple primary tumors in the head and neck. Stuttgart: Georg Thieme, 1990: 1–25.

133. Warren S, Gates O. Multiple primary malignant tumours: a survey of the literature and statistical study. Am J Cancer 1932; 51: 1358–14.

134. Hordijk GJ, de Jong JMA. Synchronous and metachronous tumours in patients with head and neck cancer. J Laryngol Otol 1983; 97: 619–21.

135. Gluckman JL, Grissman JD, Donega JO. Multicentric squamous cell carcinoma of the upper aerodigestive tract. Head Neck Surg 1980; 3: 90–6.

136. Pasche R, Savary M, Monnier PA. Multifocalité du carcinome épidermoide sur les vois digestivus superieure et respiratoris distales: technicité du diagnostic endoscopique. Acta Endosc 1981; 11: 277–80.

137. Shapshay SM, Hong WK, Fried MP, et al. Simultaneous carcinomas of the esophagus and upper aerodigestive tract. Otolaryngol Head Neck Surg 1980; 88: 373–7.

138. de Vries N, van der Waal I, Snow GB. Multiple primary tumours in oral cancer. Int J Oral Maxillofac Surg 1986; 15: 85–7.

139. de Vries N, Snow GB. Multiple primary tumours in laryngeal cancer. J Laryngol Otol 1986; 100: 915–18.

140. Wagenfeld DJH, Harwood A, Bryce DP, et al. Second primary respiratory tract malignancies in glottic carcinoma. Cancer 1980; 46: 1883–6.

141. Wagenfeld DJH, Harwood AR, Bryce DP et al. Second primary respiratory tract malignant neoplasms in supraglottic carcinoma. Arch Otolaryngol 1981; 107: 135–7.

142. Moore C. Smoking and cancer of the mouth, pharynx and larynx. J Am Med Assoc 1965; 191: 283–6.

143. de Vries N, de Lange G, Drexhage HA, et al. Immunoglobulin allotypes in head and neck cancer patients with multiple primary tumours. Acta Otolaryngol. (Stockh) 1987; 104: 187–91.

144. de Vries N, de Waal LP, de Lange G., et al. HLA-antigens and immunoglobulin allotypes in head and neck cancer patients with and without multiple primary tumors. Cancer 1987; 60: 957–61.

145. Atkins JP, Keane WM, Young KA, et al. Value of panendoscopy in determination of second primary cancer. Arch Otolaryngol 1984; 110: 533–7.

146. McGuirt WF. Panendoscopy as a screening examination for simultaneous primary tumors in head and neck cancer: a prospective sequential study and review of the literature. Laryngoscope 1982; 92: 569–76.

147. Leipzig B, Zellmer JE, Klug D. The role of endoscopy in evaluating patients with head and neck cancer. A multi-institutional prospective study. Arch Otolaryngol 1985; 111: 589–94.

148. Savary M, Passche R, Monnier P. Endoscopic screening for multiple squamous cell carcinoma of the upper digestive and respiratory tracts (Oncologically oriented upper aero-digestive panendoscopy). In: Wigand ME, Steiner W, Stell PM, eds. Functional partial laryngectomy. Conservation surgery for carcinoma of the larynx. Berlin: Springer, 1984: 51–9.

149. Batsakis JG. Tumors of the head and neck. Clinical and pathological considerations. Baltimore: Williams & Wilkins, 1979.

150. Barnes L. Surgical pathology of the head and neck. New York, Basel: Marcel Dekker, 1985.

151. Abemayor E, Kessler DJ, Ward P, et al. Evaluation of poorly differentiated head and neck neoplasms. Arch Otolaryngol Head Neck Surg 1987; 113: 506–9.

152. Henzen-Logmans SC, Balm AJM, van der Waal I, et al. The expression of intermediate filaments and MAM-6 antigen in relation to the degree of morphologic differentiation of carcinoma of the head and neck: Diagnostic implications. Otolaryngol Head Neck Surg 1988; 99: 539–47.

153. Stell PM, Morton RP, Singh SD. Cervical lymph-node metastases. The significance of the level of the lymph node. Clin Oncol 1983; 9: 101–7.

154. Saka SM, MacDonald DG. Sampling of jugulo-digastric lymph nodes in oral cancer. J Oral Pathol Med 1989; 18: 123–4.

155. Looser KG, Shah JP, Strong EW. The significance of "positive" margins in surgically resected epidermoid carcinomas. Head Neck Surg 1978; 1: 107–11.

156. Zieske LA, Johnson JT, Myers EN, et al. Squamous cell carcinoma with positive margins. Arch Otolaryngol Head Neck Surg 1986; 112: 863–6.

157. Batsakis J. Surgical margins in squamous cell carcinomas. Ann Otol Rhinol Laryngol 1988; 97: 213–14.

158. Remsen KA, Lucente FE, Biller HF. Reliability of frozen section diagnosis in head and neck neoplasms. Laryngoscope 1984; 519–24.

159. Scholl P, Byers RM, Batsakis JG, et al. Microscopic cut-through of cancer in the surgical treatment of squamous carcinoma of the tongue. Prognostic and therapeutic implications. Am J Surg 1986; 152: 352.

160. Union Internationale contre le Cancer (International Union against Cancer). TNM classification of malignant tumours, 4th ed, fully revised. Heidelberg: Springer, 1987.

161. American Joint Commitee on Cancer (AJCC). Manual for staging of cancer. 3rd ed. Philadelphia: JB Lippincott, 1988.

162. Kirchner JA. Staging of cancer of the larynx. In: (Englisch) Oncology of the head and neck. vol 5. 1978: chapter 35.

163. Boysen M, Natvig K, Winter Fö J, et al. Value of routine follow-up in patients treated for squamous cell carcinoma of the head and neck. J Otolaryngol 1985; 14:211–14.

164. Croll GA, van den Broek P, Tiwari RM, et al. Vertical partial laryngectomy for recurrent glottic carcinoma after irradiation. Head Neck Surg 1985; 7: 390–3.

165. Heeringa A, de Vries N, Snow GB, et al. Laryngeal cancer and lung cancer in the same patient: a retrospective study. Eur J Surg Oncol 1988; 14: 209–11.

166. Rodriquez E, Castella J, Puzo C. Lung cancer in patients with tracheostomy due to cancer of the larynx. Respiration 1984; 46: 323–7.

167. Bertram JS, Kolonel LN, Meyskens FL Jr. Rationale and strategies for chemoprevention of cancer in humans. Cancer Res 1987; 47: 3012–31.

168. Fallon BG. Chemoprevention of second malignancies in patients with squamous cell carcinoma of the head and neck. In: de Vries N, Gluckman JL, eds. Multiple primary tumors in the head and neck. Stuttgart: Georg Tieme, 1990; 30–49.

169. Hong WK, Lippman SM, Itri LM, et al. Prevention of second primary tumors with isotretinoin in squamous cell carcinoma of the head and neck. New Engl J Med 1990; 323: 795–801.

170. de Vries N. Euroscan. EORTC study on chemoprevention with vitamin A and or n-acetylcysteine. Eur Cancer News 1988; 1: 1–4.

2 Surgery for Head and Neck Cancer

P. M. Stell, D. A. Bowdler

Conventional Surgery as a Single Modality

The Developmental History of Surgery for Head and Neck Cancer

Surgery for squamous carcinoma of the head and neck must address three problems: firstly, extirpation of the primary tumor, secondly, control of the metastases to the lymph nodes of the neck, and thirdly reconstruction of the defect arising from excision of the primary tumor. The first of these was largely developed in Europe in the second half of the nineteenth century, the second in continental Europe and North America in the early part of the twentieth century, and the third in Great Britain and North America over the last 50 years.

The development of excisional surgery of the major structures of the head and neck, in the second half of the nineteenth century depended on two major developments in medical technology: general anesthesia, and histopathology.

General anesthesia began to develop around the year 1840: the first general anesthetic using ether was administered by Morton in Boston, Massachusetts in 1846, and that using chloroform by Simpson in Edinburgh in 1847. This development in medical technology depended on general advances in science, chloroform in particular being a by-product of the German chemical industry, having been first discovered by Liebig in 1831.

The microscope was first developed by a Dutchman, von Leeuwenhoek, in about 1660, as a single-lens instrument. Compound microscopes using a two-lens system were developed later. However, these systems could not be used for the examination of tissue until about 1855 when it was found that tissues could be stained and counterstained using the recently discovered aniline dyes.

Thus, after about 1855, both histopathological diagnosis and general anesthesia became widely available, allowing excisional surgery of major structures to develop, so that most excisional procedures for head and neck cancer began to develop in Europe, in the second half of the nineteenth century.

Excisional surgery for laryngeal cancer can be divided into three main groups: total laryngectomy, vertical partial laryngectomy, and horizontal partial laryngectomy. It is often said that the first total laryngectomy was carried out for syphilis by Watson in Edinburgh, in 1865. This is completely untrue: Watson described the larynx, trachea, and bronchi of a patient who had died from syphilis. The only operation carried out during life was tracheostomy.

The first total laryngectomy was carried out on 31 December 1873 by Billroth on a 39-year-old man with a tumor of one vocal cord. An initial attempt was made, after the induction of anesthesia using a Trendelenburg cannula, to carry out a vertical hemilaryngectomy. However, the tumor proved to be too extensive for this, and a total laryngectomy was carried out. The patient was deliberately left with a pharyngocutaneous fistula to which was fitted a speaking valve designed by Gussenbauer.

Vertical partial laryngectomy for cancer was first done about 1851 by Gurdon Buck of New York, although the first laryngofissure had been done by a Belgian, Brauers in 1834. Horizontal supraglottic laryngectomy is of a much later date and really depends on the lateral pharyngotomy first described by Trotter, an Englishman, in 1920. This procedure, however, was mainly developed by an Argentinian, Alonzo, in the 1940s. It was popularized in the English-speaking world notably by Ogura (1) and Som, working in the United States in the 1960s.

Absolon (2) has provided us with a history of surgery for oral malignancy. Glossectomy was carried out sporadically during the eighteenth century, notably by Heister, the most famous surgeon of his day (1743). During the nineteenth century it was realized that the intraoral route was unsatisfactory and the external approach was put on a firm footing by the Germans—notably Billroth and Czerny—about 1860. Midline mandibulotomy was introduced in about 1836 by Roux, but the current procedures was laid down in 1875 by Langenbeck, who divided the mandible opposite the first molar tooth for access, ligated the lingual artery, and removed the enlarged regional lymph nodes, in addition to carrying out a glossectomy.

Surgery for cancer of the hypopharynx and cervical esophagus belongs almost entirely to the twentieth century, because it was impossible in the early days to reconstruct the defect left by resection of the hypopharynx. Thus a resection of the cervical esophagus was carried out by Czerny in 1877, but the patient was left with a cervical esophagotomy. During the early part of the twentieth century occasional attempts were made to close the defect, but the matter was not put on a serious footing until Wookey, a Canadian, described a staged technique using local cervical skin flaps in about 1945. This technique had many difficulties including prolonged hospital stay, fistulae, and recurrence of the tumor before the repair was complete. The next two major advances occurred almost simultaneously: the first was the description by Bakamjian of the deltopectoral flap for reconstruction of the hypopharynx after total pharyngolaryngectomy. The second was the demonstration by Ong that it is possible to transfer the stomach to the neck through the mediastinum by the so-called "gastric pull-up." The latter has the great advantage of being a one-stage procedure, and of rarely being complicated by a fistula or a stenosis, but does have a high operative mortality rate. The next step forward was the development of the musculocutaneous flaps, and the workhorse of these, the pectoralis major flap, proved to be very useful as a one-stage procedure for replacement of the hypopharynx. Like all other methods based on skin repair there is a high incidence of stenosis and fistula formation, and the use of this technique for extensive carcinomas of the cervical esophagus is limited because the esophagus cannot be resected lower than the thoracic inlet. The most recent and the most promising method, is replacement by a jejunal loop with microvascular anastomosis of the vessels in the neck. Provided that a reasonable margin can be obtained around the tumor, this technique appears to give the best long-term results of operative mortality, and complications such as stenosis and fistula (3).

As regards resection of the upper jaw, a handful of reports of local excision of maxillary tumors begins with that described by Wiseman, the surgeon to Charles II in 1676, followed by three or four further reports during the eighteenth and very early nineteenth century. The first formal resections of the maxilla and its bony attachments was done by Gensoul in Lyons in 1827, and by Syme and Lizars, both of Edinburgh in 1829. Surgery for cancer of the upper jaw continued to be refined by the French down to about 1930: they were mainly responsible for classifying the anatomical origin of cancers of the upper jaw and for tailoring procedures to the various anatomical levels of tumor. The most notable contribution was lateral rhinotomy which began to be developed by Michaux, a French-speaking Belgian in 1848, but which was finally popularized by Moure in 1902.

Before the mid-1800s, operations capable of controlling metastatic cancer of the cervical glands were not available. Chelius in 1847 stated that once cancer from a primary lesion in the head and neck had spread to the cervical glands, control of the disease is impossible. In 1847, Warren of Boston tried to remove metastatic cancer of the neck, and in 1880, Kocher described an operation in which the tongue was removed through a submandibular approach after first dissecting the lymphatic glands. In 1900, Henry Butlin recommended dissection of the cervical lymphatics using the Kocher incision, and also discussed elective excision of lymph nodes for cancer of the oral cavity. Von Bergmann and von Bruns (1904) advised the removal of lymph nodes of the neck invaded by cancer from primary tumors of the oral cavity. Their operation was not a systematic procedure but was described as an extensive removal of these glands. The first description of a standardized anatomical dissection of the lymph nodes was that of George Crile (4) in 1906. He argued that the proximity of the cervical lymph nodes to the internal jugular vein, the sternocleidomastoid muscle and the spinal accessory nerve made it imperative to carry out a radical en bloc removal of these structures (5).

A further classic paper was that in 1947 of Hayes Martin (6) who reported on experiences at Memorial Hospital in New York with the en bloc radical neck dissection fully describing this technique and its complications. He, too, emphasized that anything less than en bloc resection would hamper the excision of the cervical lymphatic system and compromise control of the cancer.

Principles of Single Modality Therapy

Surgery when used as the sole form of treatment has two tasks: firstly to encompass the primary tumor, and secondly to control metastatic lymph nodes in the neck. The principle of both these forms of excisional surgery is determined by surgical anatomy and surgical pathology.

The anatomical limits of the sites of head and neck cancer are defined by the UICC and the AJC and include the oral cavity (including the lips) the paranasal sinuses, the salivary and thyroid glands, the naso-, oro- and hypo-pharynx, and the larynx.

The UICC (7) and the AJC have now agreed a definition for the T, N, and M stage of tumors at these sites. The primary tumor is given a T staging which depends on anatomical boundaries at some sites (e. g. the larynx) and on size at others (e. g. the mouth). The nodes are classified on size, numbers and laterality.

The anatomy of head and neck cancer has been most extensively investigated in the larynx. In the larynx the main anatomical structures to be considered are the compartments and potential spaces. The most important of these are the preepiglottic and paraglottic spaces. The pre-epiglottic space is bounded above by the hyoepiglottic ligament, in front by the thyrohyoid membrane, and posteriorly by the fixed part of the epiglottis. Inferiorly it comes to a point where the epiglottis is attached by the Broyle tendon to the thyroid cartilage. Tumors of the epiglottis are attached by the Broyle tendon to the thyroid cartilage. Tumors of the epiglottis readily spread through the foramina normally present in the epiglottis to invade this space, which must be excised routinely in the surgical treatment of all cancers of the supraglottic region. Furthermore, cancers of the base of the tongue can spread downwards into this space from above, and recurrence in this space is a common cause of failure for surgery of the base of the tongue.

The paraglottic space, or rather potential space, lies lateral to the true and false cords. Its lateral relation is the thyroid cartilage, medially it is bounded by the vestibular fold and the quadrate ligament and more inferiorly by the conus elasticus, which is covered by the mucosa of the sublgottic space. Superomedially the paraglottic space is continuous with the pre-epiglottic space, and superiorly it is bounded by the vallecula and the aryepiglottic fold. Its lateral relation is the mucosa of the medial wall of the piriform fossa posteriorly, and the thyroid cartilage anteriorly. Inferolaterally the space is bounded by the cricothyroid ligament. Its importance is that tumors of the piriform fossa or vestibular fold can spread within it, making partial surgery hazardous.

The important tendons and ligaments are the vocal ligament, the cricovocal membrane (conus elasticus), the vestibular ligament (quadrate membrane), and the anterior commissure tendon. The middle two can be important in limiting the spread of cancer; the last is an important route of spread of cancer into the thyroid cartilage.

Whole-organ serial sectioning provides an ideal method of studying the growth and spread of laryngeal tumors.

There are a number of physical barrieres within the larynx, which tend to limit the spread of tumor, and these form a number of anatomic compartments — the more important ones include the Reinke space, the pre-epiglottic space (PES), and the paraglottic space.

The conus elasticus is the histopathological boundary between the glottic and subglottic regions, and the lateral angle of the laryngeal ventricle is the boundary between the glottic and supraglottic regions. Vertical extension of glottic tumors to the supraglottic and/or subglottic regions is much more frequent than horizontal extension to the opposite hemilarynx. Glottic tumors tend to be confined for long periods by the laryngeal cartilaginous framework. When these tumors spread outside the larynx, they do so through the points of weakness in the laryngeal framework. Tumors involving the anterior commissure region of the larynx penetrate the cricothyroid membrane after extending subglottically. More than 75% of the glottic tumors extending outside the larynx use this portal of exit. These tumors often invade and penetrate the adjacent lower border of the thyroid cartilage. Further posteriorly, glottic tumors spread laterally to penetrate the cricothyroid space and extend outside the laryngeal framework, particularly those large glottic tumors extending to the supraglottic and subglottic regions. Here too, the adjacent thyroid ala and upper border of the circoid cartilage are often invaded and penetrated.

Vocal cord fixation is almost always due to invasion of the thyroarytenoid muscle. In more than half of these cases the tumor extends outside the laryngeal framework.

Tumors arising in the supraglottic region tend to have "pushing" margins. A quarter of these supraglottic tumors extend into the glottic region and nearly half invade the pre-epiglottic space (PES), the majority having arisen at the base of the epiglottis. Invasion of the preepiglottic space is uncommon in tumors arising in other regions.

Tumor arising in the subglottic region tend to be "ulcerofungating" and present themselves clinically only when far advanced. They tend to spread circumferentially and eventually involve the glottic region and/or the hypopharynx.

Multiregional tumors invade many adjacent structures, frequently extend outside the larynx and often had metastasized ot the cervical nodes at the time of surgery (8).

The pathology of carcinoma of the hypopharynx has been investigated mainly by Harrison (9). He showed that the submucosal spread of postcricoid carcinoma was on average 10 mm superiorly and 5 mm inferiorly. The other direction of spread was laterally into the thyroid gland, and into the membranous tracheoesophageal wall.

We owe the development of knowledge of the pathological anatomy of the tumors of the nose and sinuses entirely to the French. In a series of papers during the second half of the nineteenth century they developed the concept of tumors at three levels (the supra-, meso-, and infra-structure) and described the histological types and rates of spread of tumors at these sites. They tailored partial operations for tumors at these three levels.

The pathological anatomy of mouth cancer has been investigated chiefly by MacGregor's team (10). He has studied the anatomy of both the dentate and the edentulous mandible. The mandible is divided into the alveolar segment (which is covered by mucoperiosteum and is the only intraoral part of the mandible), and the lower segment covered solely by periosteum. The mandible derives its blood supply from the inferior alveolar vessels, and from the soft tissue attachments: the latter almost all lie on its lateral surface derived from muscular and soft tissue insertions, whereas on the medial surface the only source of blood supply is from the attachment of the mylohyoid muscle.

In the edentulous mandible, two anatomical events are of pathological importance: firstly, atrophy of the alveolus brings the mental foramen near the floor of the mouth: secondly, foramina remaining on the rest of the alveolus after loss of the teeth are a ready source of spread of tumor into the mandible. The spread of the tumor inferiorly is limited by the atachment of the mylohyoid muscle.

The cervical lymph nodes constitute about one-third of all the lymph nodes found in the body. They are arranged in several groups, notably the jugular chain, but other groups are the submental, the submandibular, and posterior triangle nodes.

It has been appreciated for a very long time that one of the hallmarks of squamous carcinoma of the head and neck is its propensity to metastasize to the lymph nodes in the neck. The frequency of such metastases at first presentation varies from almost nil for glottic T1 cancers to about 75% for extensive tumors of the piriform fossa. Fortunately the lymph node chains in the neck form a highly efficient barrier to spread of cancer, and the cancer remains localized to the head and neck for many months even after the development of such metastases. However, the development of a lymph node metastasis is the single most important prognostic event in head and neck cancer, and only one patient in three with a histologically invaded lymph node metastasis in the neck survives for 5 years.

The principle of radical neck dissection is that the entire lymph-bearing areas bounded by the mandible above, the clavicle below, the midline, and the anterior border of the trapezius must be removed, including the sternomastoid muscle, which is often invaded by a contiguous node, and the internal jugular vein, which too is similarly invaded.

Recent pathological studies have shown that two factors are important in the outcome of treatment of lymph node metastases to the neck: the number of nodes invaded and the concept of extracapsular disease (11). The chance of cure diminishes with increasing number of nodes and with the presence of cancer outside the capsule of a lymph node. In reality, the latter encompasses two separate entities: firstly, a tumor which has metastasized to a lymph node and then grows to burst out of the capsule, and secondly a tumor deposit in soft tissue with no relation to a lymph node. The latter is usually fatal.

The outcome for surgery for head and neck cancer is determined by a variety of factors related to the host, to the tumor, and to its treatment. The main host factors are the age and sex of the patient and his (or her) general condition.

There is controversy about the importance of these factors. Some say that older patients fare better, some that they do worse, and some that tumors grow more rapidly in the young. Age certainly has an effect in that older patients are more likely to be untreatable, more likely to die of intercurrent disease, and more likely to develop a second tumor. If these factors are taken into account, age does *not* affect the outcome, that is there is no biological effect of age on the behavior of the tumor. It is very difficult to assess the effect of sex because head and neck tumors vary widely between the sexes. For example glottic T1 cancer arises almost exclusively in men, and postcricoid cancer in women. When such effects are taken into account, sex has no bearing on prognosis.

The patient's general condition may be classified by a variety of schemes, the most popular being the Karnofsky (12) and the ECOG scheme (Table 2.1). However, these are "self fulfilling prophecies": they measure how far the progress of the disease has undermined the patient's general condition. It is obvious that a patient whose disease is far advanced will not survive long. What these systems do *not* tell us is the effect, if any, of generalized disease on the behavior of the patient's cancer.

The tumor factors bearing on prognosis are expressed by the TNM system, already referred to above. Whilst survival in general worsens with increasing T stage, this is largely due to the fact that increasing T stage is associated with increasing frequency of lymph node metastases. When the confounding effects of the latter is allowed for by multivariate methods of analysis, the effect of T stage is not marked.

The presence of palpable lymph node metastases affects survival drastically, particularly if they are multiple or large (greater than 6 cm in size). The current N classification agreed by both the UICC and the AJC is shown in Table 1.1. The importance of this clinical classification is overshadowed by the pathology of the lymph nodes.

Distant metastases, i. e. below the clavicle, are unusual in squamous carcinoma of the head and neck, being found in 1.6% of the author's series of over 3000 patients with squamous carcinoma. They are of course rapidly fatal.

The importance of the histological grade of the tumor is controversial for several reasons: inter- and intra-observer variation, variations in the grade of the same tumor at different parts and at different times, variations between the grade of the primary tumor and the node metastases, and the fact that most tumors at any one particular site are usually of one grade, e. g. most vocal cord cancers are well differentiated. Other more complex systems (e. g. Jacobson) have been developed to take account of structure, differentiation, mitotic index, and tumor−host relationship, e. g. vascular and perineural invasion. They appear to be more reliable predictors of outcome, but have not been widely used.

Another fruitful field which is currently developing rapidly is cell biology. The ploidy of head and

Table 2.1   Karnofsky scale and WHO performance scales

Karnofsky
scale performance

100	Normal, no complaints, no evidence of disease			0	Able to carry out all normal activity without restriction
90	Able to carry on normal activity, minor signs or symptoms of disease	Able to carry on normal activity, no special care is needed			
80	Normal activity with effort, some signs or symptoms of disease			1	Restricted in physically strenuous activity but ambulatory and able to carry out light work
70	Cares for self, unable to carry on normal activity or do active work				
60	Requires occasional assistance but is able to care for most of his needs	Unable to work, able to live at home, cares for personal needs, a varying amount of assistance of needed		2	Ambulatory and capable of self-care but unable to carry out any work; up and about more than 50% of waking hours
50	Requires considerable assistance and frequent medical care				
40	Disabled, requires special care and assistance				
30	Severely disabled, hospitalization is indicated although death is not imminent			3	Capable of only limited self-care; confined to bed or chair more than 50% of waking hours
20	Very sick, hospitalization necessary, active supportive treatment necessary	Unable to care for self, requires equivalent of institutional or hospital care; disease may be progressing rapidly		4	Completely diabled; cannot carry on any self-care; totally confined to bed or chair
10	Moribund, fatal processes progressing rapidly				
0	Dead				

neck tumors has been measured in several small series, with conflicting results. It appears, however, that diploid tumors have a better prognosis than aneuploid tumors, but that the latter respond better to chemotherapy and perhaps radiotherapy. Cell kinetics too is in its infancy. The potential doubling time of only a few tumors has been measured but it appears that this too may be relevent to treatment, notably fractionation of radiotherapy.

Patients with carcinoma of the head and neck who have a positive reaction to recall antigens have a better short-term prognosis than those who are anergic. Patients with impaired reaction to DNCB have a high rate of recurrence and multiple primary tumors. Measurement of the alpha-2-HS glycoprotein probably assesses the same mechanism. Finally a decreased or absent number of circulatory T-lymphocytes correlates with increasing stage of disease (13).

Another important determinant of outcome is the development of a second metachronous tumor, the two commonest sites being elsewhere in the upper respiratory tract and the lung (14). Such tumors always develop in structures of the same epithelial type, i. e. the upper and lower respiratory tract and the esophagus. In the lung almost all tumors are squamous cell, half being central and half peripheral. Unfortunately, the worthwhile yield of follow-up endoscopy is low and should probably be restricted to those at high risk, e. g. men with a tumor in the lower part of the mouth and all patients with supraglottic tumors. Also the patient's genetic make-up (e. g. Km(l)) and immunologic status may predict this event. Methods to reduce the incidence of a second tumor include stopping smoking, and possibly the administration of vitamin A or *N*-acetyl cysteine. The chance of such a second tumor developing increases with time, with the age of the patient, and with continued smoking. For some unexplained reason the development of a second tumor appears to be more common in the United States than in the United Kingdom.

The Failure of Single Modality Therapy

Treatment for cancer of the head and neck may fail for a variety of reasons, listed below.

Patient's Unsuitability

The patient may be unsuitable for treatment because of advanced disease, poor general health, or more commonly both combined; such patients are seldom included in reports of large series of cases. The proportion of patients untreatable in a personal series of 3000 previously untreated squamous carcinomas of the head and neck is shown in Table 2.2).

Table 2.2 Proportion of untreated patients

Site	No. of patients untreated (%)
Oral cavity	11.1
Larynx	2.5
PNS	6.7
Ear	7.4
Hypopharynx	24.1
Oropharynx	19.2
Nose and sinuses	10.4
Total	11.9

Surgical Mortality

This tends to be dismissed lightly by surgeons, and it is interesting to compare the vague approach of clinicians to hospital mortality rates with the precise approach developed by medical statisticians to the calculation and quoting of survivals rates. Five-year survival rates are usually quoted because it is generally recognized that if a patient is alive and apparently free of disease 5 years after an operation for squamous cancer of the head and neck, be is almost certain to be cured. In contrast, figures of operative mortality are often fudged, and there is no generally acceptable definition of the time period that should be used for calculating operative deaths. Death of a patient during the procedure is very rare, so that true operative deaths are rare. However, deaths directly due to the surgery and its effects are quite common after major head and neck surgery and increase in frequency up to at least 30 days. The recent confidential report of perioperative mortality carried out in the United Kingdom recommends including all deaths within 30 days of an operation as being due to the operation itself. The hospital mortality rate in a personal series to include death at any time after operation of over 1800 major resections for cancer of the larynx, hypopharynx, oropharynx, and mouth is ·122 (6.7%).

Recurrence at the Primary Site

The ability of either radiotherapy or surgery, when used alone to control the primary tumor, decreases with increasing size of the tumor, the decrease being more marked for radiotherapy. However, the pattern of factors differs between these two methods: it is said that radiotherapy tends to fail in the center of tumor and surgery at the periphery although careful pathological studies show that this is not so. This is one of the bases of combining radiotherapy and surgery dealt with elsewhere.

Recurrence within the Neck

Later lymph node metastases to the neck may be controlled by radical neck dissection in about 30% of cases provided the neck has not already been disturbed. However, a later metastasis in a neck which has already been dissected is almost always fatal, although the insertion of tubes which are afterloaded with radioactive iodine offers the hope that a few of these patients may be salvaged.

Distant Metastases

It used to be thought that distant metastases were uncommon, and indeed they are at presentation, being found in 1.7% of the author's series. In the early years of this century the distant metastatic rate was said to be 1%. It is probable that the ability to control the primary tumor and the lymph node metastases is improving, but this improvement has been annulled by an increasing incidence of distant metastases. Metastases at post mortem are found in a varying proportion of cases, but 50% is a reasonable average figure. The sites affected in decreasing order of frequency are the lung in 80%, the mediastinal nodes in 60%, the skeletal system (lumbosacral spine and ribs) in 35% and the liver in 25%. The metastatic rate varies with site, the glottis being the site with the lowest proportion of metastases, and the nasopharynx the greatest. Eighty percent of patients with distant metastases also have uncontrolled locoregional disease (15).

Later development of a second primary tumor elsewhere has been described above.

Advances in Surgery

Advances in Ablative Procedures

Base of Skull Surgery

Tumor of the upper respiratory tract may invade two parts of the base of the skull: firstly, the floor of the anterior cranial fossa and secondly, the floor of the middle cranial fossa. It is not intended here to discuss those tumors which are of otological interest such as acoustic neuromas.

Surgery of the Middle Cranial Fossa

The main problem here is a squamous carcinoma arising within the external auditory meatus or the middle ear invading the floor of the middle cranial fossa.

Lewis (16) has been the surgeon mainly responsible for developing petrosectomy. The highlights of the procedures, mainly taken from Lewis' descriptions, are as follows:

1. Preliminary packing of the lateral sinus. The lateral sinus is exposed by routine cortical mas-

toidectomy about 10 days before the main procedure and the sinus packed off tightly with a BIPP gauze. This induces thrombosis in the venous lake in which the bone lies, and drastically reduces bleeding at the main procedures.

2. Incision and exposure. If the auricle is to be preserved, a U-shaped incision is made and the auricle is reflected upward. However, the auricle is usually sacrificed and a large circular incision to include the auricle and any invaded skin is then made around the ear.

3. Temporal craniotomy is made early in the procedure to assess invasion of the dura and the apex of the petrous pyramid. Invasion of a small part of the dura is not an indication of non-resectability, but invasion of the petrous apex is. CSF may be removed at this point by a malleable needle to allow the dura and brain to be separated from the underlying bone.

4. Parotidectomy with tagging of the peripheral branches of the facial nerve if a graft is to be carried out.

5. Division of the temporomandibular joint and zygomatic arch.

6. Division of the styloid process to define the position of the carotid artery.

7. Division of the posterior border of the mastoid process posterior to the lateral sinus.

8. Division of the floor of the middle ear and the bulb of the jugular vein.

9. Transection of the petrous pyramid lateral to the internal carotid artery and medial to the arcuate eminence using a Stryker saw or curved chisels.

10. Reconstitution of continuity of the facial nerve either by facial–hypoglossal anastomosis or by a cross-face graft. In practice these are not often successful and local procedures to take a tuck in the facial muscles are probably better.

11. Cover of the soft tissue defect, firstly by a scalp flap, which is easy but does not provide bulk, secondly by a pectoralis major flap, which provides bulk but reaches the defect with difficulty or not at all, or thirdly by a free rectus abdominis or latissimus dorsi flap, which are very reliable and versatile and provide well vascularized muscle to plug the defect, control infection, seal CSF leaks, and provide skin cover.

Surgery of the Anterior Cranial Fossa

The second problem concerns tumors of the anterior skull base. Craniofacial surgery for tumor resection was introduced in 1941 by Dandy, a neurosurgeon who advocated the concept of extending the resection of orbital tumors into the central nervous system where they most frequently failed.

The craniofacial concept was not applied to the treatment of tumors of the nasal sinuses until Smith published a case in which, for the first time, a neurosurgeon working in conjunction with a head and neck surgeon successfully resected en bloc an antroethmoidal orbital tumor, including the cribriform plate, ethmoid roof, and the anterior wall of the sphenoid in the specimen. This new technique was only attempted slowly, but Ketcham et al. reported a series of seventeen anterior craniofacial resections in 1963. During the next 10 years, Ketcham and his colleagues wrote three further articles reporting details of complications and survival, and showing a dramatic increase in survival from 15 to 50%.

Despite its effectiveness in improving survival, the operation had a significant associated morbidity and mortality. Initial efforts in refining craniofacial surgery were directed toward correcting the major complications, notably osteomyelitis of the bone flap, and brain trauma due to frontal lobe retraction. In their last article, Ketcham et al. described the use of a single, central frontal bur hole instead of a frontal bone flap to avoid creating any areas of nonvascularized bone to prevent what they found to be the main source of operative morbidity.

Two schools of thought then formed concerning the best approach. The first continued the dual approach technique by a separate bifrontal craniotomy in conjunction with a separate lateral rhinotomy. The second was modified to allow a dual approach, i. e. a minicraniotomy in association with a lateral rhinotomy, through a single transfacial incision. The difficulty with these techniques is that they both create a nonvascularized anterior bone flap that has led to a loss of the flap in 20% of cases. Because of this persistent problem Panje (17) has developed a modification of Ketcham's transfacial intracranial approach to the anterior skull base. To improve on the technique, and yet maintain the concept of en bloc removal of the anterior skull base neoplasm, the following four specific areas were addressed:

1. Intracranial exposure of the anterior skull base without any need for frontal lobe retraction
2. Development of a vascularized bone flap that would retard infection
3. Improvement of transfacial exposure of the anterior skull base so as to allow proper exposure for en bloc tumor removal through one incision regardless of size or orbital encroachment
4. Avoidance of facial and oral mutilation

The transfacial approach to the anterior cranial fossa for tumor removal provides excellent surgical exposure, improved postoperative appearance, and a minimum of complications. The technique is different from previously reported combined craniofacial ablative procedures in that the head and neck surgeon and the neurosurgeon approach the anterior fossa mass through the same facial incision, thus avoiding the need for a separate craniotomy incision.

The formation of a vascularized nasofrontal bone flap allows for better wound healing regardless of preoperative and postoperative radiotherapy and/or chemotherapy (17).

Modified versus Radical Neck Dissections

The classical excisional procedure for malignant cervical nodes is the radical neck dissection described by Crile (4) in 1906. This operation achieves a good survival of about 35% but at the cost of significant morbidity. The most obvious is the shoulder syndrome (18) consisting of pain in the shoulder joint, limitation of abduction of the shoulder, drooping of the shoulder, and prominence of the scapula. In the last 25 years attempts have been made to develop less mutilating procedures without compromising oncological safety.

In 1966 Bocca reported 100 conservative neck dissections and compared the results with 100 classic radical neck dissections. There was no differences in survival of the two groups. Bocca's procedure entailed careful dissection of the cervical fascia and the removal of all fibrofatty tissue in the neck containing the lymphatic system, but with preservation of the sternocleidomastoid muscle, internal jugular vein, spinal accessory nerve, the cervical plexus, and usually the submandibular gland.

At about the same time Jesse and his collegaues developed a similar procedure. They were stimulated by the question as to why certain important structures (such as the carotid artery, the vagus, phrenic, hypoglossal, and lingual nerves, and the supraclavicular trunks of the branchial plexus) could be spared and yet other structures (such as the sternocleidomastoid muscle, spinal accessory nerve, and jugular vein) must be eradicated. The advantages of a modified neck dissection with preservation of the accessory nerve, jugular vein, and sternocleidomastoid muscle are as follows:

1. Preservation of neck and shoulder girdle function
2. Better cosmetic contour of the neck
3. Protection of the internal carotid artery
4. Capability of performing bilateral procedures with fewer complications
5. The procedure acts as a staging operation for determining the prognosis, the need for a more extensive procedure, and the need for postoperative X-ray therapy (5).

The rationale of doing this less-than-radical neck dissection is that control of cancer in the neck in selected cases, such as the N0 and N1 neck, is as good as with radical neck dissection but with less trauma. One of the main purposes is to reduce the incidence of the "shoulder syndrome". However, this syndrome is not invariable after classical radical neck dissection, nor is it prevented by preservation of the accessory nerve. A study by Leipzig (19) demonstrated that only 60% of patients demonstrated a significant shoulder syndrome after classical dissection, whereas 30% of patients whose accessory nerve was preserved showed this feature. Shoulder function can be preserved in whole or in part in some patients by preserving the branches from C3 and C4 to the trapezius muscle (20).

All surgeons who are interested in head and neck cancer at the present time agree that the purpose of neck dissection, radical or modified, should focus on the complete excision of all metastatic disease in the neck and must include in the removal the less essential structures, the associated lymph nodes, cervical fascia, and fibrofatty connective tissue. If necessary, other structures remaining should be sacrificed if their removal will make possible more complete excision of metastatic cancer.

Laser

The laser has been available as a surgical tool for 20 years, and the scope of treatment options has not yet been fully explored. In head and neck surgery the main type of laser in use is the carbon dioxide laser. However, due to more recent technological advances in delivery of the beam via quartz−glass fibers, the neodymium: Ittrium aluminum Garner Laser (Nd: YAG laser) and the argon ion laser are becoming increasingly useful in specific situations, because of their individual characteristics.

The carbon dioxide laser emits invisible light with a wavelength of 10.6 µm, which is within the infrared range. The light beam is absorbed in the tissues, especially by water, where it is released as thermal energy, resulting in the vaporization of tissue. There is minimal scatter of the beam when it strikes the tissue and therefore minimal penetration of the surrounding tissue, leading to its description as the laser "knife". The beam is aimed by using a low power helium−neon (He−Ne) laser guide which emits a red beam of light. The role of the CO_2 laser for benign pathology of the head and neck, such as juvenile papillomatosis, subglottic stenoses, laryngeal webs, choanal atresia, and lingual tonsils, is well recorded, though there remains controversy as to whether it is the best means of treatment of these conditions.

Its role in cancer surgery is still emerging. It has been used for excisional biopsy and staging of early laryngeal carcinomas before radiotherapy. An extension of this use is as a curative tool in some cases (21), where clearance is demonstrated. However, normal oncological principles for tumor excision must still be adhered to, so that its use remains controversial, and will need further validation by controlled clinical trials. Perhaps a more useful application in the larynx, is for advanced lesions, when the patient presents with stridor and progressive asphyxia where it is used to debulk such lesions thus avoiding either an emergency tracheostomy or emergency laryngectomy (13). It permits elective investigation of the patient radiologically and histopathologically before deciding on a treatment policy. This concept has been taken a stage further by debulking of large exophytic tumors as a routine adjunct to definitive radiotherapy (22).

Its use in extralaryngeal malignancy has also been advocated especially for carcinoma of the tongue where, due to its limited thermal damage and reasonable coagulatory effect, it gives a good clean bed for grafting. However, once again no compromise in margins of clearance can be accepted so that its use is limited to small superficial lesions. Other uses include the debulking of large obstructive nasopharyngeal tumors.

The CO_2 laser has also been successfully used to palliate patients with tracheobronchial malignancies (23), which has been facilitated by the development of reflective mirror bronchoscopic delivery systems. However, whilst it effectively varporizes tumor, and, due to its shallow penetration, carries only a minimal risk of puncturing the trachea or bronchi, it carries a high risk of perioperative hemorrhage due to its relatively poor coagulatory effect in comparison with other laser systems: many tracheobronchial lesions are highly vascular and unless effectively coagulated before excision, bleed into the lung fields.

For this reason these lesions are more effectively and safely treated by the Nd:YAG laser (24). The Nd:YAG laser emits an invisible light beam at 1.064 μm wavelength and can be transmitted through quartz–glass fibers which are passed via a rigid or flexible bronchoscope. A He–Ne laser is used to aim the Nd:YAG laser. The beam scatters on impact with the tissues resulting in deep penetration of between from 6 to 10 mm, in comparison with the CO_2 laser which penetrates only up to 0.5 mm. Due to this penetration, it coagulates blood vessels as well as vaporizing tissue. Thus it has become the laser of choice for tracheobronchial lesions, but due to its depth of penetration it also carries a greater risk of perforation of the trachea or bronchi, as well as causing more necrosis and edema. Due to the different properties of these lasers, it has been suggested that combination treatment, using the Nd:YAG laser initially as a coagulation, followed by the CO_2 laser as a vaporizer, would be the best option (25).

Whichever option is chosen, it is generally used as a palliative measure, and is only suitable for intraluminal lesions. Sadly, if there is total occlusion with distal collapse, the results are disappointing: the patient's condition deteriorates by creation of an additional dead space. It is also used to control persistent uncontrolled hemoptysis.

A more recent proposal is the use of the Nd:YAG laser to canalize tracheobronchial tumors as an adjuvant to high dose local irradiation via an afterloading catheter (26), or external beam (27).

Hematoporphyrins and the Laser

A relatively new and still largely experimental field of treatment is photoradiation therapy (PRT) or photodynamic therapy (PDT) (28). Much work has been carried out in laboratory models and animals but clinical studies have been reported only recently with any frequency. The basis of treatment is the cytotoxic effects of light as described by Raab in 1900 (29) in acridine-dye sensitized *Paramecium*. The sensitzer generally used is a hematoporphyrin derivate (HpD). One of the active agents is thought to be di haematoporphyrin ether (DHE) or Photofrin II. When either is exposed to blue light it fluoresces, leading to the proposal that they could be used in the early detection of carcinomas. With red light a photochemical reaction excites the porphyrin, releasing singlet oxygen which is thought to be the main cytotoxic agent, though other free radicals, including hydrogen peroxide, hydrogen, and superoxide are also implicated. Damage occurs mainly at the outer cell membrane, mitochondria, and lysosomes of cells, but there is also thought to be a direct action of PRT on the vascular stroma of the tumor.

The selective effect of sensitizers relies on certain characteristics of the agents. They should be nontoxic, be taken up preferentially by tumor cells with a resultant high tumor to normal tissue ratio, and be activated by a light wavelength that produces good penetration and photochemical efficiency. In fact HpD is taken up by many tissues including the skin, liver, and tumor, but by 72 hours most has been excreted through bile and urine except from the skin and tumor where it is preferentially retained. The skin retention causes problems since bright light must be avoided for up to a month.

The cytotoxic action is most marked at 405 nm but there is limited penetration whereas red light at 630 nm has good penetration but with a slightly reduced cytotoxicity. Therefore the light source generally used is an argon ion laser that pumps a rhodamine B dye laser which together produce a light of 630 mm wavelength. The main problem with this system is the loss of power of up to 75% between the argon laser and the final beam. Alternatives such as the gold vapor laser and the copper vapor laser are being considered.

The argon pumped dye laser has been used in a number of different sites including the skin, bladder, stomach, breast, and brain. It has been used to palliate and treat tracheobronchial malignancies (30) but its mode of action results in extensive necrosis and edema so that obstruction as a result of treatment is always a risk. It has also been used in head and neck sites especially the skin and tongue. The responses, where conventional methods had already failed to achieve palliation, have been encouraging (31) but it is too early to evaluate the role of this modality of treatment. One suggestion is that it could have a role to play in debulking tumors before radiotherapy.

Progress in Reconstruction and Rehabilitation

Voice Restoration

Restoration and rehabilitation of function is an important part of management following extensive resection of malignancies of the head and neck. After total laryngectomy, both swallowing and speech are affected, though swallowing soon returns to a relatively normal state. However, the normal mode of speech can never be restored and alternative methods need to be found. This challenge has been addressed ever since the first laryngectomy by Billroth in 1873. Gussenbauer (32) designed a custom-made external prosthesis for this patient which connected the tracheostoma to the pharynx, and created a resasonable voice. A variety of methods of voice restoration have been suggested since that time, particularly since the Second World War, but broadly speaking, they fall into five categories:

1. Esophageal speech
2. External fistula with a prosthetic device
3. Electrical intraoral or neck vibrator
4. Pneumatic intraoral device
5. Internal fistula with or without a prosthesis

At least one in three patients fail to develop esophageal speech (33), and a further proportion have inadequate communication skills with esophageal speech. It is for this reason that many methods of voice restoration propose the concept of diverting exhaled pulmonary air into the esophagus or pharynx to act as a "bellows" or injection system for the articulators.

The earliest surgical methods relied on creating a pharyngeal or esophagocutaneous fistula which could be connected to the tracheostoma by an externally worn prosthesis. Several different methods of producing fistulae were described (34–36) as well as many different types of prostheses to be used in conjunction with them. But all had a high complication rate due to salivary leakage and also tract stenosis, and they have now been discarded.

In the late 1960s and early 1970s several methods of voice restoration were described based on an internal tracheopharyngeal fistula or tracheoesophageal fistula (37–39). The term neoglottis was coined for these methods. However, once again they were associated with a high level of failure to produce effective speech, except in the hands of their originators. In addition, there was a high rate of stenosis and salivary leakage, often requiring multiple surgical revisions. Furthermore, most of the techniques described require extensive preservation of the trachea or even parts of the larynx. Therefore there was always a temptation to risk an oncological compromise in the surgical resection of the larynx for the sake of voice restoration. Due to the development of new techniques these methods have largely fallen out of favor.

The most significant advances have been in the last decade, beginning in the early 1980s when Singer and Blom (40) described a new indwelling valved prosthesis that could be inserted quite simply into an endoscopically created tracheooesophageal fistula or puncture. Since then the main thrust of developments in voice restoration has been along the lines of modifications or new designs of valved prostheses, including such examples as the Panje button, the Groningen prosthesis, and the Bonelli speech prosthesis among others.

The principle for all the prostheses is essentially the same. A small but direct fistula into the esophagus is created in the back wall of the tracheostoma. One of the many valves available is inserted into the fistula either immediately or after a few days when the tract has become more clearly defined, a catheter having been left in the tract. In the early days, salivary leakage and displacement of valves was common and once a valve is displaced spontaneous closure of the fistula rapidly follows. However, most prostheses now incorporate an esophageal flange to retain them in position, and some a tracheal flange in addition. The actual valve components come in various forms but are basically one-way valves which permit the flow of air from the lungs into the esophagus and pharynx, whilst preventing backflow of saliva and food into the trachea.

There are, however, still complications (41) including salivary leakage, inhalation of valves, granulations of the fistula, and inability to use the valve. However, the complications are generally less serious and less common, with a far higher success rate in terms of effective speech production than other techniques.

One of the major problems associated with valved prosthetic speech is the need to clean the valve or to change it at regular intervals, as secretions tend to block the lumen and make voice production difficult. Therefore the patient's understanding and motivation is extremely important if they are to learn to cope with the difficulties of self-management of these valves. In addition, patients must have good manual dexterity and good vision, otherwise they cannot manage effectively many of the commercially available valves.

The present situation, therefore, in voice restoration is that of providing valved speech either as a primary surgical procedure or as a delayed procedure with or without giving the patient the opportunity to develop esophageal speech. Important parts of a voice restoration progam include careful selection criteria and effective and enthusiastic follow-up of patients to try to head off problems before they get out of hand. In those patients who fail to develop either valved or esophageal speech, or in whom either or both methods of communication are rejected, electrical vibrators, either intraoral or neck devices, provide an acceptable alternative method of communication which is uncomplicated though a little cumbersome. Certainly these devices are especially useful when patients fail to reach the criteria of selection for valved speech.

The development of the Bivona stomal breathing valve is very useful for patients, releasing their hands during conversation, which would otherwise be needed for stomal occlusion.

Development or more "patient friendly" valves would seem to be the way forward at present though the experimental field of computerized voice production promises to be interesting and potentially very useful. There is, however, no place for elaborate surgery to construct various fistulae for nonprosthetic speech at the present time, as the risks are too high in comparison to other available modalities of speech restoration.

Musculocutaneous Flaps

The development of musculocutaneous flaps has depended on an increased understanding of the physiology of the blood flow to the skin. Most of the skin derives its blood supply from small musculocutaneous vessels which arise from the segmental artery lying deep in the muscles, penetrate the muscle and enter the skin perpendicular to its surface, supplying only a small area of skin.

Segmental Vessels

These vessels have perfusion pressures similar to those in the aorta. They are related to the course of underlying nerves and not to that of the bony skeleton, they run deep to muscle masses and are accompanied by large veins and their associated nerves. They also provide the perforator vessels to the muscles. An example is the thoracoacromial artery, which provides circulation to the major portion of the pectoralis major muscle.

Perforator Vessels

These vessels supply the circulation to the muscles, and also provide communication between the deeper segmental vessels and the cutaneous vessels.

An example is the intercostal perforators from the internal mammary artery, which provide circulation to the medial portion of the pectoralis major muscle and to the base of the deltopectoral flap.

Cutaneous Vessels

There are two varieties of cutaneous vessels: musculocutaneous and direct cutaneous. Musculocutaneous vessels are the innumerable small, delicate vessels passing from the segmental vessels through the muscle and extending through the subcutaneous tissue to provide circulation to the overlying skin. These vessels are found throughout the body where skin lies over a muscle mass. In contrast, direct cutaneous vessels are in direct communication with the perforator vessels. They run superficial to muscle masses and supply a discrete region of overlying skin directly. An example is the axial cutaneous vessels from the intercostal perforators at the base of a deltopectoral flap which has been described previously.

The blood supply to muscles may be subdivided into five types (42):

Type I: one vascular pedicle. Muscles with this vascular pattern include the medial gastrocnemius, the lateral gastrocnemius, rectus femoris, and tensor fascia lata. None of these is in use in the head and neck.

Typ II: dominant vascular pedicle(s) and minor vascular pedicle(s). The larger dominant vascular pedicles will sustain circulation to these muscles after their elevation as a flap when the smaller minor pedicles are divided. This is the most common pattern of circulation observed in human muscle. Muscles with this vascular pattern which are used in head and neck surgery, include the platysma, the sternocleidomastoid, and the trapezius.

Type III: two dominant pedicles. These pedicles have either a separate regional source of circulation or the vascular pedicles lie on opposite sides of the muscle. Regional and selective angiograms demonstrate equal filling of the arterial vessels within the muscle by these two pedicles, so that division of one pedicle may cause loss of muscle. Muscles with this vascular pattern used in head and neck surgery include the rectus abominis, serratus anterior, and the temporalis.

Type IV: segmental vascular pedicles. These muscles have multiple vascular pedicles entering the course of the muscle belly. Each pedicle provides circulation to a portion of the muscle. Division of more than two or three of these pedicles during elevation of a flap results in distal muscle necrosis.

Type V: one dominant vascular pedicle and secondary segmental vascular pedicles. Anatomic studies reveal a large vascular pedicle within the shoulder girdle to these muscles. Selective angiograms demonstrate filling of the internal vasculature of the muscle via this pedicle. However, the segmental pedicles entering these muscles at the midline of the trunk also provide a significant source of circulation of these muscles. The internal vasculature of these muscles is also filled on angiograms via these secondary segmental pedicles. These muscles may be elevated as a flap on either vascular system. Muscles with this vascular pattern include the pectoralis major and the latissimus dorsi. The workhorse is undoutedly the pectoralis major flap.

Axial and Random Muscle Flaps

Muscles themselves may also have a random or axial blood supply. Round muscles such as the sternocleidomastoid, biceps femoris, gastrocnius, and soleus have only perforating vessels providing a random supply. Usually the branches penetrate the proximal one-third of the muscle belly and continue in the deep aspect of the upper two-thirds of the muscle, while the lower third of the muscle is supplied by two or three small vessels. In contrast, flat muscles such as the pectoralis major muscle have an axial blood supply. For example, the pectoralis major is supplied by the thoracoacromial artery (a segmental vessel), which runs axially along its entire undersurface and provides perforator vessels to the muscle along its course. Other flat muscles such as the trapezius and latissimus dorsi also have these axial segmental vessels.

Flat muscle flaps can be thought of as axial myocutaneous flaps. Only those portions of the muscle along the vascular axis that are necessary need be elevated, allowing some of the muscle to be left behind, if desired. Round muscle flaps can be thought of as random myocutaneous flaps and need to be completely elevated. They cannot be split because the muscles do not have segmental vessels and would become devascularized. Each one of these myocutaneous flaps can also be completely freed of origin and insertion. As with the cutaneous flaps, this flap can be left attached only by the arteriovenous pedicle and transported on its vascular axis of rotation as an island myocutaneous flap, or it can be transplanted by microvascular techniques as a free myocutaneous flap (43).

The following description of the musculocutaneous flaps in common use in head and neck surgery is taken from an excellent review by Ariyan (43).

Latissimus Dorsi

The oldest myocutaneous flap to be described is the latissimus dorsi, which dates back to the turn of the century. It is a flat muscle arising from the posterior aspect of the lower six thoracic vertebrae, the lumbar vertebrae, and the sacral vertebrae, as well as from the posterior iliac crest. It converges into a tendinous insertion on the intertubercular groove of the humerus. The vascular pedicle to the muscle is the thoracodorsal artery and its accompanying vein, which course axially along the direction of the fibers from the tendinous insertion.

The advantage of this flap is that it can transport tissue on a long vascular pedicle with a good arc of rotation. Its major disadvantages are the change of position of the patient to expose the donor site, and tunneling of the flap through the area of the anterior chest, which is itself a good donor site for flaps.

Pectoralis Major

The pectoralis major is a flat, fan-shaped muscle covering the upper chest. The muscle fibers run horizontally in the upper portion, and in the lower portion they run obliquely along a course to the shoulder from the sternum, the xiphoid process, and the lower ribs.

The muscle receives a large segmental blood supply from the thoracoacromial artery running along the undersurface of the pectoralis major in an axis from the shoulder to the xiphoid process.

The pectoralis major flap has the advantage of being an axial myocutaneous flap that may be elevated for some distance on its vessels alone (although it is elevated with a strip of overlying muscle to ensure safety and provide bulk). Because of the excellent blood supply, this flap can provide vascularity at the recipient site. It also has sufficient bulk to fill cavities, to augment contour, and to provide structural support. If this myocutaneous flap is elevated on a narrow muscle pedicle, it can serve to replace the contour of the sternocleidomastoid muscle and restore symmetry to the neck after a radical neck dissection. In addition, if the muscle pedicle is elevated without the overlying skin, a skin "paddle" at the end of the muscle can be transported to the recipient site under the neck flaps in one stage, without the need for a later division and inset of the flap. Unless an extraordinarily large flap is elevated, the donor site is usually closed primarily, by means of advancing the adjacent skin.

Sternocleidomastoid

The sternocleidomastoid (SCM) muscle is a round-muscle that arises from two tendinous fascicles attached to the sternum and the medial one-third of the clavicle, passes obliquely across the side of the neck, and is inserted on the lateral surface of the mastoid process.

The three sources of circulation to the SCM muscle enter the belly through nutrient arteries at various sites, and there is no axial distribut of vessels along the undersurface of the muscle. One muscular branch from the occipital artery enters the superior portion of the muscle just below the mastoid region. The supply to the inferior portion of the muscle is provided by a branch of the thyrocervical trunk. Midway between its origin and insertion the SCM is supplied by a branch of the superior thyroid artery as well as by smaller vessels from the adjacent strap muscles.

As a result of this triple blood supply, a musculocutaneous flap can be designed with a paddle of skin that is attached to the end of a pedicle of SCM muscle, elevated from the neck, and based on either the superior or inferior blood supply.

The advantages of this flap are that it allows one-stage reconstruction of oropharyngeal defects of moderate size, that it employs local tissues, and that the donor sites can be closed either by local transposition flaps or by local advancement of neck skin, which eliminates the need for skin grafts. In addition, this musculocutaneous flap can be used successfully even if the neck has been irradiated, provided that the skin to be used is soft and supple and shows no evidence of radiation edema or induration.

A major objection to the use of this SCM flap is that it violates the principles of radical cancer resection. For many years, this muscle has been routinely sacrificed as part of the classical radical neck dissection. The investing layer of the cervical fascia over the anterior cervical triangle splits into anterior and posterior sheets to envelope the SCM, then converges again to cover the posterior cervical triangle. As such, the muscle can be dissected with only the anterior sheet of this enveloping portion of the fascia. The muscle can then be elevated from the posterior layer, which is left in its bed in continuity with the anterior and posterior cervical triangles. In this manner, the contents of the underlying neck structures are left undisturbed.

Trapezius

The trapezius is a flat, triangular muscle of the back of the neck and shoulders. Its muscle fibers originate from the occiput and the spinous processes of all the thoracic vertebrae; the muscle is inserted on the lateral third of the clavicle, the acromion, and the scapular spine. This muscle has three blood supplies: the upper neck portion of the muscle is supplied by a segmental branch of the occipital artery; the distal portion is supplied by a branch of the suprascapular artery at the shoulder tip; and the transverse cervical artery supplies the base of the muscle and transverses dorsally along the lateral portion of the spine.

This flap has the advantage of providing a good amount of neck skin without prior delaying procedures. Its disadvantages are: the donor site needs to be skin grafted; the flap can only cover the neck up to the midline on the ipsilateral side (if the flap is not lengthened with delays); and if it is used for intraoral covering, the base of the flap is too bulky for primary closure and requires a controlled orocutaneous fistula.

The choice of which flap to use is determined by many factors including the condition of the patient, the complexity of the defect, and the skills available. As regards the latter factor, it must be assumed that all the necessary skills are available including the ability to perform microvascular surgery; the surgeon doing this type of surgery must be capable of carrying out the full range of techniques, otherwise his decisions will be compromised, and the patient may not have the optimum treatment. There is a range of techniques varying in complexity and cost from the use of a split skin graft at one end to the use of a free revascularized microvascular free flap transfer at the other end. The simplest, most reliable and shortest technique must always be used. The use of split skin, however, is now confined almost entirely to the repair of the defect produced by harvesting of a flap (if this defect cannot be closed primarily which is the best solution) and to resurfacing superficial defects within the mouth.

Free Flaps

Perhaps the most significant single advance in reconstructive surgery of the head and neck in the last 10 years has been the explosion in the development and use of free revascularized grafts. This has been due largely to improved technology of both microscopes and microinstruments, as well as advances in the actual techniques of making the anastomoses, with a high rate of success. It has made possible the transfer of tissues specifically suited to a specific defect. Previously it was necessary to use axial flaps such as the deltopectoral or forehead flaps with their disfiguring results and inevitable multistage procedures. The advent of the musculocutaneous island flaps occurred at much the same time as the beginning of the free revascularized graft explosion, and due to the relative simplicity of raising these flaps and the fact that they can be used as a one-stage procedure even for the hypopharynx, they remain popular. However, despite the versatility they do not fulfil all the criteria for all the defects that occur in the head and neck. They have a limited length of pedicle and are inevitably bulky in comparison to many of the present-day alternatives. In addition, when large paddles of skin are raised, they leave a cosmetically unpleasant scar on the chest wall. The complications associated with its use in certain sites make it almost unacceptable as a choice when compared to viable alternatives, for example for replacement of the hypopharynx following total pharyngolaryngectomy. Nevertheless, along with other local pedicled flaps, it remains a very useful tool in reconstruction, and in many patients with defects who would not be suited to a free revascularized graft, it is still the method of choice.

The pectoralis major musculocutaneous flap continues to be the backbone of head and neck reconstruction but its role has been seriously undermined by the development of free revascularized grafts, which have replaced it at many anatomical sites in those centers which have developed microvascular expertise. However, by using conventional techniques, a surgeon can complete both resection and reconstruction, without becoming overtired. In contrast, free revascularized grafts require a longer operation, so that the surgeon who has done the resection is not the best person to complete the revascularization. Thus it is generally necessary to have a team for this type of surgery which can prove to be a logistical problem particularly outside larger centers. The other danger, as with any new technique, is overuse.

When used with circumspection, free revascularized grafts provide an invaluable addition to the armamentarium of reconstructive techniques in the head and neck. It is perhaps wisest to use two or three types of flaps only, as there is a certain amount of technical expertise required in the raising of some of the free grafts. In certain resections, their use has become the treatment of choice, and as expertise becomes more widespread, they will probably become the universal choice. It would be useful to consider a few examples of their application and the advantages that they confer on the patient and his subsequent recovery.

Reconstruction of the hypopharynx following total pharyngolaryngectomy has always proved a challenge to the reconstructive surgeon. Earlier methods of reconstruction included deltopectoral flaps, pectoralis major myocutaneous island grafts, and a plethora of other skin grafts and miscellaneous techniques (3). However, even with pectoralis major flap reconstruction, the complication rate, in terms of fistula and stenosis and thus prolonged hospitalization and functional rehabilitation, is inacceptably high (44). For tumors which can be resected with a good margin, thus avoiding the inevitably increased morbidity and mortality of a stomach pull-up, the jejunal flap transfer with microvascular revascularization provides a far superior alternative (45, 46).

There are few intra-abdominal complications and in the neck the loop provides a much more physiologically compatible material with which to reconstruct the hypopharynx, though the technique is not totally free of complications (47). A mucosa-to-mucosa anastomosis ensures a low fistula and stenosis rate, and rapid rehabilitation. Speech can be developed with a valved system such as the Blom—Singer valve.

Free jejunal loops can also be used in areas which have traditionally been difficult to reconstruct effectively due to the multiplane nature of the defect, such as the palate, the nasopharynx and oropharynx (48). The loop can be opened along its antimesen-

teric border and divided into two or three separate or connecting paddles of jejunum so that it can be manipulated to these three-dimensional defects. No skin flaps, including free revascularized skin grafts, permit this arrangement. Recreation of mucosal continuity again ensures fewer complications such as fistula formation. An equally effective free revascularized graft for this type of defect is the omentum.

Free revascularized omentum, when harvested and based upon the right gastroepiploic vessels, provides a variable sized, malleable, well vascularized defect filler, than can be molded to fit almost any defect. Its particular advantage over other known alternatives is its vascularity (49), and its long pedicle so that the anastomosis can be made outside an irradiated field. This feature can be utilized in difficult cases of fistula closure. Some fistulae can be very resistant to closure using conventional or free skin flaps, but omentum is highly successful in achieving a seal even in a heavily irradiated field with infection. However, this needs further evaluation before gaining full acceptance as a technique of fistula closure.

Free revascularized skin grafts offer the choice to the surgeon of whether or not to have bulk, muscle, and bone. For example, if only lining is required for an intraoral defect, a forearm flap provides a perfect solution. If, however, more bulk is required, a rectus abdominus or latissimus dorsi free graft can be used, and where bone is required to repair a mandibular defect, composite iliac crest free grafts or trapezius with spine of scapula can be used.

Undoubtedly the developments in this field of reconstructive surgery have made the success rate of revascularized grafts highly acceptable, generally having about 95% patency rates. This, along with the wide choice of grafts, allows specific tailoring of the donor graft to the defect that requires repair.

Mandibular Reconstruction

The mandible is an important structure in the support of dentition, and contributes to speech, the swallowing mechanism, the patency of the airway, and facial appearance. Loss of bone, therefore, is detrimental to these functions, particularly loss of the anterior arch. However, reconstruction of the mandible remains difficult, especially after extensive intraoral resection following radiotherapy. The problems that contribute to these difficulties are the immense stresses that are applied to the mandible during deglutition and the risk of infection of the graft due to contamination by saliva, atrophy of the mandible, loss of osteoblasts after irradiation, and the high degree of mobility of the temperomandibular joint. The two main directions of development have been alloplastic materials and bone, either homologous or autogenous.

Various types and forms of allopastic implants have been used, including Kirschner wires, meshes, trays, and plates. Latterly, the materials used have been relatively bioinactive metal alloys such as vitallium and titanium. However, vitallium is not very malleable so that the shape has to be fairly accurate for the defect to be filled. Titanium is more malleable and is probably the preferred alloy. However, the problems have always been those of infection and intra-oral exposure. The latter requires that the implant be removed. They have been used in conjunction with the alloplastic implants in the form of trays following trauma (50), but the success rates were not high following cancer surgery. In addition due to the metal it was difficult to assess new bone formation by radiology and also to calculate the dose of postoperative radiotherapy. Nonmetallic trays of Dacron−urethane have been designed to overcome these two problems.

The other problem with free bone grafts in alloplastic trays has been of maintaining a good vascular supply into the region of the graft. Owing to the poor results, interest has been turned to other alloplastic methods, in particular those using plating systems. The OA plating system is a metallic plate malleable in three dimensions; therefore it is sometimes referred to as the three-dimensional bendable defect bridging plate or 3DBDB. It is applied to the outer surface of the mandible, and at least three or four screws are used to support the fixation of each mandibular section. Owing to its lateral position it is less likely to become exposed within the mouth and it can be carried out quickly with reasonable cosmetic results. The initial idea was to use these plates as temporary splints whilst healing occurred, but when used in conjunction with bulky soft tissue flaps which cover them on the intraoral aspect, they have been found to provide a good long-term solution to mandibular reconstruction without recourse to delayed bone grafting (51). They have also been used in conjunction with solid sections of either homologous or autogenous bone grafts. The former have not proved reliable and are no longer used, although the theoretical advantage of being able to preform the shape remains attractive. Autogenous bone has been more successful, being harvested either from the iliac crest, rib, or spine of scapula, but again the complication rate is high and other methods have superseded them. Other infrequently used methods of using free bone grafts include cryogenically devitalized bone (52) and perioperatively irradiated mandible (53), but they have not gained wide acceptance.

The logical progression of free bone grafts was to harvest them in continuity with the soft tissue used in the repair, hopefully with an intact blood supply. The two main osteomusculocutaneous pedicled flaps described are the pectoralis major island flap with rib (usually the fifth or sixth) and the trapezius osteomusculocutaneous flap with the spine of the scapula (54, 55). Unfortunately, except for a few isolated reports (17), the acceptance rate was low; furthermore, only limited lengths of bone could be harvested making these grafts inappropriate for large defects.

Fortunately, the development of free revascularized flaps (56, 57) has revitalized the basic concepts of pedicled osteomusculocutaneous flaps, and new sources of bone with skin and muscle have been identified over the last decade. The advantages of free revascularized flaps is that they can be moved from sites where adequate lengths of bone can be harvested, as well as providing good soft tissue cover, either for the intraoral repair, the external repair or both. The most commonly employed integral free osteomusculocutaneous grafts are the iliac crest graft, the radius−forearm flap, and the free scapular osteomusculocutaneous flap.

Each has advantages: the iliac crest has good bulk with an osseous component that closely matches the curvature of the mandible, but the donor site is painful postoperatively and the graft may be too bulky. The radius forearm flap is simple to harvest and provides a good relatively thin intraoral lining where not too much bulk is required, but only about 10−12 cm of bone can be harvested, and there is always a risk of fracture of the remaining radius. The radial graft can be divided into segments and secured with the OA plating system to achieve adequate contouring. The free scapular osteomusculocutaneous flap has the advantages of providing good bone length but the position of the patient must be changed during the operation. In the end the choice is individual, depending on experience with a particular flap and which bone conforms best to reconstruction in each surgeon's hands.

The results of revascularized osteomusculocutaneous flaps have been very encouraging with far more patients having a successful outcome than with earlier techniques but, however, the procedures are time-consuming and not appropriate in all patients due to factors such as age, general health, and vascular status, i.e. the condition of donor or graft vessels. These grafts are generally secured in position with plating systems.

At present, therefore, the best options for mandibular reconstruction are free revascularized osteomusculocutaneous flaps or malleable plating systems, alone or in combination.

Maxillary Prosthetics

The defects created by palatal and maxillary resections for malignant disease need to be inspected at regular intervals in order to exclude a recurrence. Consequently closure of the defect with surgical flaps is contraindicated but prosthetic rehabilitation is often complex, especially when a very large cavity is created or where the soft palate has been removed. The main complications of ineffective closure of the defect relate to swallowing and speech. There is nasal leakage of food and fluid, and a nasal voice that is poorly understood. It is therefore the function of the prosthesis to make a tight seal with the edges of the defect, especially in those areas which move, such as the palate, to avoid these complications. At the same time it must be easily removable and equally easily retained.

The main directions of progress have been in surgical measures to assist retention, and in prosthetic materials and design, with particular emphasis on retention methods.

Certain surgical measures are now recognized to enhance the success of obturator retention. Perhaps the most useful technique is the careful application of split skin grafts to the inside of the denuded cheek and which is initially held in place by the obturator. A scar band forms at the mucocutaneous junction and this band provides useful retention band for later obturators. Another useful retaining band is the palatal remnant: as much as possible of the palatal shelf should be preserved so that it extends into the cavity. In order to provide adequate epithelial cover for the obturator, a greater margin of palatal epithelial is preserved and folded over the palatal shelf, thus producing a much more resistant epithelial surface than respiratory epithelium. A more controversial measure, in terms of oncological compromise, is the preservation of as much of either the anterior or posterior part of the maxilla, depending on the site of primary tumor. The rationale applies particularly to dentulous patients in whom the preservation of teeth in these areas, are very useful for retaining the obturator. The resection line should, if possible, pass through a tooth socket and not through the interproximal line, so that the tooth adjacent to the resection line has good bony support, thus contributing to the retention of the plate and obturator. An important factor in dislodging the obturator can be the coronoid process of the mandible, which should be removed therefore, especially when the pterygoid plates have been resected. This also minimizes pain on deglutition. Contraction of the cavity during healing may make insertion of the obturator difficult and prone to extrusion unless it is modified. To this end, and to preserve facial symmetry, the patients are taught to administer self physiotherapy to the healthy cavity, as well as scrupulous oral hygiene.

Of greater importance, however, is the progress in the technology and theory that an experienced prosthodontist can bring to the building of a working prosthesis. This work begins before operation and is particularly important for the dentulous patient, since the teeth where possible will be used to support the prosthesis in position. It is in the area of care of carious teeth that great advances have been made: although teeth must often still be removed before operation, preservation of teeth for fixation is much more feasible than previously. Therefore it is important to give the prosthodontist as much time as possible to optimize the condition of the mouth. Dental impressions are taken before surgery in a standard manner, to allow the first or perioperative obturator to be built up in time for the surgery. The extent of surgery, if known, should be explained to the prosthodontist before surgery so that, for example, if the soft palate is lost, he can create a palatal extension to compensate for this loss. Indeed in this area of restoration great advances have been made in achieving adequate closure of the nasopharynx during speech and deglutition, by creating custom-made extensions designed on the basis of dynamic testing of the patient's functions, in particular of velopalatine competence, by videofluroscopy, and by nasoendoscopy. Both these investigations provide a dynamic picture of the palatal movements, and allow the palatal extension to be seated and placed to give maximal closure at times of need, thus preventing nasal leakage of food and fluid.

During the operation, the primary obturator is fixed, the nasal extension acting as a support for the split skin graft and as tamponade for the cavity. The methods of fixation vary according to the dentition, the teeth being used in dentulous patients. Traditionally, zygomatic wires have been used in patients without teeth, but an easier and more acceptable method is the use of palatal screws into the vomer or remaining alveolus.

The prosthodontist now spends considerable time modifying the interim obturator whilst the cavity heals, and only when that process is complete can the final model be designed. It is a common misconception that the cheek is held out by the obturator which can therefore prevent contraction – this is untrue since contraction tends to extrude the prosthesis. Thus regular modification along with physiotherapy are essential in maintaining good function.

The cavity is often very extensive needing a large obturator. In order to facilitate the fixation, hollowed-out obturators can be made to diminish their weight, however, this not universally popular due to retention of secretion in the bowel of the obturator.

The main area of progress at present in this field, is in the methods of fixation of the obturator. Few problems are encountered in patients with good dentition, but in edentulous patients the problems are far greater. Therefore the direction of interest now is towards the newer methods of fixation, including magnetic inserts which are osseointegrated and can hold the obturator in position and by fixation bars which are fixed to osseous integrated screws. However, in general terms the success of obturation of a maxillary defect depends on the amount of bone that can be preserved and what teeth can be retained.

References

1. Ogura JH. Supraglottic subtotal laryngectomy and radical neck dissection for carcinoma of the epiglottis. Laryngoscope 1958; 68:983

2. Absolon KB, Rogers W, Bradley J. Some historical developments of the surgical therapy of tongue cancer from the seventeenth to the nineteenth century. Am J Surg 1962; 104:686.

3. Missotten FEM. Historical review of pharyngo-oesophageal reconstruction after resection for carcinoma of pharynx and cervical oesophagus. Clin Otolaryngol 1983; 8:345.

4. Crile GW. Excision of cancer of the head and neck. J Am Med Assoc 1906; 47:1780.

5. Lingman RE, Shellhamer RH. Surgical management of tumors of the neck. In: Thawley SE, WR Panje, eds. Comprehensive management of head and neck tumors. Vol 2. Philadelphia: WB Saunders, 1987:1325.

6. Hayes Martin D, Del Valle B, Erlich H. Neck dissection. Cancer 1951; 4:441.

7. UICC International Union Against Cancer. 4th ed. London: Springer, 1987.

8. Oloffson J, Nostrand AWP. Growth and spread of laryngeal and hypopharyngeal carcinoma with reflections on the effect of preoperative irradiation. Acta Otolaryngol (Stockh) (Suppl) 308.

9. Harrison DFN. The pathology and management of subglottic cancer. Ann Otol 1971; 80:6.

10. MacGregor IA. In: McGregor IA, McGregor F. Cancer of the face and mouth. London; Churchill Livingstone, 1986.

11. Snow GB, Annyas AA, Van Slooten FA, Bartelink H, Hart, AAM. Prognostic factors of neck node metastases. Clinical Otolaryngol 1982 7:192.

12. Karnofsky DA, Burchenall JH. In: McLead CM, ed. The clinical evaluation of chemotherapeutic agents in cancer. New York: Columbia University Press, 1949:191.

13. Davis RK, Shapsay SM. Pretreatment airway management in obstructing carcinoma of the larynx. Otolaryngol Head Neck Surg 1981; 89:209.

14. deVries N, Gluckman JL. The magnitude of the problem. In: deVries N, Gluckman JL, eds. Multiple primary tumors in the head and neck. Stuttgart: Georg Thieme 1990: 1−29.

15. Batsakis JG. Metastatic neoplasms to and from the head and neck. In: Tumors of the neck. 2nd ed. Baltimore: Williams & Wilkins, 1979: 249−50.

16. Lewis JS. Squamous carcinoma of the ear. Arch Otolaryngol 1973; 97:41

17. Panje, WR, Dohrmann SJ, Pitcock JK, et al. The transfacial approach for combined anterior craniofacial tumour ablations. Arch Otolaryngol Head & Neck Surg 1989; 115:301−7.

18. Nahum AM, Mullally W, Marmor L. A syndrome resulting from radical neck dissection. Arch Otolaryngol 1961; 74:424.

19. Leipzig B, Suen JY, English JL, Barnes J, Hooper H. Functional evaluation of the spinal accessory nerve after neck dissection. Am J Surg 1983; 146:526.

20. Jones TA, Stell PM. The preservation of shoulder function after radical neck dissection. Clin Otolaryngol 1985; 10:89.

21. Blakeslee D, et al. Excisional biopsy in the selective management of T_1 glottic cancers: a three year follow-up study. Laryngoscope 1984; 94:448.

22. Feldman M, et al. Applications of carbon dioxide laser surgery and radiation. Arch Otolaryngol 1983; 109:240.

23. Oswal V, Flood LM, Ruckley RW. Use of bronchoscopic CO_2 laser in palliation of obstruction tracheobronchial malignancy. Laryngol Otol 1988; 102:323

24. Hulks, G, Thomson NC. Laser Treatment of tracheo-bronchial tumours. Scott Med J 1988; 33:323.

25. Parr GW, Unger M, Trout RG, Atkinson WG. One hundred neodynium−YAG laser ablations of obstructing tracheal neoplasms. Ann Thorac Surg 1984; 38:374

26. Macha HN, Koch K, Stadler M, Schumacher W, Krumhaar D. New technique for treating occlusive and stenosing tumours of the trachea and main bronchi: endobronchial irradiation by high dose iridium-192 combined with laser conalisation. Thorax 1987; 42:511.

27. Wolfe WG, Sabiston DC. Management of benign and malignant lesions of the trachea and bronchi with the neodymium−yttrium aluminium−garnet laser. J Thorac Cardiovasc Surg 1986; 91:40.

28. Manyak MJ, Russo A, Smith PD, Glatstein E. J Clin Oncol 1988; 6:380

29. Raab O. Über die Wirkung fluorescirender Stoffe auf Infusorien. Z Biol 1900; 39:524.

30. Vincent RG, Dougherty TJ, Rao U, Boyle DG, Potter WR. Photoradiation therapy in advanced carcinoma of the trachea and bronchus. Chest 1984; 85:29.

31. Carruth, JAS, McKenzie AL. Preliminary report of a pilot study of photoradiation therapy for the treatment of superficial malignancies of the skin, head and neck. Eur J Surg Oncol 1985; 11:47.

32. Gussenbauer C. Über die erste durch Th. Billroth am Menschen ausgefuhrie Kehlkopf-Exstirpation und die Anwendung eines Kunstlichen Kehlkopfes. Arch Clin Chir 1874; 17:343.

33. Watts RF. Total rehabilitation of laryngectomies. Laryngoscope 1975; 85:671.

34. Briani AA. (1952). Reabilitazione fonetica di laringectomizzati a mezzo della corrente aerea espiratoria pulmonae. Arch Ital Ital Otol 1952; 63:469.

35. Conley JJ. Vocal rehabilitation by autogenous vein graft. Ann Otol Rhinol Laryngol 1959; 68:990.

36. Edwards N. Post-laryngectomy vocal rehabilitation. J Laryngol Otol 1974; 88:905.

37. Asai T. Laryngoplasty after total laryngectomy. Arch Otolaryngol 1972; 95:114.

38. Staffieri M. Laringectomia totale con ricostruzione di glottide fonatoria. Communicazione preliminare. Bull Soc Med Chir Bresciana 1970; 24:406.

39. Pearson BW, Woods RD, II, Hartman DE. Extended hemilaryngectomy for T_3 glottic carcinoma with preservation of speech and swallowing. Laryngoscope 1980; 90:950.

40. Singer MI, Blom ED. An endoscopic technique for restoration of voice after laryngectomy. Ann Otol Rhin Laryngol 1980; 89:529.

41. Lund VJ, Perry A, Cheeseman AD. Blom−Singer puncture (practicalities of everyday management). J Laryngol Otol 1987; 101:164.

42. Mathes SJ, Nahai F, Clinical applications for muscle and musculocutaneous flaps. St Louis: CV Mosby 1982.

43. Ariyan S, Cuono CB. Myocutaneous flaps for head and neck reconstruction. Head Neck Surg 1980; 2:321.

44. Surkin MI, Lawson W, Biller HF. Analysis of the methods of pharyngo-oesophageal reconstruction. Head Neck Surg 1984; 6:953.

45. Jurkiewicz MJ. Reconstructive surgery of the cervical oesophagus. Thorac Cardiovasc Surg 1984; 88:893.

46. McDonough JJ, Gluckman JL. Microvascular reconstruction of the pharyngo-oesophagus with free jejunal graft. Microsurgery 1988; 9:116.

47. Gluckman, JL, McCafferty GJ, Black RJ, et al. Complications associated with free jejunal graft reconstruction of the pharyngo−oesophagus − a multi institutional experience with 52 cases. Head Neck Surg 1985; 7:200.

48. Buckspan GS, Newton FD, Franklin JD, Lynch JB. Split jejunal free tissue transfer oropharyngoesophageal reconstruction. Plast Reconstr Surg 1986; 77:717.

49. Harris K. Clinical application of free omental flap transfer. Clin Plast Surg 1978; 5:273.

50. Boyne PJ. Restoration of osseous defects in maxillo-facial casualties. J Am Dent Assoc 1969; 78:767

51. Gullane PJ, Holmes H. Mandibular reconstruction − new concepts. Arch Otolaryngol Head Neck Surg 1986; 112:714.

52. Cummings CW, Leipzig B. Replacement of tumour involved mandible by a cryosurgically devitalized autograph: human experience. Arch Otolaryngol 1980; 106:252.

53. Hamaker RC. Irradiated autogenous mandibular graft in primary reconstruction. Laryngoscope 1981; 91:1031.

54. Conley JJ. Use of composite flaps containing bone for major repairs in the head and neck. Plast Reconstr. Surg 1972; 49:522.

55. Snyder C. Mandibulofacial restoration with live osteocutaneous flaps. Plast Reconstr Surg 1979; 64:14.

56. Duncan MJ, Manktelow RJ, Zuker KM, Rosen IV. Mandibular reconstruction in the radiated patient: the role of osteocutaneous free tissue transfer. Plast Reconstr Surg 1985; 76:829.

57. Soutar DF, Scheken LR, Tanner NSB, McGregor IA. The radial forearm flap: a versatile methode of intra-oral reconstruction. Br J Plast Surg 1983; 36:128.

3 Radiotherapy for Head and Neck Cancer

P. M. Busse, S. B. Bader

Introduction

Within months of the 1896 discovery of X-rays by Roentgen, patients with a variety of malignancies had already received therapeutic radiation. Among the early patients were several with advanced carcinomas of the head and neck. Although the acute side effects were considerable and the patient outcome poor, much interest was generated regarding this new use of X-rays. Anecdotal use flourished but it was not until 1919 at the Radium Institute of Paris that modern concepts regarding the use of radiation therapy as a curative modality began to emerge (39, 42). Experimental evidence by Regaud indicated that radiation given as multiple fractions was as effective in achieving a biological endpoint (cessation fo spermatogenesis) as single fraction radiation but without excessive skin damage. This principle of fractionated radiation was subsequently applied to tumors arising in the oropharynx, oral cavity, nasopharynx, and larynx by Henri Coutard (15, 16). Despite severe limitations in radiation equipment and the advanced nature of disease treated, he was able to achieve 7-year survival rates of 17 to 27%. This remarkable achievement lead others, most notably Baclese, to expand upon this experience, gradually modifying treatment parameters such as fraction size, overall dose, treatment fields, etc., to where radiation therapy has become a major modality in the treatment of most tumors of the head and neck. Perhaps the most important technical innovation in the field of radiation therapy was the development and eventual widespread availability of Cobalt and linear accelerators with energies exceeding 1 million volts. The improved dose characteristics of these higher energy machines lead to considerably less treatment breaks due to severe acute skin reactions. Further technical refinements such as radiation therapy simulators, higher energy linear accelerators, electron-beam therapy, individualized field blocks, and patient immobilization have improved the ability to maximize dose to the target volume while minimizing dose to normal tissue. The delivery of 70 Gy or more can now be delivered to certain sites of primary disease with an acceptable level of tolerance.

Advancements in clinical techniques and understanding of the radiobiology of tumors paralleled improvements in radiation delivery. Concepts such as the relationship of tumor control with tumor size rather than histology, shrinking treatment volumes, elective irradiation of clinically occult disease, and a combined modality approach have dramatically changed the way radiation therapy is practised (25). While improvements continue to be made in the optimization of radiation dose delivery through the use of charged particles, computer-controlled radiation therapy, CT-assisted treatment planning, etc., the next advances in the therapeutic efficacy of radiation will come from an improved understanding of tumor biology and the incorporation of this knowledge into new radiation treatment strategies. Recent advances in radiobiology and in the radiotherapy of head and neck cancers will be reviewed following a presentation of the general principles of head and neck radiotherapy and the expected clinical results of treatment.

General Principles of Head and Neck Radiotherapy

The goal of both radiation therapy and surgery is to eradicate the primary site of disease as well as any regional spread. To accomplish this requires detailed information of the anatomical extent of the primary lesion and knowledge of its pattern of local invasion and regional spread. A thorough head and neck examination which includes careful inspection and palpation of the oral cavity and oropharynx, indirect laryngoscopy or fiberoptic endoscopy, and examination of the neck is essential. It is useful for treatment planning as well as for follow-up to document all observable tumor on anatomic diagrams. Whenever possible, pretreatment tattoos denoting the boundaries of disease should be done. Depending upon the anatomic site, radiographic studies using computed tomography, magnetic resonance imaging (MRI), plain films, barium swallow, or tomograms provide additional information on the location and spread of disease and facilitate the design of treatment fields.

Because of the variety of distinct anatomic sites within the head and neck region each with its own unique lymphatic drainage and anatomic relationships, a small change in tumor location can have a large impact on the size and design of radiation fields. These are well documented and described in several detailed texts (26, 51, 63, 90). It is not within the scope of this chapter to describe in detail the treatment approaches used for the multiple anatomic sites, however, there are some common principles that form the basis for all radiotherapy of the head and neck.

The first and perhaps most important principle is the delivery of a tumoricidal dose to the primary site. As with surgery, the importance of knowing the full extent of disease cannot be overstated. Except for the most limited tumors, e. g. a T1 glottic carcinoma, the principle of shrinking fields is employed (Fig. 3.1). The first target volume encompasses not only the tumor, but also areas of suspected subclinical disease. Typically this volume is treated to 45–50 Gray (Gy) following which a series of one or two successively smaller fields is used to bring the primary site to the target dose which can vary from 60 Gy to greater than 70 Gy depending upon the size of the tumor usually reflected in the T stage. The biological basis for this is the delivery of radiation to progressively smaller target volumes based upon the amount of disease thought to be present within that volume.

A second principle is the treatment of apparent or suspected regional disease. The incidence of lymphatic spread is related to the site and size of the primary lesion, and its degree of differentiation. Notable exceptions are early stage tumors confined to the true vocal cords and those involving the paranasal sinuses. The incidence of occult lymphatic involvement was determined from two sources: studies of the frequency of pathologically positive lymph nodes detected during prophylactic neck dissections in patients with clinically N0 disease, as well as studies determining the frequency of relapse in the neck after treatment of the primary site and observa-

tion of an untreated neck. The radiation dose required to control subclinical disease is known due to careful observations of Fletcher and others. Patients who were felt to harbor occult regional disease were treated with elective irradiation to the cervical lymph draining areas. As can be seen in Table 3.1, radiation is effective in preventing the development of lymphadenopathy. The frequency with which patients eventually develop clinically apparent adenopathy diminishes to 5% or less as the dose increases from 30 Gy to 50 Gy (25).

Radiation alone is effective management for clinically apparent as well as occult regional disease, however, larger doses are required. For patients with limited disease, i. e. less than 3 cm, 60 Gy carries a greater than 90% probability of long-term control. As the amount of regional disease increases, the probability of control diminishes even with doses approaching 70 Gy (Table 3.2). Dose guidelines for the treatment of lymph nodes ranging in size from 1 to 6 cm have been established (Table 3.3) from retrospective analyses of dose and regional control

Table 3.1 Percent control of subclinical disease as a function of dose [modified from Fletcher (25)]

Radiation dose (Gy)	No. of patients	Disease control (%)
30–40	50	60–70
50	356	>90
60	65	>90

Table 3.2 Lymph node control vs. continuous or split-course irradiation [modified from Mendenhall (48)]

Lymph node size (cm)	Continuous course (controlled/treated)	Split course (controlled/treated)
<1.0	5/5	2/2
1.0	29/35 (83%)	19/23 (83%)
1.5–2.0	43/49 (88%)	20/24 (83%)
2.5–3.0	14/19 (74%)	10/18 (56%)
3.5–6.0	14/20 (70%)	10/17 (59%)
>7.0	0/2	0/5

Table 3.3 Dose guidelines for squamous cell carcinoma metastatic to the cervical lymph nodes [modified from Million (51)]

Lymph node size (cm)	Radiation dose 10 Gy/week (Gy)	Radiation dose 9 Gy/week (Gy)
<1	60	65
1.5–2.0	65	70
2.5–3.0	70	75
3.5–6.0	75	80

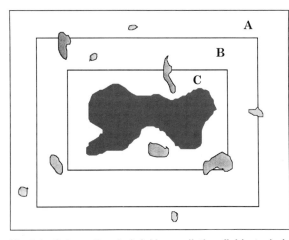

Fig. 3.1 Schematic of shrinking radiation fields technique. The initial field, A, reflects the large target volume required to encompass gross and subclinical deposits of disease. The radiation dose sufficient to control small deposits of tumor is 45–50 Gy following which the field size can be reduced, B. With tumor shrinkage, a second reduction can further minimize the treatment volume, C

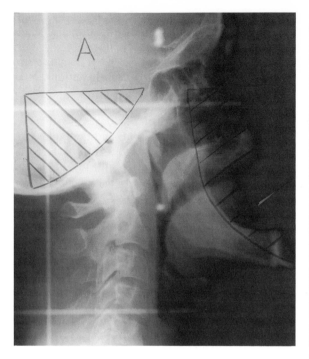

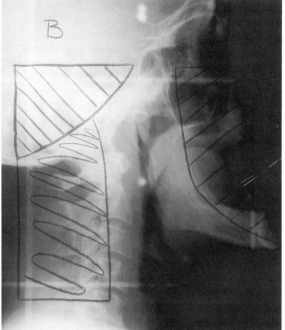

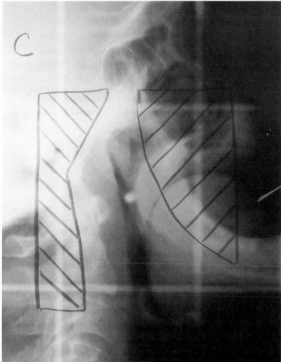

Fig. 3.2 **Radiation treatment fields of a patient treated for a T3N0M0, stage III, carcinoma of the posterior pharyngeal wall. A.** First treatment volume which includes the primary site, areas of contiguous spread and regional lymphatics. **B.** Cord block placed at 45 Gy to limit the dose to that structure. The reduced field anterior to the block is treated with an additional 10.8 Gy. **C.** Final reduced field which includes the original tumor volume plus a several centimeter margin, this is treated to a final dose of between 68–70 Gy.

conducted at institutions such as the University of Florida (48, 51). Histology may play some role in the probability of local–regional control as comparably staged lymphoepitheloma appears to be effectively managed with a 10% reduction in overall dose (51).

An example of the radiation therapy treatment volumes used for a locally advanced carcinoma of the posterior pharyngeal wall is shown in Figure 3.2). The principle of shrinking fields is used with the first

course depicted in Figure 3.2A. The primary site as well as all areas thought to harbor occult contiguous spread are included. Regional lymphatics are also included in the first course treatment volume. Because of the midline location of the tumor, bilateral treatment is necessary. Both right and left fields are treated each day, 5 days per week, 1.8–2.0 Gy per fraction. The total dose for the first course is 45 Gy after which a block is added to the posterior portion of each field in order to limit the dose to the spinal cord (Fig. 3.2B).

An additional 10 Gy is then delivered to this reduced treatment volume. In order to bring the primary site to the final target dose, between 68–70 Gy, an additional set of treatment fields are planned, much smaller than the previous two treatment volumes (Fig. 3.2C). Since this small volume is treated a high dose, it is essential to have an accurate knowledge of the extent of the primary not only to assure that all of the disease is being treated but also to exclude uninvolved tissue from the treatment field.

A third principle of head and neck radiotherapy is the recognition of normal tissue tolerance. This includes acute as well as late toxicities. The daily radiation dose per fraction, total dose, overall treatment time, and treatment volume are variables which have an impact on the probability of local tumor control as well as normal tissue toxicity. As will be discussed later, there is considerable interest in optimizing these parameters in order to increase the therapeutic index for radiation. It is not disputed that for any M0 tumor of the head and neck enough radiation could be delivered to local and regional sites to have complete assurance of tumor control within the field of radiotherapy. The fact that this is not achieved in every case is due to constraints on the total and daily radiation dose imposed by normal tissues. The normal tissue reactions to radiation therapy have as their bases the loss of reproductive capacity of a stem cell population. These reactions are broadly subdivided into acute and chronic injuries, a reflection of the rapidity with which the population of cells normally repopulates itself. The most troublesome acute reactions in the treatment of head and neck cancer are mucositis followed by erythema and desquamation of the skin. Fortunately, acutely reacting normal tissues have a tremendous capacity for self renewal, and if the daily fraction size is low enough, a full course of radiation can be given without a treatment break. The acute reactions become problematic when the planned course of therapy is seriously interrupted. With appropriate supportive care, however, acute reactions to radiotherapy do not result in serious long-term morbidity.

Late reactions to radiotherapy are the real limiting factors in the delivery of high doses of radiation. These have many manifestations and the biology of their development is complex. As with acute reactions, the underlying mechanism is the loss of mature cells as a result of the depletion of progenitor cells. The probelm is exacerbated by radiation damage to the microvasculature. Examples of chronic radiation-induced morbidity include: mucosal necrosis, cartilage necrosis, osteonecrosis, fibrosis, salivary gland dysfunction with associated dental caries, spinal cord injury, etc. Although information concerning the biological response of these tissues to radiation is accruing and dose regimens are being designed based on these data, most of the information concerning the total and daily dose limits of radiation are from retrospective analyses of complication rates of treated patients. Since the limits on increasing radiation dose are set by late normal tissue reactions, improvement in local control must derive from ways to increase the therapeutic ratio for radiotherapy. This could be accomplished by several means, including unconventional fractionation regimens, radiation sensitizers, hyperthermia, combined chemotherapy and radiation, etc. These and other novel treatment strategies will be reviewed later in this chapter as advances in radiotherapy.

Clinical Outcome with Conventional Radiation Therapy

Data on local control and disease-free survival from a number of large series are presented for the major head and neck sites in Tables 3.4 to 3.8. These data

Table 3.4 **Results of conventional radiation therapy for squamous cell carcinoma of the oral cavity**

T stage	Institution	No. of patients	Dose (Gy)	Local Control (%)	NED (%)	Follow-up (years)
T1	MGH (89)	179	65–70		83	3
	Univ. Florida (51)	28	65	89		min. 2
	MDAH (26)	101	60–70	96		5
T2	MGH	364	65–70		57	3
	Univ. Florida	52	65–70	63		min. 2
	MDAH	177	70	84		5
T3	MGH	38	70–80		19	3
	Univ. Florida	49	80–85	43		min. 2
	MDAH	126	80	67		5
T4	MGH	9	75–80		9	3
	Univ. Florida					min. 2
	MDAH	54	80	28		5

Table 3.5 **Results of conventional radiation therapy for squamous cell carcinoma of the oropharynx**

T stage	Institution	No. of patients	Dose (Gy)	Local Control (%)	NED (%)	Follow-up (years)
T1	MGH (89)	55	65–70		75	3
	Univ. Florida (51)	21	60–65	86		min. 2
	MDAH (26)	52	63–70		56	5
T2	MGH	189	65–70		59	3
	Univ. Florida	43	60–65	77		min. 2
	MDAH	136	65–70		47	5
T3	MGH	161	70–80		22	3
	Univ. Florida	47	64–68	62		min. 2
	MDAH	132	70–75		38	5
T4	MGH	49	75–80		6	3
	Univ. Florida	32		16		min. 2
	MDAH	40	75–80		18	5

Table 3.6 **Results of conventional radiation therapy for squamous cell carcinoma of the nasopharynx**

T stage	Institution	No. of patients	Dose (Gy)	Local Control (%)	NED (%)	Follow-up (years)
T1	MGH (89)	52	70		60	3
	Univ. Florida (51)	4	65	100		min. 2
	MDAH (50)	34	60	97		min. 2
T2	MGH	58	70		48	3
	Univ. Florida	5	65	90		min. 2
	MDAH	101	60	84		min. 2
T3	MGH	12	70		17	3
	Univ. Florida	10	70	90		min. 2
	MDAH	45	70	73		min. 2
T4	MGH	12	70		17	3
	Univ. Florida	20	70	50		min. 2
	MDAH	70	70	71		min. 2

Table 3.7 **Results of conventional radiation therapy for squamous cell carcinoma of the supraglottic larynx**

T stage	Institution	No. of patients	Dose (Gy)	Local Control (%)	NED (%)	Follow-up (years)
T1	MGH (89)	73	65		75	3
	Univ. Florida (49)	12	56–65	92		5
	MDAH (26)	34	60	91		5
	PMH (34)	87	50*	71		5
T2	MGH	109	65–68		50	3
	Univ. Florida	26	63–65	77		5
	MDAH	69	70	83		5
	PMH	44	50*	68		5
T3	MGH	85	65–70		38	3
	Univ. Florida	14	69–71	64		5
	MDAH	45	70	73		5
	PMH	30	50*	56		5
T4	MGH	107	65–70		26	3
	Univ. Florida	11	69–71	18		5
	MDAH	33	70	58		5
	PMH	168	50*	48		5

* Fraction size, 2.5 Gy.

T stage	Institution	No. of patients	Dose (Gy)	Local Control (%)	NED (%)	Follow-up (years)
T1	MGH (89)	723	65−70		90	3
	Univ. Florida (51)	90	56−65	92		min. 2
	MDAH (26)	332	60−70*	89		3
T2	MGH	173	65−70		69	3
	Univ. Florida	49	63−65	67		min. 2
	MDAH	175	60−70*	74		3
T3	MGH	65	70		32	3
	Univ. Florida	19	68−71	58		min. 2
	MDAH	+				3

* Doses of 60 Gy for superficial lesions, 65 Gy for small exophytic lesions, 70 Gy for bulky lesions.
+ Total laryngectomy.

are not exhaustive but serve to demonstrate the degree of disease control which can be expected following conventional radiation. For early stage head and neck sqamous cell carcinomas, radiation therapy with single daily fractions of 1.8−2.0 Gy and total doses of 60−70 Gy can achieve local control in more than 80% of patients with surgery reserved as salvage. As the tumor burden increases, however, the local control rate with single-modality radiation diminishes to less than 20% for many T4 tumors. The biological factors for this are complex but the predominant underlying cause is simply an increase in the number of clonogens. Although local control could be improved with an increase in total radiation dose, the chronic morbidity associated with such treatment is unacceptable.

As previously mentioned, advances in the treatment of head and neck cancers with radiotherapy and an increase in the therapeutic index of radiation will come from an improved understanding of tumor biology and the incorporation of this knowledge into new radiation treatment strategies. Progress in these areas has occurred in a coordinated fashion and will be reviewed together under the mantle of advances in radiotherapy.

Advances in Radiation Therapy

Advances in Radiobiology

The biological effects of radiation therapy have as their bases the loss of reproductive integrity of the cell. This is true for tumor cells as well as normal tissue. The lethal lesions, on the molecular level, have yet to be completely defined. Considerable attention has been focused on unrepaired double strand breaks, however, the series of events which begin with the deposition of energy, the production of free radicals which interact with DNA, and the ultimate death of the cell are at best poorly under-

stood. Following a sufficiently high dose of radiation, cells suffer what is known as mitotic death. That is, as cells enter into mitosis, irrespective of the cell age in which they were irradiated, they fail to progress past mitosis and eventually become pycnotic or lose the integrity of the cell membrane. This frequently does not occur in the first mitosis as reproductively moribund cells occasionally undergo several cell divisions before mitotic death. An example of this is the lineage of a lethally irradiated cell shown in Figure 3.3 (85). An important clinical ramification of this phenomenon is that a tumor can be reproductively dead but still have normal appearing, metabolically active, dividing cells (76). If an irradiated tumor were to be biopsied before the cells had undergone the requisite number of divisions it would be impossible to distinguish viable from reproductively dead tumor. The rate at which a tumor regresses is frequently referred to as radiosensitivity, a term unfortunately confused with radiocurability. A number of diverse factors impact on tumor regression i. e., the relative proportion of tumor to connective stroma, the growth fraction of the tumor, and cell cycle transit time to name a few. Tumors which have a large tumor to stroma ratio and high mitotic rate will regress with treatment much faster than those with the opposite characteristics. While clinically gratifying, a rapid tumor regression does not necessarily translate into disease control.

The most important factor which determines the likelihood that a tumor will be controlled by radiation (radiocurability), is the number of clonogens present at the start of radiation. Since any dose of radiation kills only a proportion of cells rather than an absolute number, the probability that all clonogenic cells have been rendered reproductively dead depends upon the surviving fraction after a given dose of radiation, the number of radiation fractions, and the initial number of viable tumor cells at the outset. Other factors, such as the degree of

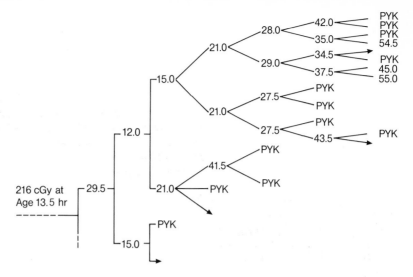

Fig. 3.3 Pedigree analysis of an L 59 mouse fibroblast cell irradiated with a single dose of 2.16 Gy at cell age 13.5 hours. These data are from time-lapse microcinematographic analysis of irradiated single cells. Following irradiation, a variable number of divisions occur before mitotic death. The numbers indicate the duration of a division cycle in hours. [From Thompson and Suit (85)]

cellular radiosensitivity, cell-age distribution, DNA repair, hypoxia, and repopulation also play a role in radiocurability albeit to a less well defined degree. The latter factors and their influence on radiocurability will be reviewed separately.

Cellular Radiosensitivity

After the first X-ray survival curve was published for HeLa cells (66), information on the survival curve parameters from a large number of cell lines became available. The degree of radiosensitivity was thought to be reflected in the slope of the exponential region of the survival curve quantified by a value called the D_O (Fig. 3.**4**). Unfortunately, this is a reflection of the single hit inactivation of a very few cells. Furthermore, the D_O correlates poorly with the clinical behavior of tumors. A notable exception is a group of patients with recurrent squamos cell carcinomas of the head and neck (95). The D_O exhibited in the survival curve from these tumors is significantly greater (i. e. the slope of the survival curve is less steep) than tumors which were controlled with radiation. This could be due to an increased repair capacity for potentially lethal damage although other reasons could exist.

Attention has recently been focused on quantifying the radiation response of the initial portion of the survival curve. This has clinical relevance since almost all radiation therapy is given through multiple fractions of less than 3–4 Gy. A large number of cell lines, derived from human tumors, have been examined by Fertil and Malaise (24) in an attempt to relate the relative clinical responsiveness to various parameters used to quantify cell killing in the low dose, 0–4 Gy, region of the survival curve. Their analysis revealed that, based on survival curve parameters, tumor cell lines could be grouped into three

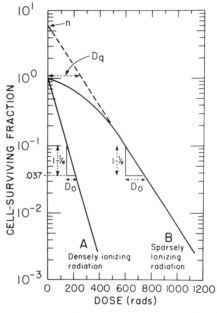

Fig. 3.4 Idealized X-ray cell survival curves. The surviving fraction of cells is plotted on a logarithmic scale against radiation dose on a linear scale. For lymphoid cell populations and cells irradiated with densely ionizing radiation, curve A demonstrates the radiation response. Squamous cell tumors of the head and neck region would respond to radiation similar to curve B. A shoulder is seen before cells become exponentially inactivated. The magnitude of the shoulder is quantified by n, the extrapolation number and D_q. The magnitude of the slope is expressed by D_O, the amount of radiation necessary to reduce the surviving fraction by $1 - 1/e$. [From Hall (33)]

catagories which reflected their clinical behavior. Squamous cell carcinomas fell into the group which exhibited an intermediate degree of cellular radiosensitivity. A prospective application of this approach or of the D_O to predict for radiotherapy failures in head and neck carcinomas has yet to be carried out. It is possible that despite large differences in intrinsic cellular radiosensitivity, other factors such as tissue oxygenation and repopulation may be far more important in determining tumor control.

Cell Age

The survival of irradiated cells is not uniform throughout the cell cycle. The age response, first described for synchronously dividing HeLa cells (84), reveals pronounced fluctuations in a cell's sensitivity to radiation that is dependant on cell age or its position in the cell cycle (Fig. 3.5). The most sensitive cell age is mitosis followed by the end of G1. Peaks of resistance are seen in late S/G2 and in mid-G1. The G1 resistance is seen only if the cell line has an appreciable G1 duration. If the transit time in G1 is short, the age–response function during this period appears flat (74). The large differences in survival seen at different cell ages prompted in vivo experiments and clinical trials that attempt to induce partial cell synchrony and deliver radiation at a specific time when the number of tumor cells that are in a sensitive cell age is maximal. Unfortunately this approach has not met with much success as a meaningful degree of tumor synchrony has not been achieved.

Radiation repair

The repair of radiation damage is an important biological phenomenon which negatively affects radiocurability. Almost all cells possess the capacity for such repair albeit to different degrees. The first description of repair in a mammalian cell system was by Elkind and Sutton (21). The phenomenon observed was a reduction in reproductive cell death which occurred when a given dose of radiation was split into two fractions separated by several hours. This process occurs fairly rapidly and is usually complete by 4–6 hours. The magnitude of the repair is related to the size of the shoulder of the single-dose X-ray survival curve an example of which is shown in Figure 3.4. Since the shoulder region was initially thought to be due to the accumulation of X-ray damage and hence sublethal, this repair process was termed "sublethal damage repair" (SLDR). This type of repair has a large impact on clinical radiation therapy as most radiation is delivered in daily fractions which fall in the shoulder region of the survival curve. A major determinant in the design of radiation programs containing multiple daily fractions (hyperfractionation) is the time interval between radiation doses and its relation to the time necessary for the repair of radiation damage.

Another type of radiation repair that has been extensively studied is potentially lethal damage repair (PLDR). This was first described by Philips and Tolmach (64). The phenomenon can be summarized as the dependency of survival on the postirradiation conditions, e. g. cell density; DNA, RNA, protein synthesis inhibition, cell age, etc. (44). The damage introduced by radiation is thought to be potentially lethal and subject to modification by the cell either by fixation in which case the cell would be killed, or by repair which would result in cell survival. PLDR is reflected in a shift in the slope of the exponential region of the survival curve and could be important clinically, particularly with large radiation doses.

Although these types of radiation repair are operationally quite distinct in experimental systems, it is possible that the same molecular events may be responsible for both sublethal and potentially lethal damage repair. Further elucidation of the mechanism of DNA damage repair will come from an understanding of the molecular biology of the process.

Hypoxia

Hypoxia, is one of the most important of the factors which affect radiation survival and is present in all tumors large enough to be detected. Because of the erratic and deficient vasculature within and about tumors, the oxygenation of tumors is compromised and large areas of central necrosis may develop within regions of relatively hypoxic cells. Cells located more than 180–200 µm from a capillary, the diffusion distance of oxygen are hypoxic (86). Cells which reside adjacent to areas of anoxia are felt to be chronically hypoxic. This is in contrast to acute or

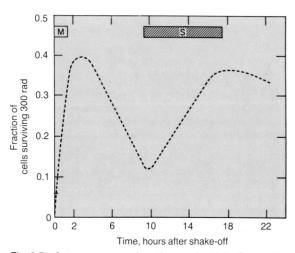

Fig. 3.5 **Age-response function of HeLa S3 cells.** Idealized curve of the response of HeLa cells irradiated with single doses of 3 Gy at various times following mitosis. M denotes mitosis, S denotes the duration of the DNA-synthetic portion of the cell cycle. [From Hall (33); modified from Terasima and Tolmach (84)]

reversible hypoxia where the oxygen tension is altered is due to intermittent blood flow within a tumor (12, 13, 53, 87). Cells irradiated during a period of intermittent hypoxia exhibit survival characteristics similar to chronically hypoxic cells. The relative radiosensitivity of cells as a function of the partial pressure of oxygen is shown in Figure 3.**6**. When the partial pressure falls to less than 20 mm Hg, cells become progressively more resistant to radiation (17). The effect of this change in radiosensitivity is depicted in the single dose survival curves for cells irradiated in vitro under aerobic and hypoxic conditions (Fig. 3.**7**). In the exponential portions of the curves, hypoxic cells are from two and a half to three times more resistant to radiation than their fully oxygenated counterparts.

In an effort to overcome the relative radioresistance of hypoxic cells, a search was made for compounds which would have electrophilic properties similar to oxygen but with greater diffusion distances. One class of compounds which has been extensively investigated are the nitroimidazoles of which metronidazole is the parent compound. Various derivatives have been developed and tested in vitro for radiosensitization, however, the clinical utility has been limited by neurotoxicity. The clinical trials with nitroimidazole radiosensitizers will be reviewed later. The importance of hypoxic cells in tumor biology and the degree to which this relatively resistant subpopulation affects tumor control is the subject of considerable experimental and clinical investigation.

Repopulation

In an unperturbed state, the number of clonogens in a tumor doubles in roughly 6–8 weeks. Factors such as the fraction of cells in cycle, cell cycle transit time, and cell loss all affect this rate. Since the duration of a conventional course of radiation therapy is also approximately 6–8 weeks, the increase in the number of clonogens would at most only double during therapy. In order to account for these additional cells, an additional two to three treatment fractions would have to be added. Unfortunately, evidence from experimental and clinical studies show that cell doubling is not constant at the unperturbed rate during a course of radiation therapy but rather accelerates towards the end of treatment (97). Barendsen and Broese (4) found that the time required for the doubling of clonogenic tumor cells in a rat rhabdomyosarcoma cell line was reduced from 4 days to 1.5 days after treatment with radiation. Changes were seen with respect to an increase in growth fraction, decreased cell loss factor, and decrease in cell cycle time. The accelerated growth seen may be due to activation of quiescent clonogenic cells previously deprived of nutrients and oxy-

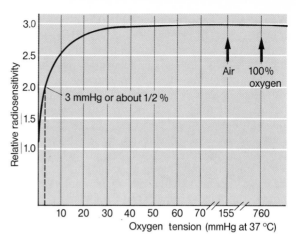

Fig. 3.**6** **Idealized oxygen dependency curve for radiosensitivity.** The survival of cells irradiated under anoxic conditions is set at 1, fully oxygenated cells are three times more sensitive to the same radiation dose for an oxygen enhancement ratio (OER) of 3. A minimal increase in the oxygen tension is sufficient to dramatically change the relative radiosensitivity. [From Hall (33)]

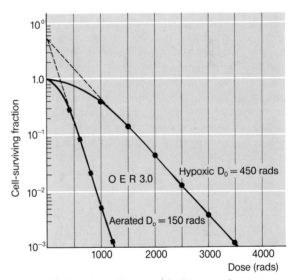

Fig. 3.**7** **Single-dose X-ray survival curves for mammalian cells irradiated under aerated and hypoxic conditions.** [From Hall (33)]

gen as well as a shortening of the cell cycle transit time. Similar changes in cell proliferation have also been seen in human tumors. The clinical data which support rapid tumor repopulation will be reviewed.

Advances in Therapeutic Radiation

For early stage tumors of the head and neck, conventional radiation therapy with doses of from 1.8 to 2.0 Gy per fraction, one fraction per day, 5 days per week results in tumor control rates of 70% or better with an acceptable level of acute and chronic toxicity (Tables 3.**4**–3.**8**). These results compare favorably to those with surgery alone. Patients with advanced disease, T3 or T4 primary lesions or N1N3 regional disease, fare less well. Attempts to improve cure rates by simply increasing the overall dose to the primary site or to involved lymphatics have not met with much success as the probability of late radiation damage to normal tissue increases dramatically as conventional treatment doses exceeds 70 Gy. Higher control rates could be achieved but the incidence of long-term complications would be unacceptable. The delivery of a radical dose of radiation therapy is greatly determined by the rate of repopulation of a rapidly renewing normal tissue population (acute reactions) and the degree of eventual cell loss in nonregenerating or slowly renewing normal tissue (late reactions). The effect of a course of radiation therapy on each of these classes of normal tissue can be quite different. Acutely responding tissues are affected by treatment time and overall dose, late tissues by dose per fraction. The magnitude of an acute reaction does not necessarily predict the degree of a late reaction.

The development of conventional radiation therapy has been an empiric progression which has sought to strike the optimal balance between the severity of acute and chronic reactions and tumor control. To circumvent the limitations of conventional radiation therapy, alternative dose schedules have been developed in order to take advantage of differences in survival between tumor and normal tissue. In its simplest form, the advantages achieved in normal tissue sparing by fractionating a course of radiation are even greater when the daily dose of radiation is divided over two or more treatments per day (hyperfractionation). One caveat is that the time between fractions must be sufficient to allow complete recovery which for experimental in vitro systems is complete in 2−4 hours (21). Clinical evidence from hyperfractionation suggests late reacting tissue may have a slightly longer time course to complete repair, approximately 6 hours. Considerable data need to be accrued on the effects of different fractionation schedules for various normal tissues. It is hoped that this information will provide an alternative to the empiric design of current treatment regimens.

Appropriately designed, prospective, randomized clinical trials evaluating the efficacy of nonstandard fraction regimens are few. Most of the information available is from single institution studies where an altered fractionation schedule was compared to that institution's historical controls. Nevertheless, this approach may represent an improvement over standard treatment. The following is a review of the available clinical experience with hyperfractionation.

The University of Florida has been using hyperfractionation with 1.2 Gy per fraction bid since 1978. Initially, 1.25 Gy per fraction was used, however, the severity of acute side effects was such that many patients required a treatment break. The total dose given was 74.40 Gy in 62 fractions over 6 weeks, which represented 10−15% higher dose than historically given with 1.8−2.0 Gy fraction sizes given once per day. The interfraction interval was 4−6 hours for all patients. Their experience with 144 patients with advanced head and neck cancer has been reported (60). Acute, severe mucosal reactions have occurred in 20% of patients. Fifteen patients required nasogastric tube feeding, 2 required a treatment break, and 4 were hospitalized for dehydratation. Although 20% higher daily dose was given, and the severity of acute reactions more frequent, 99% of patients were able to complete the prescribed therapy without a break. Late complications of moderate to severe grade occurred in 8% of patients. The incidence of severe complications was related to total dose and site of the primary. No severe late complication occurred in 33 patientes given 74.40 Gy or less; while 1/37 (11%) of patients treated with 76,80 Gy to the hypopharynx or larynx suffered moderate to severe side effects. None of the 14 patients with tumors of the nasopharynx treated to this dose suffered severe side effects. Of 19 patients who received 74.80−81.60 Gy external beam prior to a radium implant, no patient suffered a severe side effect. Local control was 10−20% higher than historical controls treated at the same institution for all patients except those with T2 tonsil and T3 supraglottic laryngeal tumors who had similar rates of control. This experience has led to the use of prophylactic gastrostomy in patients with marginal nutritional status, and the limitation of total dose to the larynx and supraglottic larynx to 74.40−76.80 Gy. Bulky paryngeal lesions are treated to 76.80−79.20 Gy, with the last 15.00−20.00 Gy, delivered to a smaller field that excludes the majority of the larynx.

The EORTC has recently reported their results of a randomized trial of hyperfractionation versus conventional fractionation for orophyaryngeal carcinoma (38). In this trial, 366 patients with T2T3 N0N1 lesions were randomly assigned to receive 70 Gy in 35 fractions over 7 weeks versus 80.5 Gy in 70 fractions over 7 weeks (1.15 Gy per fraction separated by at least 6 hours). Because the overall treatment time in the two treatment arms was the same, this trial evaluated the effect of pure hyperfractionation rather than an accelerated treatment schedule. An analysis of 293 patients with a median follow-up of over 3 years revealed a significant improvement in local and regional control favoring hyperfractionation: 59% versus 43% at 3 years, and 57% versus 37% at 5 years. Though the overall dose was 15% higher, no difference in late complication rates has been observed. Furthermore, there is a trend in overall survival at 3 years favoring the hyperfractionation arm at 57% versus 43%.

The Radiation Therapy Oncology Group (ROTG) conducted a phase III randomized trial for stage III–IV cancers of the larynx, pharynx, oral cavity, and paranasal sinuses which compared conventional fractionation of daily 1.80–2.00 Gy fractions to 66.00–73.80 Gy total dose with 1.20 Gy bid to 60.00 Gy with fractions separated by 3–6 hours (45). Predictably, complete response rates, locoregional control, and overall survival were not different between the two arms. There were more cases of severe acute reactions in the hyperfractionation arm (23% vs. 13%), however, interruption of therapy occurred in similar proportions of the two groups. There were no differences in the rates of late complications between the two groups. Some of the differences in acute and late toxicities appeared to be related to the interval between the two daily fractions. When the interval was 4.5 hours or less, the incidence of severe acute mucositis was 28% this is in contrast to 5% for greater than 4.5 hours. The incidence of late fibrosis was 40% for patients with the shorter interval, versus 27% for patients with the longer interval. A criticism of this trial is the lower overall dose in the hyperfraction arm. Because of this, no conclusion can be drawn regarding efficacy, however, the toxicity data as they relate to the treatment interval are interesting and support the use of at least in 6-hour interval between fractions in order to minimize the effects on late reacting normal tissue.

In the clinical trials above, the overall treatment times for the hyperfractionation schedules are roughly the same as for conventional treatment. The primary benefit of hyperfractionation therefore is to reduce the risk of late normal tissue injury thus allowing a higher overall dose to be given with the accompanying improvement in local control. Some hyperfractionation regimes take advantage of a reduced overall treatment time, termed accelerated hyperfractionation, which has important biological implications for the tumor as well as normal tissue. The primary rationale is to limit the potential for clonogen repopulation during a protracted course of fractionated radiaton therapy. The phenomenon of accelerated clonogen repopulation following radiation therapy has previously been discussed. The evidence that this may be an important factor in reducing local control is inferred from clinical data on time to recurrence, the results from split course radiation therapy trials, and the experience in protracted treatment schedules. Unperturbed tumors have a median clonogen doubling time of 2 months which is also roughly the time for the tumor to double in size as well (14, 75, 97). For most radiation series in head and neck cancer, recurrences are seen most commonly in the first 6 months (26). If a small number of clonogenic cells survive radical treatment, at least thirty doublings would have to occur before a clinically detectable mass would be seen. This would imply a cell doubling time of 1 week.

Several institutions have reported diminished clinical efficacy with split-course radiation schedules. The experience from the University of Florida (59) found a 10–15% decrease in local control rates for patients treated with split-course versus continuous radiation with similar techniques and overall doses. Holsti and Mantaya (37) found in a randomized trial conducted in Finland that 10% additional dose given to the split-dose patients gave an equivalent local control and survival results. Overgaard found surprisingly similar results in a retrospective review of larynx cancer patients treated in Denmark (57). He found that an additional 20% total dose was required for a 3-week break in treatment in order to achieve a local control equivalent to that achieved with continuous radiation. Fowler (27) has estimated that 6 Gy is required to decrease the number of clonogens in a tumor by a factor of 10 thus a 12-Gy increase in dose would kill 100 additional clonogens, which over 3 weeks would require a doubling time of 3–4 days to achieve.

The effect of overall treatment time on estimates of tumor cell repopulation was recently reviewed by Withers et al. (97). They analyzed the radiotherapy results of a large number of head and neck cancer patients with respect to the total dose required to control 50% of tumors (TCD50) in relation to the overall treatment time. The significant finding was that the TCD50 remained constant for treatment times under 4 weeks, however, once the duration of therapy exceeded this, the TCD50 rose rapidly. With this information, it was possible for them to calculate a clonogenic cell doubling time of 3–4 days, a value remarkably consistent over a wide range of studies. The clinical relevance of this degree of repopulation is that in order to achieve the same degree of local control, an additional 0.6 Gy per day is required for treatment durations greater than 25 days to compensate for this repopulation of clonogens.

There are several ways to circumvent this problem of repopulation. One is to add additional fractions to the end of a course of radiation therapy, the other is to shorten the overall treatment time through the use of multiple fractions per day.

This is called accelerated hyperfractionation. Several different treatment strategies have been used in clinical trials, these include thrice daily fractions, accelerated hyperfractionation with a planned break, and concomitant boost schedules, i. e., treatment to primary site twice per day. The results of these trials are presented below.

One of the earliest experiences with three fractions per day (tid) accelerated hyperfractionation was reported by Svoboda (77) on patients with advanced breast and head and neck cancer. For head and neck cancer patients, 50–55 Gy was delivered over 10–13 days. The fractions were separated by 3–4 hours; and patients were treated continuously without a break. In an update of that experience in 59 patients (79), the CR rate was 86%, and 3-year survival 44%. They found that for larger volumes the fraction size needed to be limited to 1.6–1.75 Gy. Five severe and four moderately severe late reactions were reported. This experience is to be contrasted with that reported by Peracchia and Salti who treated 47 patients with head and neck cancer using 2.00 Gy tid to total doses of 48–54 Gy over 9–11 days with 4-hour intervals between fractions. Among the 22 patients with follow-up greater than 24 months, mucosal radionecrosis occurred in 55%. The survival was only 14% at 2 years.

Morgan (52) reported on 15 patients with stage III–IV lesions of the larynx treated with 1.1–1.5 Gy tid and a minimum of 3 and a maximum of 4 hours between fractions. A dose of 45 Gy over 10–12 days was given before a boost of 15 Gy to the primary site. Local control was achieved in 13 cases. Severe late complications occurred in 4 cases, including one with radiation myelitis. Three patients had severe soft tissue necrosis, all received greater than 65 Gy. Saunders and Dische (69, 70) have used 1.4 Gy tid with a 6-hour interval of 42 Gy, followed by a boost of 8.40 Gy in 12 consecutive days. Of 15 patients with head and neck cancer, all 15 showed a complete regression of their primary tumor, and 5/7 had a complete response of treated nodes. The early reaction was maximal by day 16–20, with complete resolution by day 42. No patient required tube feedings, but as part of the protocol, all patients remained hospitalized for 2 weeks following radiation therapy until the acute reaction peaked. The follow-up is relatively short, so only tentative conclusions can be made about the late effects.

Accelerated split-course schedules for head and neck cases have been used by Wang at the Massachusetts General Hospital (MGH) since 1979 (91). In his protocol, 1.6 Gy bid is employed with a minimum interval of 4 hours between fractions to 38.4 Gy followed by a planned 2-week treatment break. Radiation therapy is then resumed with 1.6 Gy bid to a total overall dose of 64 Gy over 6 weeks. His experience with accelerated hyperfractionation for supraglottic carcinomas (92) has been compared to an historical control from the same institution using a conventional treatment schedule of 66–72 Gy in 7½ weeks in the 4 years prior to 1979. The 3-year actuarial local control rate was 76% for the group treated bid and 50% in the group treated with conventional daily fractionation. By stage, patients with T1 and T2 lesions had local control rates of 88% versus 63% and for T3 and T4 lesions, it was 66% and 33%. The late effects at the time of publication were insignificant. No undue skin changes, fibrosis, or necrosis has occured in the

patientes treated bid. An improvement in local control for nasopharyngeal (94) and oropharyngeal tumors (93) using this approach has also been reported. In the latter study, improved results were seen in patients treated with a bid/bid schedule (hyperfractionation before and after the treatment break) versus bid/bid (hyperfractionation followed by once daily after the break) which was used in the early part of the hyperfractionation program at the MGH. The radiation techniques and overall dose were similar between the two treatment groups. This experience is not randomized, and the bid/bid patients have shorter median follow-up, so firm conclusions on the overall benefit of this approach would be premature. However, it does suggest that improved results of local control may be obtainable with accelerated fractionation with acceptable acute and late toxicities. An interesting observation of the oropharyngeal trial is the improved results with bid given in the latter half of radiation therapy. This is consistent with the observation of Withers et al. (97) where tumor call repopulation escalates around the fourth week of treatment. Accelerated hyperfractionation may, and should theoretically, have its greatest impact when given during this period, i.e. the latter part of a course of radiation therapy.

A third treatment strategy to reduce the overall treatment time has been used for selected patients at the M.D. Anderson Hospital (MDAH) (40). This treatment plan consists of a concomitant reduced field boost to gross disease for patients with early postoperative recurrences or with rapidly growing primary or nodal masses. All patients received conventional fractionation of 9–10 Gy/week using standard field arrangements. A concurrent boost of 1.20–1.50 Gy per fraction was delivered 3–6 hours after the first treatment 2–3 times per week for 3–5 weeks. The usual timing of initiation of the boost was the second or third week of treatment. Patients with enlarging nodular masses were boosted in an AP/PA manner, whereas primary tumors were treated with reduced lateral fields. The total dose ranged from 69–75 Gy. The results of treatment for this poor prognostic group was a local and regional control rate of 65% at 2 years, and a survival of 55%. Severe late reactions were related to overall dose, and to whether or not patients underwent neck surgery after radiotherapy. These results have prompted the initiation of a randomized trial at the MDAH using three different concurrent boost schedules at the beginning, middle and end of treatment for total doses of 69–72 Gy.

Some generalized statements can be made regarding these experiences with accelerated hyperfractionation: (1) the volume is radiated by tid regimens must be limited for acute reactions to be tolerable; (2) it is essential to allow adequate time between fractions for complete recovery in late responding tissues usually 6 hours; (3) high doses per fraction, e. g. 2.0 Gy, result in an unacceptable high incidence of late complications; (4) overall doses are limited by this approach. Although a large number of patients have been treated with a wide variety of unconventional dose schedules, the global experiences with hyperfractionated radiotherapy suffers from the paucity of prospective randomized trials where adequate daily and total doses were given and an adequate period of time was allowed between fractions to allow for complete recovery. Clearly some impressive results have been reported, whether or not these will stand up in an the appropriate trial remains to be determined. The RTOG is in the process of designing and conducting a series of prospectively randomized trials evaluating different schedules of hyperfractionation and accelerated hyperfractionation (46). An ongoing study conducted by the EORTC (22 851) randomizes patients to either conventional fractionation with 1.8−2.0 Gy per fraction, one fraction per day to 70−72 Gy or 1.6 Gy per fraction, three fractions per day to 72 Gy in 5 weeks. The results of these trials are eagerly awaited.

Hypoxia and Hypoxic Cell Sensitizers

The effect of oxygen on radiation sensitivity has been known for over 50 years. Oxygen is a potent radiation sensitizer by nature of its electrophilic properties that lead to free radical formation. The relatively long-lived radicals which are formed interact with DNA and lead to damage which if not repaired is ultimately lethal. The magnitude of the oxygen effect is quantified by a value called the oxygen enhancement ratio (OER) which is the ratio of radiation doses needed to achieve a given biological effect, e. g., 1% cell survival, in the presence and absence of oxygen. This had been found to be from 2.5 to 3.0 for large single fractions in a variety of experimental tumors and normal tissues. Since the tissue pO_2 required for full radiosensitivity is quite small, approximately 3 mmHg (Fig. 3.**6**), a small increase in the oxygen delivery to a tumor could yield large therapeutic gains.

Indirect evidence exists that oxygen delivery may be a factor in local tumor control. A number of studies have shown hemoglobin level to be an independent prognostic factor for local control in patients treated with radiation therapy (7, 9, 10, 36, 56, 80). At present the physiological basis for this phenomenon is unclear. Animal models have been developed which test the importance of acute and chronic anemia during radiation therapy. These models, however, are not thought to reproduce adequately the complexities of human tumors in situ. One prospective clinical trial has evaluated the impact of anemia on response to radiation. In this study patients with cervical cancer and hemoglobin levels below 12.5% were randomized to either receive therapeutic red cell transfusions or no transfusions during radiation therapy (9). Patients who were transfused as well as those patients who presented with hemoglobins greater than 12.5% had a significancy lower local recurrence rate.

Because of the latter clinical data, an effort is made to maintain hemoglobin concentrations above an accepted minimum during radiation in order to enhance the oxygen-carrying capacity of the blood and reduce tissue hypoxia. However, the point at which a patient needs to be transfused is subject to individual interpretation. An untested but commonly used minimum hemoglobin concentration is 10%. The potential gain in local control which might be realized with red cell transfusions must be weighed against the associated risk of hepatitis, HIV infection, allergic reactions, etc.

In addition to the maintenance of a minimum hemoglobin concentration during radiotherapy, the deleterious effects of a low intratumoral oxygen tension have been counteracted by a number of divergent investigational means. These include the concurrent administration of hyperbaric oxygen, electrophilic molecules, or using bioreductive chemotherapeutic agents which are selective for hypoxic cells, e. g. mitomycin C.

Randomized trials in head and neck cancer using hyperbaric oxygen and radiation therapy suggest an advantage in both local control and survival for the treatment group receiving hyperbaric oxygen (35). However, this approach is extremely cumbersome and necessitates the use of unconventional fraction sizes and less than optimal radiation delivery.

Although oxygen is the best radiosensitizer, the difficulty encountered in increasing oxygen delivery to tumors led to the development of electrophilic molecules which could act like oxygen and increase the radiosensitivity of hypoxic cells. The first class of such compounds were the 5-nitroimidazoles of which metronidazole was the parent compound. The clinical utility of this drug was hampered by its neurotoxicity which limits both the single and cumulative doses that can be delivered. This led to the search for other nitromidazoles which would have similar sensitizing capabilities but less neurotoxicity (less liphophilicity). Misonidazole, a 2-nitromidazole, was developed in the 1970s and based on encouraging preclinical results, was rapidly placed into clinical trial (28, 65).

Dische (20) has reviewed many of the controlled trials of misonidazole that have been conducted in patients with head and neck cancer (Table 3.**9**). These trials are very heterogeneous with respect to the dose and scheduling of both radiation and misonidazole and a summated impression of their results is difficult. The reason for this variability in study design was the fear of unacceptable neurotoxicity

Table 3.9 **Misonidazole: controlled clinical trials** [modified from Dische (20)]

Study	No. of patients	Case material	Treatment regimen*	Assessment of local tumor control
Sealy (71)	97	Advanced oral cancer	3	No benefit at 1 year
Sealy (72)[+]	64	Advanced oral cancer	3	Benefit to misonidazole and hyperbaric O_2 (local control and survival significant)
Bataini (8)	56	Oral cavity Oropharynx	4	No benefit
DAHANACA (54)	494	Pharynx Larynx	1 and 3	Both regimes gave similar results; the only subset which benefited was males with pharyngeal carcinoma
Archangeli (47)	25	Secondary carcinoma Neck nodes	5	Complete study including hyperthermia and hyperfractionation; difficult to interpret
MRC (47)	164	Oropharynx Larynx	3	No benefit
Cattan (11)	71	Locally advanced tumors	5	No benefit
Giaux (30)	56	Buccopharyngeal	3	No benefit
Bataini (8)	45	Larynx Hypopharynx	1	No benefit
MRC (47)	93	Oropharynx Larynx	1	No benefit
Gil Gayarre (31)	40	Head and neck sites[+]	1	Early benefit to misonidazole
EORTC (22)	523	Head and neck sites	5	No benefit
RTOG (23)	306	Head and neck sites	2	No benefit

* **Treatment regimen:** 1, small dose of misonidazole combined with conventional radiation; 2, high dose of misonidazole combined with conventional radiation; 3, high dose misonidazole combined with high dose hypofractionated radiation; 4, high dose misonidazole combined with high and low dose hyperfractionated radiation; 5, high dose misonidazole combined with hyperfractionated radiation.

[+] Misonidazole was combined with hyperbaric O_2.

[+] Includes some cases of cervical carcinoma.

due to misonidazole and the need to stay within a cummulative dose of $12 \, g/m^3$. Different schedules of misonidazole and radiation were developed in an effort to maximize the number of radiation fractions during which effective doses of the sensitizer were administered. Trial designs included small daily doses of misonidazole combined with conventional fractionation, high dose−hypofractionated radiotherapy together with high dose misonidazole, and high dose misonidazole with hyperfractionated radiotherapy. As can be seen in Table 3.**9**, data for an improvement over radiation alone are sparse. In interpreting this apparant lack of efficacy, the limitations in misonidazole delivery must be considered.

If radiosensitizers are to be appropriately tested, new compounds with lower lipophilicity, shorter serum half-life, and equal efficacy needed to be developed in order to sensitize a larger number of fractions. A number of these less toxic compounds have emerged most notably etanidazole (SR 2508) and pimonidazole (Ro 038 799). SR 2508 is a neutral hydrophilic analogue of misonidazole with similar radiosensitizing activity but with less peripheral neurotoxicity. It is excluded from CNS tissues, but achieves high plasma and tumor concentrations. Ro 038 799 is a more potent hypoxic sensitizer than misonidazole but is relatively lipophilic. Dose-limiting acute CNS toxicity has been seen which may limit its clinical utility. The RTOG has conducted phase I−II trials with SR 2508 and is concluding a randomized clinical trial designed to evaluate the effectiveness of SR 2508 in patients with a variety of locally advanced head and neck cancers. Conventional radiation with respect to timing, dose, and fractionation size is being used. Patients receive SR 2508 three times per week for 17 doses, $2 \, g/m^2$ per dose during radiation. Data are not yet available on clinical efficacy of SR 2508, however, the reported level of toxicity has been acceptable (41).

Perflourochemicals are a class of chemicals that have been developed to increase the oxygen-carrying capacity of blood. An emulsion of these chemicals is able to efficiently transport oxygen and carbon dioxide with rapid uptake and release of O_2 at a higher partial pressure than that for hemoglobin. The emulsion particles used are smaller ($0.2 \, \mu m$ in diameter) than red blood cells (average $5−10 \, \mu m$) and have the theoretical advantage of being able to transverse a disordered tumor microvasculature and areas of partial luminal obstruction that would be inaccessible to red blood cells. Both of these factors may contribute to raise the level of oxygenation within the hypoxic areas of a tumor.

Fluosol, combined with carbogen breathing (95% O_2 5% CO_2), has been shown to enhance the response to single dose and fractionated radiotherapy in several animal tumor model systems (58, 82, 83). The amount of enhancement is equivalent to that which would be expected if tumor hypoxia were reduced from 100% to 50%. This effects has not been seen when Fluosol is combined with air breathing. Teicher and Holden (81) have studied the effects of Fluosol/carbogen breathing on a variety of chemotherapeutic agents. Most alkylating agents showed an improved effectiveness with the addition of Fluosol, whereas CDDP showed no improvement. Interestingly, a negative interaction was seen with Mitomycin-C. The latter results would be expected given the bioreductive nature of this drug which is preferentially toxic to hypoxic cells.

Head and neck cancer has been the first clinical site where fluosol has been tested. Nineteen patients with stage III and IV tumors of the head and neck have been treated in a phase I-II dose escalation study (67, 68). Fluosol was infused on the Monday of each treatment week; the first 11 patients received 8 ml/kg in 5 infusions, 3 received 8 ml/kg for 6 infusions, and 5 patients received 9 ml/kg for 5 infusions. Fifteen of 19 patients (79%) achieved a complete response within 6 weeks of completing treatment. One patient was able to be rendered disease free following an neck dissection to remove residual regional disease. Thus 84% of patients achieved a Complete response and 14/19 patients (74%) remained alive after 1 year of follow-up. Toxicity included fever and chills with the initial dose in 5 patients. Ten patients developed transient elevations in serum transaminases.

No patient developed a painful or enlarged liver or spleen during treatment of follow-up. Mucositis was seen in all patients and was observed earlier that that expected from radiation therapy alone. These preliminary results are encouraging and further studies will be required to show if an advantage to treatment with Fluosol will be found. A prospective, randomized study of Fluosol and definitive radiation for patients with previously untreated head and neck cancer is in progress.

Hyperthermia in Head and Neck Cancer

There is increasing interest in hyperthermia as an adjunct to radiation in cancer therapy. In a recent review of clinical trials involving multiple sites and histologies, the therapeutic enhancement seen with the addition of heat to radiation therapy was 2-fold or greater with respect to local control after radiation alone (55). Patients with head and neck cancer often present with large or fixed metastatic nodal disease that is difficult to control with conventional therapies of surgery and/or radiotherapy (5, 29, 48). Because of the relatively superficial nature of cervical lymphatic disease, it has leant itself to experimentation with hyperthermia in conjunction with radiation therapy. Initially, only the most superficial tumors could be adequately heated which limited the utility of the approach. However, several methods of heating have been developed including electromagnetic waves with frequencies in the ultra high frequency range (microwave), which can reliably heat tumors to a depth of 4 cm, as well as ultrasound and phased array systems which have even greater depth capabilities (reviewed in International Journal of Radiation Oncology, Biology, Physics 1989; 3). These developments, along with the use of interstitial hyperthermia, have expanded the number of patients with advanced head and neck malignancies that may benefit from this approach.

Hyperthermia to temperatures of 42 °C or greater is cytotoxic as a single modality. The magnitude of the effect is dependent upon the temperature achieved as well as the duration of the hyperthermia (18). One clinically important aspect of hyperthermia is the enhanced sensitivity of S phase cells compared with cells in the G1 phase of the division cycle (96). This is in contrast to the age response function of radiation where S phase cells are the most resistant (Fig. 3.**5**) (74, 84). The difference in cell age sensitivity between hyperthermia and radiation suggestes at least additive effects when these two modalities are administered concurrently. Heat has also been shown to selectively affect chronically hypoxic cells versus acutely hypoxic or fully oxygenated cells (19), thus targeting another cell population that is relatively radioresistant. Other effects of hyperthermia inclucde decreased DNA, RNA and protein synthesis (77).

The biological basis for enhanced cell killing with hyperthermia and radiotherapy is incompletely understood despite considerable in vitro and in vivo preclinical investigations (32, 33, 77). That the increased cell killing with hyperthermia and radiation occurs under temperature conditions which are not, by themselves, cytotoxic strongly suggests that the interaction between hyperthermia and radiation is potentially synergistic. Within the temperature ranges used clinically, possible mechanisms of interaction include the inhibition of both sublethal (6, 28) as well as potentially lethal (43) X-ray damage repair.

The sequential timing of heat and radiation appears to be important. A uniform finding in vitro is that as the interval between heat and radiation increases, the magnitude of the interaction decreases. In vivo, the optimal sequence is more obscure. The usual treatment order of radiation followed by heat is typically determined by logistical considerations rather than experimental evidence for improved efficacy.

The use of hyperthermia in conjunction with radiation therapy for cervical lymph node metastasis has been reported by several centers. Archangeli (1) treated a group of 15 patients, each with multiple N2 or N3 regional nodes, using multiple daily fractions of 2.00, 1.50, 1.50 Gy per day, 4−5 hours between fractions to total doses of 40−70 Gy. Comparably sized lymph nodes on the same patient were treated with and without hyperthermia, so each patient served as his own control. A tumor core temperature of at least 42 °C, for 40−50 minutes was generated 15 minutes after the middle fraction on days 1, 3, and 5 of each week. Complete responses were found for 17 of 20 (85%) lymph nodes treated with hyperthermia, 3 of 20 (15%) had partial responses. Lymph nodes receiving radiation only had a complete response rate of only 6 out of 13 (46%). No adverse normal tissue reactions were seen.

In a later report by Archangeli (3), the effects of thermal dose on tumor response were studied in patients with head and neck cancer treated with hyperthermia and radiation. In this controlled study, complete responses were seen in 30 of 38 lymph nodes (79%) after combined treatment versus 10 of 43 (42%) complete responses with radiation therapy alone. At 2 years, the actuarial local tumor control was 58% after hyperthermia and radiation versus 14% after radiation alone. These differences were statistically significant. The amount of heat appears to be important. After 28 months, 56% of lymph nodes heated to 124 Eq 42.5 °C (an isoeffect relationship relating the amount of heat delivered to equivalent minutes at 42.5 °C) and 92% of lesions treated to 305 Eq 42.5 °C were controlled. This was compared to a local control rate of 14% for lesions which did not receive hyperthermia. The lymph nodes treated to 56 Eq 42.5 °C responded no better than those not receiving hyperthermia, implying that a threshold thermal dose may exist for radiosensitization.

A RTOG phase I−II trial evaluating hyperthermia with definitive radiation therapy has been reported by Scott et al. (71). Between 1981 and 1986, 133 patients with tumors less than 4 cm, were entered, 41 with head and neck squamous cell carcinomas. Radiation was given 5 days per week with 1.80−2.00 Gy per fraction, to total doses of 60−70 Gy. Hyperthermia, 43 °C to the deepest part of the tumor for 60 minutes, was given twice weekly, 15 minutes postirradiation. Because of poor geometry and patient discomfort, only 32% of patients were able to undergo an average of 43 °C, for 46 minutes. A complete response was noted in 51% of

patients. Of the 20 patients who received at least 54 Gy and 9 heat treatments, 65% had a complete response. Three of 4 patients with lymph nodes less than 3 cm had a complete response, versus 18 of 36 patients with nodes greater than 3 cm. A logistic regression analysis of patients surviving at least 6 weeks post-therapy found tumor response to be related to an average temperature for all sessions greater than 43 °C as well as size of the tumor mass. This study exemplifies the difficulty in achieving an adequate degree of hyperthermia for head and neck cancer patients. With improved equipment and thermometry, the problems in delivering an adequate homogeneous dose of hyperthermia should be minimized. It is expected that advancements in heat delivery will lead to improved therapeutic results.

A number of reports using hyperthermia in conjunction radiation therapy to treat cervical lymph nodes have been published (1, 3, 55, 61, 62, 88). However, only one randomized trial of radical radiation versus radiation plus hyperthermia for neck disease is available for analysis. Valdagni et al. (89) evaluated 44 patients with N3 cervical adenopathy due to squamous cell carcinoma and randomly assigned them to treatment with radiation to a total dose of 64−70 Gy either with, or without concurrent twice weekly regional hyperthermia. The former patients were further randomized to receive either 2 or 6 heat treatments. Patients were eligible for this study if their N3 disease had a maximum cervical node diameter of 7 cm, a tumor depth of less than 5 cm and a Karnovsky score of greater than 60. Twenty-three lymph nodes were treated in the radiation alone arm, and 21 lymph nodes were treated with hyperthermia in conjunction with radiation (8 with 2 heat sessions, 13 with 6). The goal of hyperthermia was a minimum of 42.5 °C, for 30 minutes. A complete response was seen in 36.8% for radiation only versus 82.3% for radiation and hyperthermia ($p < 0.01$). Progressive disease was seen in 21% of patients treated with radiation alone versus only 11% of patients treated with the combined modality. Both arms were comparable with respect fo radiation dose and lymph node size. The effect of tumor size on local control was greatest in the radiation only arm with control achieved in 60% of nodes 3.5 to 3.9 cm, 38% of 4.0 to 5.9 cm nodes, and 17% of 6.0 to 7.0 cm nodes. In the radiation plus hyperthermia arm, 80% of all nodal sizes were controlled. The acute side effects between the 2 arms were comparable. One patient died of carotid rupture 2 months after completing the combined modality arm. No differences could be found between the 2 versus 6 treatment arms though the number of lymph nodes in each arm is small. Due to observed differences between the 2 treatment arms, the control arm of radiation alone was abandoned. However, the trial of radiation with either 2 or 6 hyperthermia treatments remains in progress. While this study can be critized for the early closure of a control arm utilizing radiation alone as well as its limited follow-up, it nevertheless demonstrates that hyperthermia may be an effective adjunct with radiation therapy in the management of patients with large, fixed, cervical lymphatic disease from head and neck cancer.

Definitive Treatment of Head and Neck Cancers with Radiotherapy: Case Selection and Future Directions

Conventional radiation therapy, i.e., one 2.0 Gy fraction per day, 5 days per week appears to be sufficient treatment for most T1 and T2 squamous cell cancers of the head and neck. The decision as to use radiation or surgery is often not straightforward. Since both have equivalent tumor control rates, the ultimate selection is frequently determined by the morbidity associated with each approach. For example, a T1 tumor of the true vocal cord could be managed by a partial laryngectomy or radiation therapy to a limited field. The two therapies do not differ with respect to disease control, however, the qualitiy of the voice is much less with surgery. If this is an important aspect of a patient's life or work, then radiation is clearly a better approach. Each anatomic site in the head and neck is different and has its own set of radiation fields and surgical procedures, which makes the experience of the radiation therapist and surgeon an important part of the decision-making process. In addition, it is also necessary to take into consideration the nature and extent of any long-term side effects, the level of function attainable after treatment, and overall performance status of the patient. The patient should, of course, be fully apprised of all therapeutic options as this is where the final decision rests.

For more advanced lesions, the therapeutic shortcomings of a single modality are generally recognized. If treatment with radiation alone is necessary, there are sufficient data to justify using twice-a-day, hyperfractionated radiation for T2−T4 tumors, irrespective of anatomic site. While the acute morbidity of this regimen may be higher, there appears to be a 10−20% improvement in disease control. This is enough of an improvement to warrant the logistical difficulties in the hyperfractionation schedule.

Considerable progress has been made over the years in the treatment of head and neck cancers with radiation therapy. The goal of organ preservation, already available for patients with early stage disease, is now a realistic expectation for patients with advanced disease through the use of combined modality approaches. These include the administration of concurrent chemotherapy and radiation or induction chemotherapy prior to radiation therapy alone and

will be discussed elsewhere. As our experience in this area matures and develops, it is expected to hold additional promise for improving the outcome for patients with advanced head and neck tumors.

References

1. Archangeli G, Barni E, Cividalli A, et al. Effectiveness of microwave hyperthermia combined with ionizing radiation: Clinical results on neck node metastases. Int J Radiat Oncol Biol Phys 1980; 6: 143−8.
2. Archangeli G, Mauro F, Nervi C. Multiple daily fractionation (MDF) in association with misonidazole (MIS): A two-year experience with head and neck cancer. In: Breccia A, Rimondi C, Adams GE, eds. Advanced topics on radiosensitizer of hypoxic cells. New York: Plenum Press, 1982.
3. Archangeli G, Benassi M, Cividalli A, Lovisolo G, Mauro F. Radiotherapy and hyperthermia. Analysis of clinical results and identification of prognostic variables. Cancer 1987: 950−6.
4. Bardenson GW, Broese JJ. Experimental radiotherapy of a rat rhabdomyosarcoma with 15 MeV neutrons and 300 Kv X-rays. II. Effects of fractionated treatments applied five times a week for several weeks. Eur J Cancer 1970: 6: 89.
5. Bataini P, Brugere J, Bernier J, Jaulerry CH, Picot C, Ghossein NA. Results of radiotherapeutic treatment of carcinoma of the pyriform sinus: Experience of the Institute Curie. Int J Radiat Oncol Biol Phys 1982; 8: 983−9.
6. Ben-hur E, Elkind MM, Bronk BV. Thermally enhanced radioresponse of cultured chinese hamster cell: Inhibition of sublethal damage and enchacement of lethal damage. Radiat Res 1974; 58:38−51.
7. Blitzer P, Wang CC, Suit HD. Blood pressure and hemoglobin concentration: Multivariate analysis of local control after irradiation for head and neck cancer. Int J Radiat Oncol Biol Phys, 1984: 10 (suppl 2): 98.
8. Brunin E, Bataini JP, Asselain B, Jaulerry C, Brugere J. Resultats preliminaires d'un essai therapeutique sur l'effet radiosensibilisant due misonidazole dans les cancers de la tete et du cou. J Eur Radiother 1983; 4: 182−8.
9. Bush RS, Jenkin RDT, Allt WEC, et al. Definitive evidence for hypoxic cells influencing cure in cancer therapy. Br J Cancer 1978; 37 (suppl. III): 302−6.
10. Bush RS. The significance of anemia in clinical radiation therapy. Int J Radiat Oncol Biol Phys 1986; 12: 2047−50.
11. Cattan. Personal communication to Dische S (48).
12. Chaplin DJ, Durand RE, Olive PL. Acute hypoxia in tumors: Implications for modifiers of radiation effects. Int J Radiat Oncol Biol Phys 1986; 12: 1229−82.
13. Chaplin DJ, PL Olive, Durand RE. Intermittent blood flow in a murine tumor: Radiobiological effects. Cancer Res 1987; 47: 597−601.
14. Charbit A, Malaise EP, Tubiana M. Relation between the pathological nature and the growth rate of human tumors. Eur J Cancer 1971; 7: 307−15.
15. Coutard H. Roentgen therapy of epitheliomas of the tonsillar region, hypopharynx, and larynx from 1920 to 1926. Am J Roentgenol 1932; 28: 313−31.
16. Coutard H. Principles of X-ray therapy of malignant diseases. Lancet 1934; 2:1−8.
17. Deschner EE, Gray LH. Influence of tissue oxygen on X-ray induced chromosal damage in Erlich ascites tumor cells irradiated in vitro and in vivo. Radiat Res 1959; 11: 115−46.
18. Dewey WC, Hopwood LE, Sapareto SA, Gerweck LE. Cellular responses to combinations of hyperthermia and radiation. Radiology 1977; 123: 463−74.
19. Dewey WC, Thrall DE, Gillette EL. Hyperthermia and radiation—A selective thermal effect on chronically hypoxic tumor cells in vivo. Int J Radiat Oncol Biol Phys 1977; 2: 99−103.
20. Dische S. Chemical sensitizers for hypoxic cells: a decade of experience in clinical radiotherapy. Radiother Oncol 1985; 3: 97−115.
21. Elkind MM, Sutton H. X-ray damage and recovery in mammalian cells in culture. Nature 1951; 184: 1293−5.

22. EORTC. Early results of the EORTC randomized clinical trial on multiple fractions per day (MFD) and misonidazole in advanced head and neck cancer Int J Radiat Oncol Biol Phys 1986; 12: 587−91.

23. Fazekas J, Pajak TF, Wasserman T,, et al. Failure of misonidazole-sensitized radiotherapy to impact upon outcome among stage III−IV squamous cancers of the head and neck. Int J Radiat Oncol Biol Phys 1987; 13: 1155−60.

24. Fertil B, Malaise EP. Intrinsic radiosensitivity of human cell lines is correlated with radioresponsiveness of human tumors: Analysis of 101 published survival curves. Int J Radiat Oncol Biol Phys 1985; 11: 1699−707.

25. Fletcher GH. The evolution of the basic concepts underlying the practice of radiotherapy from 1949 to 1977. Radiology 1977; 127: 3−19.

26. Fletcher GH. Textbook of radiotherapy. 3rd ed. Philadelphia: Lea and Febiger, 1980.

27. Fowler JF. Potential for increasing the differential response between tumors and normal tissues: Can proliferation rates be used? Int J Radiat Oncol Biol Phys 1986; 12: 641−5.

28. Gerweck LE, Gillette EL, Dewey WC. Effect of heat and radiation on synchronous chinese hamster cells: Killing and repair. Radiat Res 1975; 64: 611−23.

29. Ghossein NA, Bataini P. The role of radiotherapy in treatment of neck metastases from head and neck cancer. In: Wolf GT (ed). Head and neck Oncology. Boston: Martinus Nijhoff, 1984.

30. Giaux. Personal communication to Dische S (48).

31. Gil Gayarre M, Poveda Pierola A, Delgado Macias T, Oton Sanchez C. The use of misonidazole with multiple doses associated to external irradiation. Proceedings of the Inaugural Meeting of the European Society of Therapeutic, Radiol Oncol (ESTRO), London, 1982.

32. Hahn GM. Hyperthermia and Cancer. New York: Plenum Press, 1982.

33. Hall EJ. Radiobiology for the radiologist. 3rd ed. Philadelphia: Lippincott JB, 1988.

34. Harwood AR, Beale FA, Cummings BJ, et al. Supraglottic laryngeal carcinoma: An analysis of dose−time−volume factors in 410 patients. Int J Radiat Oncol Biol Phys 1983; 9: 311−19.

35. Henk JM, Kindler PB, Smith CW. Radiotherapy and head and neck cancer: Final report on the first clinical trial. Lancet 1977; 2: 101−3.

36. Hirst DG. Anemia: A problem or an opportunity in radiotherapy? Int J Radiat Oncol Biol Phys 1986; 12: 2009−17.

37. Holsti LR, Mantyla M. Split-course versus continuous radiotherapy. Analysis of a randomized trial from 1964 to 1967. Acta Oncol. 1988; 27: 153−61.

38. Horiot JC, LeFur R, NGuyen T et al. Two fractions per day versus a single fraction per day in the radiotherapy of oropharynx carcinoma: Results of an EORTC randomized trial. Int J Radiat Oncol Biol Phys 1988; 15 (suppl. 1): 179.

39. Kaplan HS. Historic milestones in radiobiology and radiation therapy. Semin Oncol 1979; 6: 479−89.

40. Knee R, Fields RS, Peters LJ. Concomittant boost radiotherapy for advanced squamous cell carcinoma of the head and neck. Radiother Oncol 1985; 4: 1−7.

41. Lee DJ, Wasserman T, Coleman CN, et al. A progress report of the RTOG head and neck SR-2508 trial. Int J Radiat Oncol Biol Phys 1989; 17 (suppl 1): 133.

42. Lenz M. The early workers in clinical radiotherapy of cancer at the radium institute of the Curie Foundation, Paris, France. Cancer 1973; 32: 519−23.

43. Li GC, Evans RG, Hahn GM. Modification and inhibition of repair of potentially lethal X-ray damage by hyperthermia. Radiat Res 1976; 67: 491−501.

44. Little JB, Hahn GM. Plateau phase cultures of mammalian cells: An in vitro model for human cancer. Curr Top Rad Res 1972; 8: 39−83.

45. Marcial V, Pajak TF, Chang C, Tupchong L, Stetz J. Hyperfractionated photon radiation therapy in the treatment of advanced squamous cell carcinoma of the oral cavity, oropharynx, larynx, and sinuses, using radiation therapy as the only planned modality: (preliminary report) by the radiation therapy oncology group (RTOG). Int J Radiat Oncol Biol Phys 1987; 13: 41−7.

46. Marcial V, van den Bogaert W, Horiot JC. Head and neck: Cancer research plan. Int J Radiat Oncol Biol Phys 1988; 14 (suppl. 1): 119−25.

47. Medical Research Council. A study of the effects of misonidazole in conjunction with radiotherapy for the treatment of head and neck cancers. A report from the MRC working party on misonidazole for head and neck cancers. Br. J Radiol 1984; 57: 585−95.

48. Mendenhall WM, Million RR, Bova FJ. Analysis of time−dose factors in clinically positive neck nodes treated with irradiation alone in squamous cell carcinoma of the head and neck. Int J Radiat Oncol Biol Phys 1984; 10: 639−43.

49. Mendenhall WM, Million RR, Cassisi NJ. Squamous cell carcinoma of the supraglottic larynx treated with radical irradiation: analysis of treatment parameters and results. Int J Radiat Oncol Biol Phys 1984; 10: 2223−30.

50. Mesic JB, Fletcher GH, Goepfert H. Megavoltage irradiation of epithelial tumors of the nasopharynx. Int J Radiat Oncol Biol Phys 1981; 7: 447−53.

51. Million RR, Cassisi NJ. Management of head and neck cancer. A multidisciplinary approach. Philadelphia: JB Lippincott, 1984.

52. Morgan DAL, Bradley PJ, MacLennan KA. Early results of radiotherapy for advanced laryngeal cancer using three small fractions per day. Acta Oncol 1987; 27: 437−40.

53. Olive PL, Chaplin DJ, Durand RE. Pharmacokinetics, binding and distribution of Hoechst 33 342 in spheroids and murine tumors. Br J. Cancer 1985; 52: 739−46.

54. Overgaard J, Anderson AP, Jensen RH, et al. Misonidazole acombined with split course radiotherapy in the treatment of invasive carcinoma of the larynx and the pharynx—a preliminary report of the Danish Head and Neck Cancer Study (DAHANCA) Protocol 2. Acta Otolaryngol, 1982; 386 (suppl.): 215−20.

55. Overgaard J. Rationale and problems in the design of clinical studies. In: Overgaard J, ed. Hypothermic oncology 1984. Vol. 2. London, Philadelphia: Taylor and Francis, 1985.

56. Overgaard J, Hansen HS, Jorgensen K, Hansen MJ. Primary radiotherapy of larynx and pharynx carcinoma—an analysis of some factors influencing local control and survival. Int J Radiat Oncol Biol Phys 1986; 12: 515−21.

57. Overgaard J, Hjelm-Hansen M, Vendelbo Johansen L, Andersen AP. Comparison of conventional and split-course radiotherapy as primary treatment in carcinoma of the larynx. Acta Oncol 1988; 27: 147−52.

58. Rockwell S, Mate TP, Irvin CG, Nierenburg M. Reactions of tumors and normal tissues in mice to irradiation in the presence and absence of a perfluorochemical emulsion. Int J Radiat Oncol Biol Phys 1986; 12: 1315−18.

59. Parsons JT, Bova FJ, Withers RR. A re-evaluation of split-course technique for squamous cell carcinoma of the head and neck. Int J Radiat Oncol Biol Phys 1980; 6: 1645−52.

60. Parsons JT, Mendenhall WM, Cassisi NJ, Issacs JH Jr, Million RR. Accelerated hyperfractionation for head and neck cancer. Int J Radiat Oncol Biol Phys 1988; 14: 649−58.

61. Perez CA, Emami B, Hederman MA, Straube W, Von Gerichten D, Fox S. Clinical results of irradiation combined with local hyperthermia in superficial tumors. Radiation Research Society Abstracts of papers for the Thirty-fifth Annual Meeting, 1987.

62. Perez CA, Emami B, Scott B, Hornback NB, et al. Irradiation and hyperthermia in treatment of locally advanced and recurrent head and neck tumors. In Jacobs JR, Crissman J, Valeriote FA, Al-Serraf M.: Head and neck cancer: scientific perspectives in management and strategies for cure. New York: Elsevier, 1987.

63. Perez CA, Brady LW: Principles and Practice of radiation oncology. Philadelphia: JB Lippincott, 1987.

64. Philips RA, Tolmach LJ. Repair of potentially lethal damage in X-irradiated HeLa cells. Radiat Res 1966; 29: 41−32.

65. Phillips TL, Wasserman TH, Stetz J, Brady LW: Clinical trials of hypoxic cell sensitizers. Int J Radiat Oncol Biol Phys 1982; 8: 327−34.

66. Puck TT, Marcus PI. Action of X-rays on mammalian cells. J Exp Med 1956; 103: 653−66.

67. Rockwell S. Perfluorochemical emulsions as adjuncts to

radiotherapy. Biomater Artif Cells Artif Organs 1988; 16: 519−31.

68. Rose C, Lustig R, McIntosh N, Teicher B. Clinical trial of Fluosol DA 20% in advanced squamous cell carcinoma of the head and neck. Int J Radiat Oncol Biol Phys 1986; 12: 1325−27.

69. Saunders MI, Dische S. Radiotherapy employing three fractions each day over a continuous period of 12 days. Br J Radiol 1986; 59: 523−5.

70. Saunders MI, Dische S, Fowler JF, et al. Radiotherapy employing three fractions on each of twelve consecutive days. Acta Oncol. 1988; 27: 163−7.

71. Scott R, Gillespie B, Perez CA, et al. Hyperthermia in combination with definitive radiation therapy: results of a phase I/II RTOG study. Int J Radiat Oncol Biol Phys 1988; 15: 711−16.

72. Sealy R, Williams A, Cridland S, Stratford M, Minchinton A, Hallet C. A report on misonidazole in a randomized trial in locally advanced head and neck cancer. Int J Radiat Oncol Biol Phys 1982; 8: 339−42.

73. Sealy R, Cridland S. The treatment of locally advanced head and neck cancer with misonidazole, hyperbaric oxygen and radiation. An interim report. Int J Radiat Oncol Biol Phys 1984; 10: 1721−3.

74. Sinclair WK, Morton RA. X-ray sensitivity during the cell generation cycle of cultured Chinese hamster cells. Radiat Res 1966; 29: 450−74.

75. Steele GG. Growth kinetics of tumors. Oxford: Oxford University Press, 1977.

76. Suit HD, Gallager HS. Intact tumor cells in irradiated tissue. Arch Pathol 1964; 78: 648−51.

77. Suit HD, Shwayder M. Hyperthermia: Potential as an antitumor agent. Cancer 1974; 34: 122−9.

78. Svoboda VHJ. Radiotherapy by several sessions a day. Br J Radiol 1975; 48: 131−3.

79. Svoboda VHJ. Further experience with radiotherapy by multiple daily sessions. Br J Radiol 1978; 51: 363−9.

80. Taskinen PJ. Radiotherapy and TNM classification of cancer of the larynx. Acta Radiol 1969; 287: 1−121.

81. Teicher BA, Holden SA. Survey of the effect of adding Fluosol-DA 20%/O_2 treatment with various chemotherapeutic agents. Cancer Treat Rep 1987; 71: 173−7.

82. Teicher BA, Rose CM. Effect of dose and scheduling on growth delay of the Lewis lung carcinoma produced by the perfluorochemical emulsion, Fluosol-DA. Int J Radiat Oncol Biol Phys 1986; 12: 1311−13.

83. Teicher BA, Rose CM. Perfluorochemical emulsions can increase tumor radiosensitivity. Science 1984; 223: 934−6.

84. Terasima R, Tolmach LJ. X-ray sensitivity and DNA synthesis in synchronous populations of HeLa cells. Science 1963; 140: 490−2.

85. Thompson LH, Suit HD. Proliferation kinetics of x-irradiated mouse l cells studied with time-lapse photography. Experimental methods and data analysis. Int J Radiat Biol 1967; 13: 391−7.

86. Thomlinson RH, Gray LH. The histological structure of some human lung cancers and possible implications for radiotherapy. Br J Cancer 1955; 9: 539−49.

87. Trotter MJ, Chaplin DJ, Durand RE, Olive PL. The use of fluorescent probes to identify regions of transient perfusion in murine tumors. Int J Radiat Oncol Biol Phys 1989; 16: 931−4.

88. Valdagni R, Kapp DS, Valdagni C. N3 (TNM−UICC) metastatic neck nodes managed by combination radiation therapy and hyperthermia: clinical results and analysis of treatment parameters. Int J Hyperthermia 1986; 2: 189−200.

89. Valdagni RM, Amichetti M, Pani G. Radical radiation alone versus radical radiation plus microwave hyperthermia for N3 (TNM−UICC) neck nodes: A prospective randomized trial. Int J Radiat Oncol Biol Phys 1988; 15: 13−24.

90. Wang CC. Radiation therapy for head and neck neoplasms. Indications, techniques and results. Littleton: John Wright, 1983.

91. Wang CC, Blitzer PH, Suit HD. Twice-a-day radiation therapy for cancer of the head and neck. Cancer 1985; 55: 2100-4.

92. Wang CC, Suit HD. Blitzer PH. Twice-a-day radiation therapy for supraglottic carcinoma. Int J Radiat Oncol Biol Phys 1986; 12: 3−7.

93. Wang CC. Local control of oropharyngeal carcinoma after two accelerated hyperfractionation radiation therapy schemes. Int J Radiat Oncol Biol Phys 1988; 14: 1143−6.

94. Wang CC. Accelerated hyperfractionation radiation therapy for carcinoma of the nasopharynx. Cancer 1989; 63: 2461−7.

95. Weichelbaum RR, Beckett MA, Schwartz JL, Dritschilo A. Radioresistant tumor cells are present in head and neck carcinomas that recur after radiotherapy. Int J Radiat Oncol Biol Phys 1988; 15: 575−9.

96. Westra A, Dewey WC. Variation to sensitivity to heat shock during the cell-cycle of Chinese hamster cells in vitro. Int J Radiat Biol. 1971; 19: 467−77.

97. Withers HR, Taylor JMG, Maciejewski B. The hazard of accelerated tumor clonogen repopulation during radiotherapy. Acta Oncol. 1988; 27: 131−46.

4 Biostatistical Issues in the Design and Interpretation of Clinical Trials in Head and Neck Cancer

J. W. Andersen, L. A. Kalish

Introduction

The treatment of head and neck cancer has evolved to include components of chemotherapy, surgery, radiotherapy, immunotherapy, and bone marrow transplantation. Refining strategies for the optimal sequence and timing of multidisciplinary modalities is the focus of large current and planned studies. At the same time, new combinations, new agents, and novel modalities are being investigated in smaller studies. Protocol designs need a coherent framework so that the most promising of these can move rapidly yet safely from small-scale investigations to be either incorporated into successful treatment programs or tested against standard regimens in the future. This will necessitate among other things a standardization of techniques to ensure comparability between related studies, a consistency in the nomenclature to ensure the interpretability of protocol documents and results, and a commitment of clinical and patient resources to protocol programs of sufficient size to evaluate therapies efficiently and definitively. In this chapter, we will not recommend specific therapies, but will define some endpoints commonly targeted in clincal trials and discuss their standardization. We will then provide a brief guide to some basic statistical techniques appropriate for the analysis and presentation of these endpoints and discuss the sample size needed for studies of these endpoints, both in terms of calculation for prospectively designed trials and as it relates to the interpretation of recently completed and published trials.

Study Objectives

Clinical trials are broadly characterized by "phase." Knowledge of the phase of a trial gives immediate information about the intent and size of the trial. In this section, we define studies by phase within the context of oncology trials, broadly enumerate the endpoints and suggest some design strategies.

Phase I

The main objective of phase I studies is to determine the MTD (maximum tolerated dose). This is established by entering a small number of patients at a preplanned dose and escalating the dose for the next group of patients unless an unacceptable rate of DLT (dose limiting toxicity) is seen. Generally, the dose below that which produces an unacceptable rate of DLT is designated as the MTD. The MTD is used for further testing in pilot and phase II studies. Prior to large-scale evaluation, it is advisable to add a few (< 10) patients at the MTD to further investigate toxicity both quantitatively (how much and at what severity) and qualitatively (what organs and what clinical presentations). Typically, the patient population entered in a phase I trial is heterogeneous, is not restricted to a single disease type, and is comprised of patients well enough to tolerate the toxicity of therapy but with disease so advanced or refractory that standard and experimental therapies have ceased to give relief. The investigation of the human pharmacology of the agent is often an important scientific endpoint. The quantitative and qualitative natures of the toxicity are only very broadly defined and objective response is a secondary, even anecdotal, outcome.

Phase II

The main objective of phase II studies is either to investigate the efficacy of an experimental agent (often called a pilot study) or to refine an estimate of the efficacy of a piloted agent or a new combination of standard treatments. Rapid evaluation is desirable and, in general, response is the primary outcome although in diseases with high response rates, in adjuvant settings, or where time to failure or survival are the primary outcomes, other parameters may be used. The patient population often has recurrent or refractory disease and the presumption is that efficacy in a high-risk population will translate to favorable results in an "up-front" setting. Further definition of toxicity is an additional objective of prime interest. Planned "early stopping," or termination prior to full accrual, due to clear lack of efficacy in early registrations, can be an efficient use of clinical resources, allowing the testing of more agents and limiting the number of patients treated with ineffective therapy.

Multi-arm randomized phase II studies are sometimes run by institutions and groups with rapid accrual where the administration of a sequence of small trials can be awkward. Such trials simultaneously evaluate several experimental therapies but do not contain a standard treatment control arm. While the sample sizes on any treatment are likely to be too small for useful treatment comparisons, a compelling scientific reason for conducting randomized phase II trials is that selection bias (that is, the slanting of results due to studying a nonrepresentative or "select" group of patient) is less a problem than in one-arm trials. In a randomized phase II trial, every patient must have been considered as a potential candidate for any of the treatments being tested, so results are less likely to be influenced by selection.

Phase III

The objective of phase III trials is to determine the efficacy of two or more treatments with sufficient precision to establish their relative superiority. This is done by conducting a randomized trial of sufficient size to ensure a high probability that important true differences will be detected statistically and a low probability that differences will erroneously be observed by chance. The primary endpoints may be response, duration of response, time to failure, disease-free survival, overall survival, and/or other parameters relevant to the disease site.

Phase III trials can compare experimental treatments with a "standard," compare among several experimental treatments when there is no standard efficacious therapy, or even compare among "standard" treatments when several are in clinical use. Eligibility criteria are generally quite rigorous so that the patient population is fairly homogeneous and treatment differences will not be obscured by patient variation. Randomization is used to ensure that each patient has an equal chance of receiving any of the therapies under study. Randomized treatment groups will tend to be comparable with respect to all factors which may affect outcome, thus yielding an unbiased treatment comparison and lending credibility and validity to the study results. Sequential study designs have been developed which can allow for early stopping due to early convincing evidence of a treatment difference. As with phase II trials, these designs are intended to conserve clinical resources, advance active agents rapidly, and reduce the number of patient treated with inferior agents.

Generally, anticancer agents do not receive FDA approval for general clinical use until they have undergone extensive phase III testing. There are exceptions as α-interferon in hairy cell leukemia which had such clear cut efficacy that it received approval after phase II testing. Only because the phase II trials were well planned and well executed was the evidence accepted as compelling without phase III testing. In most diseases, and head and neck cancer is no exception, advances are small, and only through well designed, well run, statistically valid clinical trials can small advances be demonstrated convincingly.

Clinical Trial Endpoints

In this section, we provide some discussion of endpoints commonly used in clinical trials, highlighting those with particular relevance to head and neck cancer, and providing some guidelines for standardization and interpretation. The emphasis will be on appropriate use of various endpoints and procedures and the statistical vocabulary needed for the discussion of analysis, study design and sample size calculations.

Toxicity. Ideally, toxicity is defined objectively as the change in a parameter from baseline or normal values (e. g. creatinine $1.5-3 \times$ normal: grade 2 or moderate) or in absolute terms as specific counts or events (e. g. WBC $< 1000/\mu L$: grade 4 or life-threatening). The cooperative groups have long had grading schemes for standardization of toxicity. However, while the grades were internally consistent, they were not consistent across groups. For example, a platelet count of $85\,000/\mu L$ would be considered "moderate" (grade 2) thrombocytopenia according to the ECOG (Eastern Cooperative Oncology Group) toxicity criteria (1) but "mild" (grade 1) according to the RTOG/EORTC toxicity criteria. Recently, in cooperation with the NCI, a multigroup effort resulted in the creation of the common toxicity criteria, or CTC (2), which consolidated the objective criteria of several groups and added other categories such as sensory and psychologic changes which are seen commonly with the biologic response modifiers (BRMs). While the CTC are quite extensive, multimodal therapies will continue to need ancillary toxicity grading schemes such as the RTOG/EORTC acute radiation morbidity scoring criteria and late radiation morbidity scoring scheme to grade modality-specific toxicities. Use of uniform grading schemes helps ensure comparability of results within an institution or group and between studies both over time and across investigators.

Response. Response is usually designated as complete (CR), partial (PR), stable disease (SD or NC for no change), or progressive disease (PD). Some reports define additional categories as minimal response (RTOG) or bone improvement (ECOG) in patients with metastatic breast cancer which identifiy "good" SD. Documentation of and adherence to objective response criteria are essential to the implementation of a good clinical trial program. The cooperative groups have standardized objective response criteria (1). As was the case with toxicity grading schemes, there is not uniformity of response coding in the literature and, more unfortunately, not always consistency among protocols within a group or institution. For example, Table 4.**1** presents the definitions of partial response for four protocols in similar patient populations from three groups or institutions. In addition to PR, RTOG defines mini-

Table 4.1 **Response criteria for partial response (PR)**

RTOG 85-27 A Phase II–III Study of SR2508 Combined with Radiotherapy for Locally Advanced Head and Neck Squamous Carcinoma.

PR: (measurable disease) Tumor shrinkage greater than 50% of the product of the perpendicular diameters of the two largest dimensions without increase in size of any other area of known malignant disease (excluding regional nodes) or without appearance of new areas of malignant disease within the treated volume.

PR: (evaluable, nonmeasurable lesions) A definite decrease in size of diseased areas amounting to an estimated 80% regression (close to complete regression) or better. This should be confirmed by at least two investigators evaluating independently, or photographs or radiographs should be submitted to the study chairman for confirmation.

83-084 Dana–Farber Cancer Institute: Induction Chemotherapy for Advanced Head and Neck Cancer.

PR: greater than 50% reduction in the sum of the products of the greatest perpendicular diameters of the lesion(s). Duration of response > 1 month during which no new lesions may appear and no existing lesion may enlarge.

ECOG P-C385 Pilot Study for the Evaluation of Simultaneous Cisplatin/5-FU Infusion Chemotherapy and Limited Radiation Therapy in Regionally Recurrent Head and Neck Cancer.
PR: Greater than or equal to 50% decrease in tumor size lasting for at least 4 weeks without increase in size of any area of known malignant disease by more than 25% or appearance of new areas of involvement.

Measurable, bidimensional: Greater than or equal to 50% decrease in size of one or more lesions (multiplications of longest diameter by the greatest perpendicular diameter) for at least 4 weeks.

Measurable, unidimensional: Greater than or equal to 50% decrease in linear tumor measurement lasting for at least 4 weeks. Palpable masses that can be measured in only one dimension may be evaluated for response by using the formula: A = on-study measurement; B = measurement after treatment; PR if $(A - B)/A \geq 0.3$.

ECOG EST-1386 Phase II Randomized Study to Compare Weekly Methotrexate to Trimetrexate given Daily × 5 in Advanced Recurrent or Metastasic Squamous Cell Cancer of the Head and Neck.

PR: a reduction by at least 50% of the product of the longest perpendicular diameters of the tumor with no new area of malignant disease appearing for at least 3 weeks.

mal response (MR). A patient with a 75% reduction in the product of the largest diameters of one of several lesions lasting > 4 weeks with a 20% increase in another lesion would have MR on the RTOG trial, SD on DFCI 83-084, a PR on P-C385, and perhaps a PR on EST-1386 depending on whether the sum of all lesions met the 50% reduction criterion. This variety in coding makes it difficult for investigators to

compare response percentages between articles and especially among abstracts where brevity is the norm and definitions are rarely given.

Time-to-event. Much data on clinical trials are concerned with estimating the duration of a biological state (survival, duration of response, time to bone marrow engraftment) which is terminated by an event (death, relapse, engraftment). "Censor" is the term used for a case followed for a time-to-event endpoint for whom the event of interest has not been observed at the time of analysis. Cases entirely lost to follow-up are generally censored at the date lost. The topics which follow are examples of time-to-event endpoints.

Time-to-treatment failure (TTF). TTF is defined for all patients as the time from entry in a study (or a given discrete treatment phase or "step" of a study) until progression, death from any cause, relapse after a response, or (rarely) nonprotocol therapy prior to documented progression or relapse. The only cases censored are those alive without relapse or progression and those lost to follow-up where there is no reason to suspect that the loss was due to worsening condition (termed "uninformative censoring"). This is an important endpoint in advanced and metastatic head and neck cancer where absolute documentation that a patient is clinically free of disease is frequently difficult and where long periods of rewarding stable disease can result from therapy.

Duration of response. This is defined as the time from documentation of response to documented progression. As noted above, the definitions of response are not uniform in the literature which implies that the duration of response may not be comparable between studies, either. Additionally, the schedule of follow-up visits can affect the apparent duration of response. RTOG 85-27 requires follow-up at 1 week and 1 month after therapy and every 3 months during the first 2 years. A phase III intergroup study, INTERG-0034, of chemotherapy with surgery and RT for resectable squamous cell carcinoma of the head and neck (SCCHN), calls for follow-up at 1-month intervals for the first year after treatment. DFCI 83-084 has no follow-up schedule in the protocol. Thus, a patient with a clinically detectable but no overt relapse 7 months after response could be credited with a 9-month duration of response on RTOG 85-27, 7 months on INTERG-0034 and some other figure on DFCI 83-084 depending on clinic schedules or self-diagnosis. Randomized studies, especially those in adjuvant settings where an observation arm might be an option, must be designed so that the follow-up schedule is comparable across treatments and over time. Otherwise, relapse will be detected earlier on the more frequently followed arm which can appear to do worse only because of differential scheduling. While similar follow-up schedules are essential for multi-arm trials, groups and institutions which conduct multiple and sequential phase II trials should consider similar standardization so that results from trial to trial will be comparable.

Disease-free survival (DFS). DFS is the time from the patient becoming disease free to time of relapse. In most disease sites, this is equivalent to the duration of CR. In adjuvant trials, all patients are by definition disease free at entry and the measurement of DFS begins at the date on-study. However, in multi-modal therapy where postchemotherapy surgery and/or radiotherapy (RT) can render a patient with PR or even SD disease free, researchers have reported DFS. DFS in this setting starts either at the date of clinical CR induced by chemotherapy and/or RT or at the date when surgery and/or RT have rendered the patient free of clinically detectable disease (i.e. with no evidence of disease or NED). The same cautions noted above about differential follow-up schedules apply. Additionally, in trials with surgery and/or RT, the conversion of cases from PR or SD to NED is in part a function of the aggressiveness and technical expertise of the surgeons or radiotherapists and, especially in randomized trials with a few institutions, it may be appropriate to take the institution or even the treating physician into account in the design and evaluation of studies that have DFS as a primary endpoint.

One problem with the interpretation of analyses of duration of response and DFS stems from the fact that they are analyses of retrospectively defined subsets. It is likely that a very aggressive treatment will have a higher response rate than a more conventional regimen. However, if the extra responders have "fragile" responses of short duration, then that arm may appear to have worse overall DFS only because of the additional fragile responses in one comparison group. For example, patients may be randomized to chemotherapy plus radiotherapy (CT + RT) or RT alone. CT + RT will have a higher overall response rate if the CT, but not RT, converts a select risk group of patients to responders. Although the percent of patients who become disease free with CT + RT is higher because of the "fragile" responses, the DFS of this subset may be worse than that of the smaller subset of patients who become disease free after RT alone. This concept has recently been discussed in the context of hematology trials (3, 4), but is particularly relevant to multimodal therapy in head and neck cancer. In particular, when a high response rate leads to poor DFS, investigators should be aware of this potential effect and treat comparisons of DFS with additional caution.

The difficulty with relying on stratified or multivariate analyses to adjust for this potential problem is that the comparison groups are determined not by pretreatment randomization but retrospectively by the fact of having responded. All factors identifying the group with "fragile" responses may not be balanced between treatments and may not be charac-

terized by data which have been collected. It has been suggested that analyses of remission durability be done among all randomized patients with time measured from the date of randomization and the duration equal either to zero (3) or the time-on protocol treatment (4) for nonremitters. How the results of such analyses would be interpreted is not covered. When interpreting analyses of duration of response or DFS, it is important to realize that the results cannot be used to predict the prognosis of a future patient at the start of therapy, since it is not yet known if that patient will respond or be rendered NED. Survival remains the least problematic, if longest to evaluate, endpoint.

Local vs. regional vs. distant relapse. In head and neck cancer as in other diseases such as primary breast cancer where total local eradication is possible through multi-modal therapy, it may be important to the interpretation of a trial to distinguish the site of relapse and to perform separate analyses to evalutate the control of local−regional and distant disease.

Survival. This is defined for all patients as the time from entry to a study until death from any cause. Patients are censored if alive at the time of statistical analysis or if lost to follow-up. However, patients with head and neck cancer are often elderly with multiple comorbidities and with histories of alcohol and tobacco abuse. In diseases with relatively long disease-specific survival, the death rate from other causes can be quite high. One way to handle this problem of "competing risks" is to censor survival for cases who died from other cancers or diseases at the date of death as though they were lost to follow-up (5, 6). For example, in a small trial in soft palate cancer (7), overall survival was 60% at 3 years but aerodigestive cancer had an estimated rate of occurrence of only 10% per year after treatment of the soft palate cancer. When deaths from this and other intercurrent diseases were taken into account, the cause-specific survival was 81% at 3 years. This adjustment must be used cautiously as the results are hypothetical (if the other causes of failure could be eliminated) and the interpretation is valid only if the competing causes of failure are totally independent of one another, a difficult assumption to verify. The analysis which counts all deaths as failures is unbiased if conservative and unadjusted survivals should be always be reported. This adjustment is never appropriate for deaths due to treatment which must always be interpreted as failure.

In order to evaluate the effect of treatment in nonrandomized trials, survival among responders is sometimes compared with that of nonresponders. The rationale is that nonresponders did not receive the potential benefit of treatment, so they constitute an appropriate control group. This reasoning is fallacious and such comparisons do not provide information with which to evaluate treatment efficacy. There are two separate biases in this type of analysis. First, for a patient to be classified as a responder, that patient must have lived long enough to be so classified. This adds a guarantee time to all survival times among responders which is not added to the survival times of nonresponders. Likewise, patients experiencing early death are de facto nonresponders. Thus, even if responders are a purely random sample of all patients, a naive analysis will tend to imply that they live longer. There are statistical methods for dealing with this bias (8, 9) but not for the second (and more important) bias. The second bias is that responders and nonresponders are not comparable subgroups and there is no statistical basis for interpreting the analysis as a comparison of treated vs. untreated patients (10). For example, patients with low risk characteristics (good performance status, small tumors, early stage disease) are more likely to respond and are more likely to live longer no matter what treatment they receive. Thus, tumor response may be a surrogate for other known or unknown patient characteristics which also are associated with longer survival and ought not be used to test whether treatment causes longer survival.

The issues discussed here are more general than comparing survival between responders and nonresponders. The same issues arise whenever outcomes are compared in subgroups which can only be defined after treatment begins (e.g. survival of patients by full dose received versus dose reductions required, or by radiotherapy according to protocol versus noncompliant radiotherapy). Retrospectively defined patient characteristics should be considered outcomes. An observed association between one outcome (response) and another outcome (survival) should not be interpreted as cause-and-effect.

Analysis of Clinical Trial Endpoints

The purpose of an analysis is to summarize the results of a given experiment and to use those results to make some generalizations or predictions about the general population from which the treated group was drawn and to which the study treatment might reasonably be applied.

A brief review of the framework of hypothesis testing may help at this point. A *hypothesis* is a statement regarding the true state of nature. In the clinical trials setting, this is generally a statement regarding treatment differences. The null hypothesis, H_0, suggests no difference (e. g. that the probability of response is the same for two treatments) and the alternative hypothesis, H_A, suggests a difference (e.g. that the probabilities of response differ for two treatments). If H_A allows for the possibility of either treatment being superior, then the test is a "two-sided" test. A one-sided test would specify an H_A which only considers deviations from H_0 in one direc-

tion (e.g. treatment A is better than treatment B). A statistical test is used for making decisions between H_0 and H_A.

If the decision is that H_0 is false when it is in fact true, this is termed a type I error (or false positive). The probability of making this error is written as $\alpha = \text{prob}(\text{reject } H_0 | H_0 \text{ true})$ and can be set by the investigator. Traditionally, the false-positive rate has been set to $\alpha = 0.05$. The *p*-value is the probability of observing the data actually seen or data which are as consistent or less consistent with H_0, given that H_0 is true. To expand, if H_0 is that there is no difference between the response rates of two treatments and response rates of 25% and 35% are observed in a randomized trial of the two treatments, the *p*-value is the probability of observing a 10% or larger difference, calculated under the assumption that H_0 is true. A "small" *p*-value, defined as being less than or equal to the prespecified α, therefore indicates that the data are not consistent with H_0 and H_0 is rejected.

Conversely, a type II error, or false negative, occurs when the decision is made that H_0 is true, when it is indeed false. The probability of this happening is called β, so $\beta = \text{prob}(\text{accept } H_0 | H_0 \text{ false})$. The power of a test, equal to $(1-\beta)$, is the probability that one will correctly reject H_0; that is, $(1-\beta) = \text{prob}(\text{reject } H_0 | H_0 \text{ false})$. It is the ability to detect a difference given that one truly exists and depends on the true magnitude of the treatment difference (the larger the difference between treatment outcomes, the more power) and the sample size (the power increases with increasing sample size).

There is a rule in statistics; the more tests you perform, the more likely it is that something, often something irrelevant, inexplicable or silly, will be significant by chance. In statistical terms, the false positive rate is greatly inflated. Therefore it is important to focus both at the design stage and at the analysis and publication phase of the study on the prime purpose of the trial: to investigate the effect of the treatment. Analysis and interpretation should concentrate on the overall association between treatment and outcome. Subset analyses should be considered exploratory, with much less weight given to their conclusions.

Analysis of Percents

Counted data (e. g. the number who responded, the number who experienced grade 4 hematologic toxicity) are generally presented as percents. Very briefly, if *s* represents the number of "successes" or observed events (responses, treatment without toxicity, successful bone marrow engraftments) and *n* represents the total sample size, then the estimated success rate or probability of success, $\hat{p}$, is calculated as $\hat{p} = s/n$, where $\hat{p}$ is called "*p* hat" and is an estimate of the true but unknown success rate, p. The proportion of "failures" (nonresponders, those who experienced toxicity) is estimated as $(1-\hat{p})$. When percents are shown, these are calculated as $\hat{p} \times 100\%$ and $(1-\hat{p}) \times 100\%$. For the remainder of these discussions, we will refer to the proportions $\hat{p}$ and p.

A very basic, very simple, and too often overlooked analysis of a single proportion is the confidence interval which gives a range of values within which p is likely to lie. The chance that the interval contains p or the confidence with which we can predict that the true underlying success probability falls in that interval is called the confidence coefficient. When we calculate a 95% confidence interval, there is a 5% chance that p falls outside that interval. In this setting, 0.05 (i. e. 5%) is α and the confidence coefficient is $(1-\alpha) \times 100\%$. When s and $(n-s)$ are both larger than 5, a symmetric 95% confidence interval is easily calculated as $\hat{p} \pm 1.96\sqrt{\hat{p}(1-\hat{p})/n}$, where $\sqrt{\hat{p}(1-\hat{p})/n}$ is the standard error of the estimate, $sc(\hat{p})$, and 1.96 is the critical value read from a table of the standard normal distribution with area $\alpha/2$ to the right of the critical value and area $\alpha/2$ to the left of minus the critical value. The standard notation for the critical value is $z_{1-\alpha/2}$. For a 90% confidence interval ($\alpha = 0.10$), $z_{1-\alpha/2} = z_{.95} = 1.64$. With this simple tool, an investigator hearing or reading the results of a study may determine quickly the relative precision (or imprecision) of the estimate by calculating the range over which the true probability likely lies. When s or $(n-s)$ is smaller than 5, exact tables and methods (11, 12) should be used because symmetric intervals based on the normal approximation given above may not be accurate.

Phase I and small pilot studies often report no occurrence of an event as one of their primary findings. It is again easy to calculate the chance that no episodes of an event (response, lethal toxicity) would have occurred given a hypothesized underlying rate, p_0. This is simply equal to $(1-p_0)^n$. For example, if five patients are treated at the MTD in a phase I study, there is a probability of $0.44 = (1-0.15)^5$ that no episodes of a toxicity will be seen if the true underlying toxicity rate is 15%. Conversely, there is only a 56% chance of seeing at least one untoward event in this small sample, which is why it is a good idea in phase I trials to treat a larger group (e. g. 10 patients) at the MTD before suggesting a given dose for wider testing.

When proportions are to be compared between two groups (e. g. treatment 1 versus treatment 2, males versus females), the data are most conveniently presented as a 2×2 table. Table 4.2 shows the usual layout for comparing two treatments where, for example, a represents the number in row 1 (outcome 1) and column 1 (treatment 1), n_1 gives the total number in row 1 summed over columns 1 and 2 (treatments 1 and 2) and n gives the total

Table 4.2   **2 × 2 table of data**

	Treatment 1	Treatment 2	Total
Outcome 1	a	b	$a+b$
Outcome 2	c	d	$c+d$
Total	n_1	n_2	n

sample size. If outcome 1 is response, then the proportion of responders on treatment 1 is estimated as $\hat{p}_1 = a/n_1$. In a similar fashion, $\hat{p}_2 = b/n_2$ and $(a+b)/n$ is the overall response rate, $\hat{p}$.

A two-sided statistical test of $H_0: p_1 = p_2$ versus $H_A: p_1 \neq p_2$ is the Pearson chi-square test:

$$\chi^2 = \frac{(ad-bc)^2}{n_1 n_2 (a+b)(c+d)/n}$$

where the p-value is read from a chi-square (χ^2) distribution with one degree of freedom. This is mathematically equal to basing the test on:

$$Z = \frac{|\hat{p}_1 - \hat{p}_2|}{\sqrt{\hat{p}(1-\hat{p})\left(\frac{1}{n_1} + \frac{1}{n_2}\right)}}$$

That is, the absolute difference (ignore the sign) divided by an estimate of $sc(\hat{p}_1 - \hat{p}_2)$. The p-value is read from a standard normal distribution as twice the area to the right of Z. This latter formula simplifies evaluation of published studies where the response probabilities and sample sizes are the only data available. When Z is at least 1.96, the p-value is 0.05 or less.

Further discussions of the analysis of proportions in clinical trials can be found in references 13–16, listed in the approximate order of mathematical complexity. Tests often used for the analysis of 2×2 (2 response categories, 2 treatments) and $R \times C$ tables (≥ 2 response categories, ≥ 2 treatments) are Pearson chi-square (shown above for the 2×2 case) and the Fisher exact test. When the outcomes have a natural order (CR is better than PR is better than NR), the Wilcoxon ($2 \times C$ or $R \times 2$) or Kruskal–Wallis ($R \times C$) (17) are appropriate and make use of the ordering. This is especially useful for analysis of toxicity where the grade is ordered qualitatively but not quantitatively (grade 2 is not necessarily twice as bad as grade 1).

Stratified Analyses and Logistic Regression

The Mantel–Haenszel procedure for stratified 2×2 tables (18, 19) is used to compare treatments while adjusting for another patient characteristic or "covariate" (say, histology or age) which itself may be associated with the outcome probabilities. The principle of stratified analysis is that the sample is split into homogeneous subgroups (strata). The treatment comparison is made separately within each stratum and the stratum-specific comparisons are combined. By doing this, the treatment comparison is made comparing "like with like" so that, for example, if by chance more poor risk patients were allocated to one treatment group, the treatment comparison will not be "confounded" by comparing mostly poor with mostly good risk patients. The procedure is most powerful when the stratum-specific comparisons are all in the same direction (e. g. treatment 1 is better than treatment 2 in all risk groups). Randomized studies are not likely to require stratified analyses since the randomized groups are likely to be balanced by covariates. However, stratified analyses are particularly useful for nonrandomized comparisons as they are more likely to be confounded or unbalanced by risk groups.

When there are many patient characteristics of interest to be adjusted for simultaneously, then the stratified analysis approach becomes cumbersome. Logistic regression (20), a form of regression function or model for dichotomous (yes/no, response/no response) outcomes, is used in this setting and has the advantage that it is just as easy, operationally, to adjust a treatment comparison for, say, five other covariates as for one. Another advantage is that the explanatory variables can retain continuous values (age, hemoglobin, etc.) or be expressed with dichotomous values (treatment A = 0; treatment B = 1). Disadvantages are that the concepts involved in modeling are less intuitive than working with raw percentages and the technique requires important mathematical assumptions which are not easy to verify. Additionally, computers are required to calculate the regression parameters and the *p*-values associated with the explanatory variables. The choice of candidate variables is important to the interpretability of the model because variables can act as "proxies" for each other (for example, stage II disease may have good performance status and stage IV have poor performance status) or be confounded with each other. Response can be associated with several variables in a complex way requiring interaction terms in the model (if, say, age is a strong prognostic factor in patients with lung metastases but not in patients without lung metastases). Clearly, the performance and evaluation of multivariate analyses need to be done with close collaboration between investigator and statistician. However, when done correctly and interpreted carefully, this can be a powerful tool for the identification of significant prognostic factors and groups of factors, and the model and the regression parameters can be used to predict response probabilities in important subgroups.

Survival Analysis

Survival analysis methodology can be applied to any data expressed as time-to-event. When absolutely all cases have been followed to the event of interest (i.e. are complete), then standard statistical methods such as the Wilcoxon and previously mentioned tests for proportions can be used. This is rarely the case. In most clinical trials, some or many cases are censored for the outcome of interest at the time of analysis. It is incorrect simply to omit the continuing cases or to pretend that censored times are complete. Either of these approaches leads to biased analyses. It is incorrect to report or analyze by the previously mentioned techniques (Pearson χ^2, Fisher exact, logistic regression) the percent of failures by some specified time or at analysis unless all cases have failed or have been followed at least that long. Special methods must be employed which take the censoring into account in a proper way. Survival analysis requires a specifically defined start and end of the relevant time period for each patient. We begin with a discussion of what that means and follow with a brief outline of commonly used analysis techniques for censored data and some cautions about the application and interpretation of these procedures.

The date of registration/randomization on a clinical trial is the preferred origin time for TTF and survival as the date is precisely known, the on-study data are current as of that date and the patients are as alike as possible. Some reports use the date of start of treatment, but that can induce bias if there is differential delay or drop-out after registration but before the start of treatment due to required therapy (e.g. RT preceeding chemotherapy or delaying treatment to improve alimentation only on one arm) or progressive disease. The date of documented response or date of achievement of a clinically disease-free state are the start of the "duration of response" and DFS, respectively. These dates are less precisely known as they depend on the frequency and completeness of the assessment. Response duration and DFS also are conditional measures since they are only defined among patients achieving a response or NED state.

Generally, entry on a clinical trial is staggered as patients accrue over time so that possible follow-up differs from patient to patient. The date of death is generally quite accurate. The date of censoring for survival and other time measures is a function of the frequency and diligence of follow-up. The date of progression or relapse is also somewhat "soft," depending on the frequency and completeness of assessment and also on the clinical features involved in the relapse. For example, disease in the oral cavity is quite obvious in relapse and patients may present in self-diagnosed progression while disease in the nasopharynx or neck require scans and other medical procedures to detect disease, and relapse may not be diagnosed until protocol-mandated tests have been performed.

The Kaplan–Meier or product limit estimator, first presented in a quite readable paper (21), is nonparametric method for estimating a survival function from censored data. It does not require the specification of a mathematical model for the failure-time distribution. Figure 4.1 illustrates a Kaplan–Meier curve for overall survival in a study of advanced head and neck cancer (22). Of 114 patients, 80 were dead and 34 censored (alive or lost to follow-up) at the time of analysis. The curve drops at each time point with at least one failure and has a circle at each time a case has been censored. The height of the survival function gives the probability of remaining alive at each time-point on the horizontal axis. Median survival is estimated as that time when the probability of survival is 50% (dotted line). Also estimable are the percents continuing at various fixed points, so that 5-year survival is approximately 32%.

Confidence intervals can be placed on these percents as $\hat{p} \pm z_{1-\alpha/2}sc(\hat{p})$. With censored data, the standard error is not $\sqrt{\hat{p}(1-\hat{p})/n}$ as for simple proportions, but must be calculated using Greenwood's formula (5, 6). However, an approximation to Greenwood's formula particularly useful for reading the literature is $sc(\hat{p}) = \sqrt{\hat{p}^2(1-\hat{p})/r}$, where r is the number of patients "at risk" (i.e. alive and uncensored) at time t (5).

Visual comparison of survival curves is instructive but does not provide a rigorous statistical comparison between treatments or subgroups to test hypotheses formulated a priori. The logrank test (5, 6, 16, 23) is the most commonly used technique for comparing survival curves. This is a nonparametric test; no assumptions regarding the form of the failure–time distributions are required. The test statistic is constructed by first calculating, at each time with at least one failure, the number of failures expected for each group under the null hypothesis of no effect (i. e. identical survival curves) and comparing that with the observed number failures at that time. The observed and expected counts are combined over time to provide an overall comparison. The logrank test is not a test of difference in medians or difference in proportions continuing at some specified time (e. g. 2-year DFS), but an overall test of difference between the survival curves. Focusing on one timepoint can be deceiving if that time is arbitrary, if censoring patterns differ between groups or if the choice of time resulted from visual inspection of the curves.

Other techniques for analysis and sample size calculations require distributional assumptions about survival time. The most basic is to assume that the failure rate or hazard is constant over time. This results in the exponential failure–time distribution in which the probability of continuing beyond time t is assumed to be of the form: $p_t = e^{-\lambda t}$, where λ is the hazard or failure rate. With estimates of two of the three (p_t, λ, t), the third is easily calculated. For example, RTOG study 73-03, which compared preoperative versus postoperative RT in advanced SCCHN (24), estimated 33% survival in preoperative RT patients at 4 years. If $0.33 = e^{-\lambda 4}$, then $\lambda = 0.28$ deaths per person–year of follow-up. We can estimate median survival, t_m (the time when half are surviving), by solving $0.5 = e^{-.28t_m}$, yielding

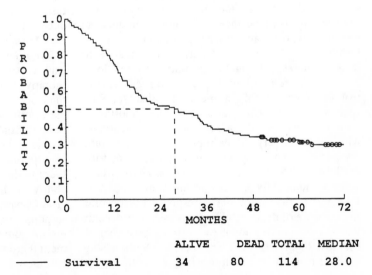

Kaplan Meier Example (80-016)

Fig. 4.1 **Kaplan–Meier curve for overall survival in a study of advanced head and neck cancer**

	ALIVE	DEAD	TOTAL	MEDIAN
—— Survival	34	80	114	28.0

$t_m = -\ln(0.5)/\lambda = 2.5$ years. This compares well with the reported 2.1 years, suggesting that modeling the survival data in this study as exponential would be quite reasonable.

There is a stratified form of the logrank test (16), but for analyses where there are many variables which have a potential association with failure time, the Cox proportional hazards model is used (5, 6, 16, 23). This is a semiparametric technique for modeling the hazard or rate of failure as a function of treatment and other prognostic factors or covariates.

Prognostic factors can be expressed dichotomously (stage III = 0; stage IV = 1), continuously (age, blood values) or with a ranked score (performance status, for example) which produces a "trend" test. However, as with logistic regression, verification of the appropriateness of the modeling assumptions, creation of the list of candidate variables, examination of interactions and colinearity, and interpretation of the results ought involve collaboration between clinician and statistician.

Study Design and Sample Size Implications

In previous sections, we have discussed statistical aspects of study design from the standpoint of broad intention, potential endpoints and their evaluation, and analysis techniques and their assumptions. A prime factor in determining the required sample size in a clinical trial is the choice of endpoint(s). We have discussed the limitations on the interpretability of some common endpoints, especially with multimodal therapy in the heterogeneous group of diseases represented by head and neck cancer. Toxicity is an important endpoint in all oncology clinical trials but, with the exception of phase I studies, very rarely is it the primary endpoint. Response may be a relevant endpoint in therapies employing combinations of chemotherapy, radiotherapy, immunotherapy, radiosensitizers, hyperthemia, retinoids, modulators of tumor hypoxia, and other tumorocidal agents. In locally advanced disease, it may be informative to distinguish response in the primary site and local control from response in the neck and regional control of disease (25). In metastatic disease, site-specific regression of metastases may be important if nonresponsive local disease is amenable to treatment with RT or surgery. Many reports in nonmetastatic disease give both response rates and rates of total eradication (NED) among those patients where surgery and/or RT were possible and were successful. DFS rather than duration of response has become the measure of the durability of remission, especially when local control involves peri- or post-chemotherapy RT or surgery. Local relapse may be distinguished from distant relapse when chemotherapy is intended to control micrometastases and/or overt disease and other modalities are targeted at local control (24). All potential endpoints considered, survival may be the only useful measure of the efficacy of complex therapy for many of these diseases.

There are many references which deal in depth with clinical trials from study design and ethics through sample size to administration and forms development (e. g. 14, 16, 26, 27, 28). In this section, we will discuss sample size with, as before, reference to the literature for computational details.

Phase II Trials

The eventual size of a phase II trial is generally modest, usually less than 50 patients. One consideration is whether to mount a single-institution trial or to take the therapy into a cooperative setting. The single-institution trial has the advantage of being more closely under the investigator's control. The patients are treated very similarly, may receive surgery or RT from very few, even only one, specialist and can be followed very closely for sequellae and even for synergistic effects (response or toxicity enhancement, for example) of subsequent salvage therapy. However, especially in a rare disease, only the largest institutions can complete prospective phase II trials of substantial size in a sensible time frame and the cooperative setting may be the most expedient vehicle. While there are more variations in and restrictions on the patient population, therapy, medical support, dose reductions, and data flow, the results from cooperative studies will be evaluable earlier and may be more representative of what will be seen when the therapy is taken into phase III testing or general practice. It is common for single-institution results to be over optimistic, the bias demonstrated in later multi-institution implementation of the same regimen (29). For example, methotrexate plus leucovorin which had produced a response rate $> 40\%$ in smaller studies, only produced a 24% response rate in EST-1373, a large ECOG randomized study (30) in SCCHN.

Another consideration is whether the focus of the trial is to ask, "is there any benefit in a new therapy"? or "is there evidence that the new is better than the old"? Studies which seek to detect or estimate efficacy are relatively straight forward to design. Studies which seek to advance to further testing an agent only if it shows compelling evidence of superiority over a standard or historic control therapy should be approached cautiously. The availability of the patient characteristics of the historic group, past definitions of and documentation of response, the precision of the estimate of the historic group's outcome, and the similarity to the experimental group are among the factors which need to be considered. The results of retrospective analyses of un- or quasi-documented treatment groups must be viewed as "soft" data as patient characteristics and outcome are generally not collected on an ongoing basis in nonprotocol settings and it is difficult to establish if there is an appropriate control population. Medical technology has changed over time affecting both staging and response coding as new techniques have supplemented and even replaced invasive surgery for documentation of disease. Even when a well documented comparable group exists from, for example, prior protocols in the same population, the sample size of the historic group needs to be sufficient that the control efficacy rates can be treated as though they are true rates, known almost without error.

Some single-arm studies are mounted because of insufficient accrual to conduct randomized studies. An example of the value of a coherent and cohesive historic datebase to conduct studies in this setting is the series of nonrandomized adjuvant chemotherapy trials for nonmetastatic osteosarcoma at DFCI/TCH (31). Sequential studies with historical controls are being used to confirm results from their prior studies and to ask additional questions which build on these results and on those of other centers. This might be a useful model to consider for studies of rare malignancies in sites such as the nasopharynx or salivary glands where the incidence is low, response and long term DFS are good, but advances in therapy are limited in part by the problems in mounting definitive randomized trials even in an intergroup setting.

When the primary objective of a phase II trial is to detect efficacy via response, a strategy employing two or more stages of accrual ought be considered (32, 33). If insufficient evidence of efficacy is observed in early accrual, that therapy is dropped and clinical and patient resources can be devoted to other promising regimens. ECOG has successfully used this strategy for years both in limited institution pilots and in group-wide phase II studies. For example, if we would be interested in testing a therapy further only if it showed evidence of a response rate of 20% or better and want a high chance of rejecting the agent if it had a true response rate of 5%, a very efficient design would be to accrue 14 patients and cease testing if there are no responses. If any respond, an additional 16 patients are added. If 3 or more responses are seen in the 30 total patients, the agent is recommended for further consideration. This strategy has a 49% chance of early stopping if the lower response rate is true, and an 93% chance of advancing the agent if the true response rate is 20%. When accrual is rapid with respect to the evaluation of response or the objective is to refine a prior estimate of efficacy, such adaptive schemes may not be appropriate and sample size is set either to obtain desired precision on the response rate estimate (i. e. to minimize the width of the confidence interval

Table 4.3 Sample size* to detect an increase from a historic control (p_0) to p_1

p_0 control	p_1 response rate wich will be detected 80% of the time				
	0.3	0.4	0.5	0.6	0.7
0.2	109	29	18	8	
0.3		135	35	15	8
0.4			150	37	16
0.5				152	37

* $\alpha = 0.05$, one-sided; $1 - \beta = 0.80$.

around $\hat{p}$) or to have high power to detect a clear improvement over standard therapy. Table 4.3 gives the sample sizes for some potential scenarios with $\alpha = 0.05$ and 80% power to detect an improvement from p_0, the historic control response probability, to p_1, the minimum response probability of interest with the experimental agent (34). Sample sizes in many single-arm head and neck studies (the article by Choksi (29) has several tables of recent phase II trials) are insufficient to detect anything but substantial increases in the response rate.

In addition to response, most phase II trials plan to evaluate DFS or survival and some have these as the primary objective. One can estimate the sample size by planning to control the width of a confidence interval on the estimated probability of continuing at some time point, $\hat{p}_t$ (2-year DFS, 5-year survival). However, as mentioned before, unless nearly all observations are complete (not censored), Greenwood's formula which accounts for censoring must be used to estimate $SE(\hat{p}_t)$. The size of $SE(\hat{p}_t)$ depends on how heavily the data are censored and, generally, if more than half the cases are censored, the estimates of $\hat{p}_t$ are very unstable (i. e. have wide confidence intervals).

In the setting where the therapy will only be advanced to further investigation if it shows evidence of improvement over a control, we can, with the assumption that survival has an exponential distribution, explicitly calculate the required sample size with knowledge of m_0, the median with standard therapy, m_1, the median with the new therapy, the desired α-level and power, and the length of the accrual period, a. Table 4.4 gives the sample sizes needed with no follow-up beyond termination of accrual to detect a 50% improvement in median survival as a function of a/m_1 (34). That is, if m_0 is 1 year, m_1 is 1.5 years, and a is 3 years, then a/m_1 is 2 and the approximate accrual is 81 cases. If these calculations are to be applied to a subset of patients, the sample size must be increased accordingly. For example, DFS can only be measured in those patients who achieve NED (i. e. gain a CR or are resectable after therapy, do not progress early or

Table 4.4 Sample size* to detect a 50% survival improvement as a function of a/m_A

a/m_A	n
1.0	134
1.5	101
2.0	81
2.5	69

* $\alpha = 0.05$, one-sided; $1 - \beta = 0.80$.

leave due to refusal or toxicity, etc.). If 30 cases are accrued based on a calculation for response estimation and 60% achieve NED, DFS will be evaluable in only 18 cases. It is clear that most phase II studies, especially those with moderately long DFS or survival, are too small and/or too short to evaluate time endpoints with any precision.

Phase III Trials

Not until a treatment has shown itself to be an improvement over current regimens will it be moved to standard clinical use. The most credible method for demonstrating increased efficacy is the randomized clinical trials. Investigators are referred to the literature (e. g. 14, 16, 26, 27) for extensive discussions on the role of the randomized trial. Those interested in current developments should consider journals as *Controlled Clinical Trials* and *Statistics in Medicine* which are aimed at both clinician and statistician.

Randomization and Stratification

As mentioned earlier, randomization is used to ensure that treatment groups will tend to be comparable with respect to known and unknown factors which may affect outcome, thus eliminating bias. However, randomization only guarantees balance "on average" and any specific trial may exhibit imbalances purely by chance. Although the chance of a major imbalance is slim, especially in a large trial, it is desireable to force treatments to be balanced with respect to factors known to be important prognostically, since being able to demonstrate comparability enhances the credibility of study results. A variety of treatment allocation procedures have been proposed to effectively guarentee such balance while retaining an element of randomization (35).

The most popular allocation method is permuted blocks within strata. In an unstratified permuted block design, each successive group or block of, say, 4 patients entering the trial is randomly allocated, 2 to treatment A and 2 to B. This ensures that the treatment totals will never be out of balance by more than a difference of 2. To carry out permuted blocks

within strata (26, 27, 36), this procedure is followed within each unique stratum defined by combinations of prognostic factor levels. By balancing treatment totals within strata, the prognostic factors will be balanced across treatment groups.

Investigations of Prognostic Factors

It is common for there to be exploratory multivariate analyses to identify predictors of outcome as a part of the evaluation of many large phase II trials and most phase III studies. It is unfortunately common for these analyses to be either not part of the initial study design and have no a priori hypotheses or to be fully retrospective and be based on data generated without standardization and collected with knowledge of the outcome data. It is also unfortunately common for investigators to perform analyses within small subsets of the patients entered and then to declare "no difference" or "no effect" on the basis of this subanalysis when the p-value is greater than 0.05. Lack of significance in these settings can be due to insufficient sample size rather than lack of relevant differences between groups. Prospective, mandatory, standardized prestudy evaluations are essential so needed data will be available on all cases and sample size ought be sufficient so definitive statements can be made about prognostic factors.

Dichotomous Endpoints in Phase III Design

In early disease and with multimodal therapy in advanced disease, achievement of a NED state may be a useful dichotomous (yes/no) endpoint which is identifiable early in a patient's course. The required sample size for a test of proportions in a randomized trial is a function of the difference in proportions we wish to be able the detect, the desired power $(1-\beta)$, and the α level and "sidedness" of the intended analyses. For a two-sided test, the total sample size for a trial with equal allocation to two treatments is approximately (15):

$$n = 2\frac{(z_{1-\alpha/2}\sqrt{2\bar{p}(1-\bar{p})} + z_{1-\beta}\sqrt{p_1(1-p_1) + p_2(1-p_2)})^2}{(p_2-p_1)^2}$$

where p_1 and p_2 are the response probabilities of the standard and experimental therapies, respectively and $\bar{p} = (p_1 - p_2)/2$. For a one-sided test, one would use $z_{1-\alpha}$ in place of $z_{1-\alpha/2}$. There are versions for power and/or sample size under unequal allocation (14, 15). Response is not likely to be the only endpoint in a trial in head and neck cancer so sequential designs with early stopping for response may not be appropriate.

Table 4.**5** gives the total sample sizes needed with equal allocation to detect response rate differences

Table 4.5 Sample size needed with equal allocation to detect response rate differences ($\alpha = 0.05$, two-sided)

p_0 control	Power	p_1 improved response rate					
		0.4	0.5	0.6	0.7	0.8	0.9
0.3	0.8	752	206	97			
	0.9	992	268	125			
0.4	0.8		815	214	97		
	0.9		1076	279	125		
0.5	0.8			815	206	90	
	0.9			1076	268	115	
0.6	0.8				752	182	76
	0.9				992	236	97

from 10–30% as a function of the control rate and power for some representative situations. Table 4.**6** adapted from Choski (29) and Clark (38), lists some recent randomized trials of induction chemotherapy for head and neck cancer with the sample sizes eventually analyzed. It is clear that the sample sizes of most were inadequate to detect even a 30% difference in response rates. Note that the sample sizes required for a two-arm randomized trial (Table 4.**5**) are not calculated by simply doubling the corresponding values for a one-arm trial with a historic control rate (Table 4.**3**). This is because the calculation for the phase II trial with a historic control is one-sided and essentially assumes that the control rate is known without error. The two-arm calculation presented in Table 4.**5** is two-sided and takes into account the fact that the control rate is subject to sampling variability. This dramatic increase in sample size is the price paid for an unbiased comparison.

Time-to-Event Endpoints in Design

In a surgical/RT adjuvant trial, time to recurrence and survival are the only measurable efficacy endpoints. In multimodal therapy with perioperative chemotherapy, neoadjuvant chemotherapy or varying combinations and sequences of modalities, response (except perhaps for parallel induction chemotherapies) and achievement of NED are interesting but not the most interpretable data. Time-to-failure among all patients, DFS (which, as has been mentioned, ought be interpreted with caution as the analysis is a nonrandomized comparison) and overall survival are the definitive measures of efficacy in almost all phase III trials in head and neck cancer and sample sizes ought be sufficient to detect relevant improvements in time to these events.

Standard sample size determinations for survival comparisons assume the distribution of survival times on each treatment is exponential. Although this assumption is rarely made when analyzing the data, the sample size formulae are simple and give good approximations. If δ is the ratio of the failure

Table 4.6 Summary of randomized trials of induction chemotherapy

Authors	No. of patients	Percent 2-year*	
	$R_x 1, R_x 2$	DFS	Survival
Stell	39, 47	–	55, 22
Head and Neck Contract	152, 291	55, 60	60, 58
Kun	40, 43	64, 59	43, 31
Schuller	76, 82	44, 30	55, 40
Toohill	33, 27	70, 70	67, 53
Martin	53, 54	42, 39	–
Carugati	38, 82	25, 33[+]	–

* Figures indicate percent DFS or survival with treatment 1, percent survival with treatment 2.

[+] 5-year DFS.

rates of two treatments, say treatment 1 and treatment 2, so $\delta = \lambda_1/\lambda_2$, then:

$$n_f = 4\frac{(z_{1-\alpha/2} + z_{1-\beta})^2}{(ln\delta)^2}$$

when n_f is the number of failures needed to detect this difference with the stated power and α level (two-sided test). λ_1/λ_2 is also the inverse of the ratio of the median survival times, thus $\lambda_1/\lambda_2 = t_{m2}/t_{m1}$. However, in most trials, not all patients are followed to failure and the total sample size needed to yield n_f at analysis is a function of the accrual rate, accrual duration, follow-up period, λ_1 and λ_2. There are tables (40, 41) and nomograms (42) to guide sample size in simple two-arm studies.

Table 4.**7** gives the total sample size and study duration needed to detect a 50% improvement in median survival for a few representative scenarios. Again, referring to Table 4.**6**, it is clear that the bulk of published randomized trials of induction chemotherapy for head and neck cancer which have been tabulated in recent review articles on the subject (29, 38) had insufficient power to detect a 50% increase in median survival (that is, an increase from 2 to 3 years or 4 to 6). In their lengthy and thoughtful discussion of the induction chemotherapy trials, Choksi et al. (29) only criticize the Toohill trial as having too few patients, suggesting for the others that the reason for lack of demonstrated efficacy was "ineffective or inadequate chemotherapy." A comparison of Tables 4.6 and 4.7 suggests that inadequate sample size decreased the interpretability and generalizability of all but one of the listed studies. The Head and Neck Contracts Program not only was planned to have adequate power to detect a 50% increase in median survival, but the investigators were also sensitive to the issue of sample size and discussed (39) the lower power of the study to detect small but clinically meaningful differences in DFS.

Trials to investigate DFS must inflate accrual to account for the percent of patients who will not become disease free. Many factors, both planned and unplanned, affect the accrual needed to maintain desired power. For instance, referring to Table 4.7, it would take 320 patients and 5.2 years to have 80% power to detect a 50% increase in median survival from 3 years with standard therapy with accrual of 100 patients per year. If there is no "standard" or the experimental regimen is expected to be more toxic, a two-sided $\alpha = 0.05$ is appropriate. This would require 380 patients (5.8 years). Or a one-sided 0.05 test may be reasonable but 90% power is more appropriate requiring 410 patients (6.1 years). Most cooperative groups now formally inflate accrual goals by 10% to account in advance for ineligible and clearly unevaluable patients. This would increase the planned sample size from 410 to 451. If the experimental regimen is complex or toxic and some patients, say 10%, will actually get the control regimen or a fraction of the experimental regimen which has efficacy similar to the control, then 557 patients (43) would be needed to preserve 90% power. If, due to the large sample size, a sequential design is planned to have a chance for early stopping if the experimental regimen is clearly more effective, the maximum sample size is inflated by approximately

another 5–10% (44, 45), although, the actual sample size may be smaller if the trial is stopped before full accrual is reached. Small randomized trials are not efficient nor informative.

Summary

This brief discussion of the design and analysis of head and neck clinical trials was not intended to be exhaustive but an introduction and review. We have categorized trials broadly by "phase" based on the nature of the endpoint(s) of interest, outlined some definitions of these endpoints, reviewed some basic principles of statistics and their applications in the analysis of clinical trials and in the evaluation of the literature, and, lastly, addressed the magnitude of sample sizes needed for credible results from prospectively designed trials. We have emphasized several issues: that standardization among related trials will improve the interpretability of the literature and help investigators plan future trials based on published data; that comparisons of DFS, while reported in much of the head and neck literature, are unbiased only in a truly adjuvant setting and that endpoints (TTF and survival) that utilize all patients avoid problems inherent in nonrandomized comparisons; and, that sample sizes in many trials have been insufficient to support the conclusions of lack of difference. Single-institution efforts and small one-arm trials are essential for the development and piloting of innovative therapies. Only large cooperative efforts (46) like the Head and Neck Contract Program (39), the Veteran's Administration Cooperative Study in Laryngeal Cancer (47) and the ongoing INTERG-0034 (48) will have the power to detect important advances in therapy.

Table 4.7 **Sample size and study duration* to detect a 50% improvement in median survival** ($\alpha = 0.05$, one-sided)

	Annual accrual			
	60		100	
m_0 Power	0.8	0.9	0.8	0.9
2	234 (5.9)	300 (7)	260 (4.6)	340 (5.4)
3	282 (6.7)	360 (8)	320 (5.2)	410 (6.1)
4	324 (7.4)	408 (8.8)	370 (5.7)	470 (6.7)

* Accrual plus 2 years additional follow-up.

References

1. Oken MM, Creech RH, Tormey DC, et al. Toxicity and response criteria of the Eastern Cooperative Oncology Group. Am J Clin Oncol. 1982; 5:649–55.
2. Common Toxicity Criteria, issued by the Cancer Therapy Evaluation Program (CTEP) on February 18, 1988. Bethesda: NCI.
3. Morgan TM. Analysis of duration of response: A problem of oncology trials. Controlled Clin Trials. 1988; 9:11–18.
4. Dixon DO, McLaughlin P, Hagemeister FB, et al. Reporting outcomes in Hodgkin's disease and lymphoma. J Clin Oncol 1987; 5:1670–2.
5. Cox DR, Oakes D. Analysis of survival data. New York: Chapman and Hall, 1984.
6. Miller RG. Survival analysis. New York: John Wiley, 1981.
7. Esche BA, Haie CM, Gerbaulet AP, Eschwege F, Richard JM, Chassagne D. Interstitial and external radiotherapy in carcinoma of the soft palate and uvula. Int J Radiat Oncol Biol Phys. 1988; 15:619–5.
8. Anderson JR, Cain KC, Gelber RD. Analysis of survival by tumor response. J Clin Oncol 1983; 1:710–19.
9. Simon R, Makuch RW. A non-parametric graphical representation of the relationship between survival and the occurrence of an event: application to responder vs non-responder bias. Stat Med 1984;3:35–44.

10. Anderson JR, Cain KC, Gelber RD, Gelman RS. Analysis and interpretation of the comparison of survival by treatment outcome variables in cancer clinical trials. Cancer Treat Rep 1985; 69:1139–46.

11. Biometrika tables for statisticians. 3rd ed. London: Biometrika, 1976.

12. Mainland D, Herrera L, Sutcliffe MI. Statistical tables for use with binomial samples. New York, 1956.

13. Harrington DP, Andersen JW. The analysis of response data in clinical trials. Oncology 1990; 4:95–106

14. Buyse ME, Staquet MJ, Sylvester RJ, eds. Cancer clinical trials, methods and practice. Oxford: Oxford University Press, 1984.

15. Fleiss JL. Statistical methods for rates and proportions. 2nd ed. New York: John Wiley, 1981.

16. Mike V, Stanley KE, eds. Statistics in medical research. New York: John Wiley, 1982.

17. Lehmann EL. Nonparametrics: statistical methods based on ranks. Oakland: Holden-Day, 1975.

18. Mantel N, Haenszel W. Statistical aspects of the analysis of data from retrospective studies of disease. J Nat Cancer Inst. 1959; 22:719–48.

19. Kleinbaum DG, Kupper LL, Morgenstern H. Epidemiologic research: principles and quantitative methods. New York: Van Nostrand Reinhold 1982.

20. Cox DR. Analysis of binary data. London: Chapman and Hall, 1970.

21. Kaplan EL, Meier P. Nonparametric estimation from incomplete observations. J Am Stat Assoc 1958; 53:457–81.

22. Clark J, Fallon B, Weischselbaum R, et al. The influence of resectability on response to induction chemotherapy and survival in advanced squamous cell carcinoma of the head and neck. Proc Am Soc Clin Oncol. 1985; 4:C-542.

23. Kalbfleisch JD, Prentice RL. The statistical analysis of failure time data. New York: John Wiley, 1980.

24. Kramer S, Gelber RD, Snow JB, et al. Combined radiation therapy and surgery in the management of advanced head and neck cancer: Final report of study 73-03 of the RTOG. Head Neck Surg 1987; 10:19–30.

25. Fallon BG, et al. Induction chemotherapy for advanced squamous cell carcinoma of the head and neck: An analysis of clinical and histopathologic correlates after a complete response to chemotherapy. In: Head and neck oncology research. Proceedings of the Second International Head and Neck Oncology Research Conference, Arlington, VA, September, 1987. Amsterdam: Kugler and Ghedini, 1988.

26. Pocock JS. Clinical trials, a practical approach. New York: John Wiley, 1983.

27. Friedman LM, Furberg CD, DeMets DL. Fundamentals of clinical Trials. 2nd ed. Littleton: PSG Publishing 1985.

28. Shapiro SH, Louis TA, eds. Clinical trials: issues and approaches. New York: Marcel Dekker, 1983.

29. Choksi AJ, Dimery IW, Kong WK. Adjuvant chemotherapy of head and neck cancer: The past, the present, and the future. Semin Oncol 1988; 15:45–59.

30. Deconti RC, Schoenfeld D. A randomized prospective comparison of intermittent methotrexate, methotrexate with leucovorin, and methotrexate combination in head and neck cancer. Cancer 1981; 48:1061–72.

31. Goorin AM, Abelson HT, Frei E III. Osteosarcoma: Fifteen years later. N Engl J Med 1985; 313:1637–43.

32. Fleming TR. One-sample multiple testing procedure for phase II clinical trials. Biometrics 1982; 38:143–51.

33. Simon R. Optimal two-stage designs for phase II clinical trials. Controlled Clin Trials 1988; 10:1–11.

34. Schoenfeld D. Statistical considerations for pilot studies. Int J Radiat Oncol Biol Phys 1980; 6:371–4.

35. Kalish LA, Begg CB. Treatment allocation methods in clinical trials: A review. Stat Med 1985; 4:129–44.

36. Zelen M. The randomization and stratification of patients to clinical trials. J Chron Dis 1974; 27:365–75.

37. Clark JR, Falloon BG, Dreyfuss AI, et al. Chemotherapeutic strategies in the multidisciplinary treatment of head and neck cancer. Semin Oncol 1988; 15:35–44.

38. Clark JR, Fallon BG, Dreyfuss AI, et al. Induction chemotherapy for advanced cancer of the head and neck. [In press in]: Head and neck cancer, vol II. Proceedings of the International Conference on Head and Neck Cancer, Boston, MA, July, 1988. Toronto: BC Dekker, CV Mosby.

39. Head and Neck Contracts Program. Adjuvant chemotherapy for advanced head and neck squamous cell carcinoma: final report of the Head and Neck Contracts Program. Cancer 1987; 60:301–11.

40. Freedman LS. Tables of the number of patients required in clinical trials using the logrank test. Stat Med 1982; 1:121–9.

41. Makuch RW, Simon RM. Sample size requirements for comparing time-to-failure among k treatment groups. J Chron Dis 1982; 35:861–7.

42. Schoenfeld DA, Richter JR. Nomograms for calculating the number of patients needed for a clinical trial with survival as an endpoint. Biometrics 1982; 38:163–70.

43. Donner A. Approaches to sample size estimation in the design of clinical trials – a review. Stat Med 1984; 3:199–214.

44. O'Brien PC, Fleming TR. A multiple testing procedure for clinical trials. Biometrics 1979; 35:549–56.

45. Peace KE, Schriver RC. p-value and power computations in multiple look trials. J Chron Dis 1987; 40:23–30.

46. Marcial VA, van den Bogaert W, Horot J. Head and neck: cancer research plan. Int J Radiat Oncol Biol Phys 1988; 14:S119–S125.

47. Department of Veterans Affairs Laryngeal Cancer Study Group. Induction chemotherapy plus radiation compared with surgery plus radiation in patients with advanced laryngeal cancer. N Engl J Med 1991; 324:1685–90.

48. Schuller D. Phase III study to determine the effect of combining chemotherapy with surgery + radiotherapy for resectable squamous cell carcinoma of the head and neck. Proceedings of the International Conference on Head and Neck Cancer, Boston, MA, July, 1988 (abstract 32).

Multimodality Therapies

5 Combined Surgery and Radiotherapy

H. T. Hoffman, C. J. Krause, F. Eschwege

Definition

Among the different strategies employed in treating head and neck cancer, "combination therapy" has been most frequently used to refer to the combined use of radiation therapy and surgery. Although combinations of other therapeutic modalities are in use which include chemotherapy and immunotherapy, the following discussion of combination therapy will be limited to radiotherapy and surgery. Additionally, we restrict our interpretation of combination therapy to those instances in which both modalities are employed in the same location to treat a tumor. With this understanding, surgical treatment of a tumor at a primary site coupled with radiotherapy to the neck would not be considered combination therapy.

Flexibility in the decision to employ combination therapy is maintained by most oncologists, who will often defer the final decision whether to use a second treatment modality until after the initial treatment is completed. When the initial treatment of a tumor is surgical, the decision to use postoperative radiotherapy may be modified by the pathologic findings in the excised specimen, such as the presence of extracapsular spread, multiple levels of nodal involvement, or evidence of aggressive biological behavior. Less commonly, a trial of preoperative irradiation may be used as the initial treatment in which the response of the tumor will determine whether surgery will follow.

Only a brief planned delay (4–8 weeks) between the two treatment modalities should be utilized to obtain the maximum benefit from combination therapy. The use of one modality to treat a recurrence after full treatment with the other should be considered salvage treatment and not combined therapy.

Historical Aspects

Early History

Clinical experience with radium in the early 1900s demonstrated its potential to not only cause tumor shrinkage, but also to cause the complete disappearance of tumor with apparent cure. The combination of surgery with radiotherapy as a planned treatment strategy logically followed with the thought that if either of two different treatments were capable of cure, perhaps the combination of those two treatments would increase the effectiveness.

Reports in the 1920s of the use of combination therapy employing preoperative radiotherapy initially showed promising results (1–3). Included among these early trials was a report published in 1929 of a large series of patients treated in Sweden for squamous cell carcinoma of the head and neck (4). This study reported that the percentage of patients with oral cancer and cervical metastases that were symptom-free after 5 years was 0% when treated with radiation alone, compared to 40% when treated with preoperative irradiation and surgery. The results of treatment with surgery alone were not reported.

The enthusiasm expressed for the use of preoperative irradiation in the 1920s waned as further experience failed to show increased survival rates when compared to the use of surgery alone and as problems with the healing of radiated tissue became apparent. As a result, in the 1930s and 1940s it became more common to employ combined therapy with radiation administerd postoperatively (5). However, long-term studies evaluating postoperative radiotherapy during this period again failed to consistently demonstrate benefit from its use. Although wound healing occurred normally in the postoperative period when radiation was administered following surgery, the use of kilovoltage irradiation available at that time still frequently caused significant morbidity from skin damage. As a result most oncologists chose to reserve radiotherapy for palliation of recurrences rather than for use in planned combination with surgery (6).

The introduction of megavoltage radiotherapy with its skin-sparing effect in the 1950s allowed for a renewed interest in the use of combined therapy for a variety of cancers (7, 6). Other recent advances in the field of radiation therapy including improvements in dosimetry, new fractionation schemes, and the use of electron beam therapy have further decreased the morbidity associated with radiotherapy. As a result, the potential for the use of irradiation as an adjuvant to surgical treatment was expanded. Although debate continues as to the indications and methods of administration of combination therapy, surgery coupled with perioperative radiotherapy has become the standard of care in most institutions in the treatment of advanced neoplasms of the head and neck.

Rationale

The basic premise behind the use of combination therapy is that the complementary effect of two treatment modalities will result in improved eradication of tumor cells. Surgery best addresses gross disease that radiotherapy cannot, and radiotherapy eradicates microscopic disease for which surgery is less effective.

It was more than four decades after its introduction into clinical use that the combination of radiotherapy and surgery was first studied in the laboratory. Among these early investigations was a study in 1960 by Agostino and Nickson who reported that treatment with 800 centigrays (cGy) before surgical resection significantly decreased the recurrence rate of cecal tumors in rats (8). Most subsequent animal studies have shown that combined modality therapy with irradiation either preceding or following surgery results in a similar decreased tumor recurrence rate when compared to the use of surgery as a single modality (9, 10). The effects of combination therapy on survival, however, have been variable and dependant to a large extent on tumor type and the animal model used (11).

Despite the large numbers of studies that have been designed to answer questions about the basic biology of radiotherapy, the mechanism whereby perioperative irradiation decreases local recurrences is not yet explained conclusively. It has been suggested that preoperative radiotherapy may exert its beneficial effect by altering the tumor bed in a manner separate from its effect on the tumor cells (11, 10). Radiation-induced obstruction of draining lymphatics is one such mechanism whereby radiotherapy may help to confine tumor cells to the primary site and resulting in less potential for tumor dissemination and regrowth (12, 13). Other theories that remain unproven include induction of an enhanced local immunity in the irradiated tissue surrounding the tumor and alteration of adjacent host tissue to make it less accepting of tumor seeding (14). Support for these theories comes from animal studies which have demonstrated that irradiation alters tissue to make it less supportive for survival of unirradiated tumor cell implants (14–16).

Although the beneficial effect of perioperative radiotherapy may be related in part to its effect on adjacent host tissue, it is generally felt that adjuvant radiation therapy exerts its primary effect by damaging the reproductive capacity of the tumor cells (11). Hoye and Smith offered support for this concept from an animal study in which irradiation was administered to a tumor in doses small enough to cause no measurable effect on tumor mass or viability (17). When these irradiated cells were implanted into unirradiated tissue, their growth was found to be decreased by 90% relative to similar unirradiated tumor cells.

Treatment Strategy

The approach to the use of combination therapy may differ between specialists and between cancer treatment centers. Dosage of irradiation, extent of surgery, and the timing of each may be influenced by the predisposition of the oncologist responsible for treatment planning. The use of combination therapy may be categorized according to the use of irradiation preoperatively, postoperatively, in a "sandwich technique," or intraoperatively.

Preoperative Radiotherapy

For theoretical reasons, radiation therapy given preoperatively offers advantages over its use postoperatively. It has been known since the early part of this century that oxygenation is a key factor in determining radiosensitivity (18, 19). Well oxygenated cells are much more susceptible to the effects of irradiation than are poorly oxygenated cells (20). It would therefore be expected that irradiation would more effectively kill malignant cells prior to surgery, before scar formation and interruption of blood supply to the tumor diminishes the cells' oxygenation (21). The malignant cells about the periphery of the tumor are generally better oxygenated than those cells at the center of the tumor, and thus are more sensitive to irradiation than is the central core. Surgical treatment conversely is well suited to remove the central bulk of hypoxic radioresistant cells (21).

It was also thought that radiotherapy would result in fewer recurrences when given before the tumor had been disturbed by surgical treatment. Several types of tumor tend to recur in healing wound edges following surgical treatment (13). In theory, irradiation administered to diminish tumor cell viability and to alter the surgical field to make it less accepting of spilled tumor cells would diminish the capacity for tumor implantation at the time of surgery (22).

Time–Dose Factors

The Dose of Irradiation

Although the protracted, fractionated method of administering irradiation was first introduced by Coutard in the 1920s, investigators continue to explore the relationship between time and the dose in treating cancer (23, 24). Single-dose preoperative radiation therapy for squamous cell carcinoma of the head and neck was used early in the twentieth century, and has been reported as recently as 1969.

Ketcham et al. at the time published results from clinical trials designed to determine optimal pre-operative radiation doses. They reported that the administration of 2000 cGy 24 hours before the excision of a primary tumor with radical neck dissection resulted in such severe surgical morbidity that the dose was decreased after treating only 3 patients. Similar complications of skin and mucosal edema, mucositis, wound separation, and complete wound breakdown developed in 3 more patients treated with 1500 cGy in a single dose preoperatively. Final adjustment of the preoperative dose to 1000 cGy allowed completion of the study in which 60 patients receiving preoperative irradiation were compared with 19 treated with surgery alone. Despite this lower dose of irradiation, a significant increase in complication rate was seen in the group treated with combined therapy. Differences between the two groups for local recurrence, metastases, and survival were not significant (25).

Powers and Ogura in 1965 reported results from animal experiments designed to help determine the optimal dose and timing of preoperative radiotherapy (11). They developed a rat tumor model employing implanted fibrosarcoma in which they found that the administration of one-third the curative dose of irradiation given immediately as a single dose preoperatively significantly increased cure rates without interfering with postoperative healing. They applied this model to clinical practice in the treatment of 30 patients with head and neck carcinoma, administering irradiation in doses ranging from 1500 to 3200 cGy fractionated over a period of from 2 to 3 weeks and completed from 9 to 16 days before surgery. They were able to demonstrate normal wound healing in the majority of patients despite the findings on excised specimens that the irradiation had been sufficient to modify the histologic characteristics of the tumors.

Oncologists at Memorial Sloan Kettering Cancer Center throughout the 1960s and into the 1970s routinely employed 2000 cGy delivered in five treatments on successive days prior to the surgical treatment of advanced head and neck cancer (26, 10). Strong and associated in Boston employed a similar treatment schedule which was chosen because of its recognized activity in reducing survival of transplanted tumor cells in animals, its minimal effect on normal tissue, and its relatively low cost (27).

Other philosophies regarding the optimal time-dose relationship for preoperative radiation therapy have been proposed. Goldman et al. stated that the largest dose of irradiation which permits healing should be used (28). They perfomed long-term studies employing 5500 cGy rads given over a 5 to 6-week period followed by surgery from 3 to 6 weeks later. These investigators noted that although this treatment regimen did increase postoperative mor-

bidity, an acceptable complication rate was obtained by using additional preventative measures such as routinely covering the carotid bulb with a levator scapulae flap. They reported that all patients eventually healed completely and that there were no deaths resulting from wound breakdown (28).

In contrast, Vandenbrouck et al. reported a high complication rate in patients with hypopharyngeal cancer following treatment with a preoperative dose of 5500 cGy (29). At this dose, 38% of the patients developed carotid hemorrhage, with an associated high operative mortality rate.

A more conservative treatment plan was employed at the University of Iowa in the 1960s, calling for the use of 4500 cGy given over 4 to 5 weeks followed by surgery 4 weeks later (30). A similar plan of 5000 cGy given over 5 weeks was adopted by oncologists at the MD Anderson Hospital (22). Fletcher and other researchers have offered evidence that this dose is sufficient to eradicate more than 90% of subclinical deposits of tumor cells in tissue that had not been operated upon (31–33). Although most centers eventually adopted a treatment plan using medium dosage (4500–5500 cGy) during the 1970s, a uniform treatment approach for preoperative radiotherapy has never been achieved.

The Timing of Surgery

Hard data in support of an optimal time to perform surgery following radiotherapy is not available. Perez and Powers demonstrated that surgery done imediately after a single dose of 1000 cGy to mice with lymphosarcoma resulted in significantly lower recurrence rates than when surgery was delayed for 1, 3, or 7 days (34). In contrast, Inch et al. demonstrated that recurrence rates following treatment of adenocarcinoma in mice with 2000 cGy were lowest when surgery was performed on the sixth postirradiation day rather than the first or the twelfth (9). Moss writes that differences between the cellular kinetics of both normal cells and cancer cells are significant enough that the optimal interval between irradiation and surgery is likely to be highly variable from one tumor type and anatomic site to another (13). As a result, information about the optimal time for surgery following radiation therapy in treatment of squamous cell carcinoma of the head and neck has been derived primarily from clinical trials.

Most oncologists feel that the best time for surgery following radiotherapy in the head and neck is as soon after completion of radiotherapy as wound healing will allow. Most investigators allow a proportionate increase in the delay before surgery as the amount of preoperative irradiation increased. In a retrospective study of a heterogeneous group of patients with head and neck cancer, Moore et al. reported the use of three different treatment

Table 5.1 **Preoperative radio-therapy time–dose schedule*** (University of Louisville School of Medicine)

Dosage	2000 cGy in 6 days	3000 cGy in 14 days	5000–6000 cGy in 5–6 weeks
Interval between completion of irridation and operation	Immediate surgery	4 weeks	6 weeks

* Schedule to determine timing of surgery following irradiation employed by Moore et al. (35).

schemes that exemplify this principle (35) (Table 5.**1**). Patients treated with 2000 cGy over 6 days received surgery immediately after completion of the irradiation. Those who received 3000 cGy over 14 days were operated upon 4 weeks later, and those who received from 5000 to 6000 cGy over 5 or 6 weeks were operated upon 6 weeks following completion of radiotherapy.

Following treatment with 5500 cGy over 5 weeks, Goldman et al. suggested waiting from 3 to 6 weeks before performing surgery (28). They state that with this dose schedule, most of the acute radiation changes will have resolved by 3 weeks and the late postradiation changes of fibrosis and obliterative endarteritis will not become important surgically until after 6 weeks have passed (36). A similar delay following radiotherapy has been used at most other institutions. It is believed that this 3 to 6 week delay in surgery is not sufficient to have a negative impact on tumor control.

A very long delay following high-dose radiation therapy has been interpreted by investigators as an alternative form of combination therapy. Buschke and Galante in 1958 reported the use of "radical preoperative roentgen therapy" in the treatment of head and neck carcinoma in which a dose of from 60 to 80 cGy was followed from 1 to 5½ months later with radical surgical treatment (37). They did note that surgery performed more than 2 or 3 months after irradiation became more difficult because of increasing fibrosis and vascular changes. Many oncologists have argued that this type of delayed operative treatment should not be considered combined therapy, but rather surgical salvage following failed irradiation. Goldman et al. point out that not only is healing impaired by the late effects of irradiation, but a new generation of tumor cells has had time to proliferate to the point that complete removal may be more difficult (36). However, the debate regarding the use of radical radiation therapy followed by surgical salvage if necessary as a planned treatment regime continues. Support for this type of treatment comes primarily from those who believe this treatment plan will preserve key structures. For instance, T3 and T4 laryngeal lesions that have been shown to have the best chance for cure with total laryngectomy may be treated with full-course radiation therapy instead. Salvage surgery will be required in most of these patients, but those who are cured with irradiation will have had their larynx preserved.

The rationale for this treatment plan is that "modern quality controlled radiation therapy is able to cure more patients" than in the past, and that "salvage surgery is also increasingly being able to compensate for some of the failures of radiation therapy" (38). Harwood et al. have utilized such a regimen in patients with T3N0 and T4N0 laryngeal cancer, with survival rates similar to those with combined therapy (39). It is not likely that patients with N+ disease would fare as well.

Flexibility in the use of combination therapy has been utilized at several institutions in which the decision whether to proceed with surgery is made after the irradiation is begun. A dose of 5000 cGy is administered in conventional fractionation as a trial to judge the radiosensitivity of a tumor. Based on the response of the tumor, a decision is made either to complete a radical course of radiation therapy or to proceed with surgical excision (40,41). This treatment plan is designed to minimize postoperative complications by selecting for those patients that will require surgery before a full radical dose of irradiations administered. Although there is laboratory evidence which correlates tumor regression with radiocurability in mice and clinical studies which correlate regression of neck metastases with an improved prognosis in humans, most clinical studies have found that it is not possible to correlate early tumor regression with radiocurability (42–46). As a result, Henk and others object to treatment plans in which the use of surgery is contingent on the response to the preoperative radiotherapy (38, 47). He writes that the term "preoperative radiotherapy" should be reserved for cases in which surgical treatment will be performed regardless of the tumors' response initial irradiation (47).

Controlled Studies

Although in recent years the trend has been changing, most published studies evaluating the effect of various treatment plans have been either retrospective in design or not well controlled. It is recognized that retrospective review and analysis of treatment results have many built-in limitations which may bias the results and lead to incorrect conclusions. Evaluation of the nature of the patients and the extent of their tumors as well as specific aspects of the treatment techniques are often quite different for the study group as compared with historical controls.

Definitive answers to questions regarding treatment methods are best obtained from prospective trials in which patients are stratified and randomized between the therapeutic regimens under investigation. Four well controlled studies that have helped to shape opinion regarding the use of preoperative radiotherapy are presented.

Strong EW, et al. (1966): Memorial Sloan–Kettering Cancer Center. Between 1960 and 1964 in a prospective study at Memorial Sloan–Kettering Cancer Center, patients were randomized to treatment with either 2000 cGy administered in five successive daily treatments to the neck prior to radical neck dissection or to radical neck dissection alone (10, 48) (Table 5.2). Although the time interval is not stated, the authors noted that surgery was performed "as soon as possible" following completion of the radiotherapy. Although there was no significant difference between the two groups with reference to complication rate, recurrence of tumor in the neck was significantly decreased in the irradiated group relative to the surgery-only group. Three-year survival rates were similar between the groups studied.

Strong MS, et al. (1978): Boston University School of Medicine. From 1967 to 1976 all patients with resectable stage II or stage III squamous cell carcinoma of the oropharynx or hypopharynx were randomized to treatment with surgery alone or with preoperative radiotherapy and surgery (27). Radiotherapy was administered to a dose of 2000 cGy over 5 consecutive days prior to surgery which was carried out "as soon as was practical," but always within 30 days of completion of the radiotherapy. Eighty-six of the patients enrolled in the study were evaluable at 3 years. Although a statistically significant increase in the incidence of distant metastases was seen in the irradiated group, there were no significant differences between surgical complications, survival, or local recurrence rates between the two groups (Table 5.3).

Terz JJ, King ER and Lawrence W (1981): City of Hope National Medical Center and Medical College of Virginia. Between 1969 and 1975, 248 patients with resectable stage II, III, and IV previously untreated squamous cell carcinoma of the oral cavity, oropharynx, and hypopharynx were entered into a trial evaluating survival and recurrence in comparing treatment with surgery with or without preoperative radiation therapy (49, 50). Preoperative radiotherapy was administered to a total dose of 1400 cGy delivered in two equal fractions 24 and 48 hours prior to surgery. Patients were randomized between the two groups studied. Complications between the two groups were similar in frequency with the exception

Table 5.**2** **Preoperative radiotherapy: effect on neck recurrence and survival*** (Memorial Sloan–Kettering Cancer Center 1960–1966)

| | No. of patients | Recurrence in the neck (12 month minimum follow-up) | | | | |
		Total	With negative nodes	With positive nodes	With nodes positive at multiple levels	Minimal 3-year survival rate
Surgery only	204	(75) 36.8%	(5/75) 6.7%	(70/129) 54.3%	(47/66) 71.4%	49.7%
Surgery with preop. XRT	144	(34) 23.6%	(0/40) 0.0%	(34/104) 33.4%	(20/54) 37.1%	46.7%

* Recurrence rates of squamous cell carcinoma in the operated neck in a prospective, randomized trial of surgery alone compared to surgery preceded by 200 cGy administered over 5 days (10).

Table 5.**3** **Preoperative radiotherapy: effect on locoregional recurrence and survival*** (Boston University School of Medicine 1967–1976)

Demonstrable metastases	No. of patients	Without disease	Locoregional recurrence	Recurrence at primary site	Recurrence in the neck	Distant
Surgery only	44	17/44 39%	18/44 41%	7/44 16%	13/44 30%	1/44 2%
Surgery with preop. XRT	42	17/42 40%	15/42 36%	4/42 10%	11/42 26%	6/42 14%

* Locoregional recurrence rates with 3-year follow-up of stage II and III squamous cell carcinoma of the oropharynx and hypopharynx in a prospective randomized trial comparing surgery alone with surgery preceded by 2000 cGy over 5 days (27).

Table 5.4 Preoperative radiotherapy: effect on locoregional recurrence and survival* (City of Hope National Medical Center and Medical College of Virginia 1969–1975)

	No. of patients	5-year disease-free survival	Locoregional recurrence (neck and/or primary site)		Demonstrable distant metas-tases	Death from second primaries
			Total	Those with histologically proven lymph nodes metas-tases		
Surgery alone	122	26%	36%	46%	8%	12%
Surgery with preoperative XRT	126	32%	22%	29%	7%	13%
		($p = 0.1$)	($p = 0.02$)	($p = 0.03$)		

* Locoregional recurrence rates of stage II, III, and IV squamous cell carcinoma of the oral cavity, oropharynx, and hypopharynx in a prospective randomized trial with 4-year follow-up comparing surgery alone with surgery preceded by 1400 cGy given in equal fractions 24 and 48 hours prior to surgery (49).

that those who received radiotherapy had a higher incidence of postoperative exposure of the mandible or mandibular prosthesis than those treated with surgery alone. Follow-up at 5 years demonstrated similar survival between the two treatment plans when calculated according to stage of disease, primary site, and lymph node status. Recurrent tumor developed more frequently in those patients who where treated with surgery alone (36%) compared to those who received preoperative radiotherapy (22%) (Table 5.4). The difference in recurrence rates was even more marked when patients with histologically positive neck nodes where compared for the surgery only group (46% recurrence rate) and the preoperative irradiation group (29% recurrence rate). The incidence of distant metastases and death from second primaries was similar in the two groups.

Hintz B, Komanduri C, et al. (1979): University of Miami. Between 1971 and 1975, 44 previously untreated patients with squamous cell carcinoma of the upper aerodigestive tract were evaluated for tumor recurrence and survival following randomization to receive treatment with surgery alone, preoperative irradiation with surgery, and irradiation alone (Table 5.5) (51). Radiation therapy was administered preoperatively to 4000 cGy over 4 weeks by external beam to the primary site and both sides of the neck. Patients treated with radiotherapy alone received additional centigrays through different techniques which included interstitial implantation of radon seeds in selected cases.

It is difficult to derive conclusions from this study because of the small numbers of patients studied and the failure to stratify them before randomization which led to an unequal distribution between site, T stage, and AJC staging among the three treatment groups. Tumor recurrence rates and patient survival were similar among the three groups tested. Postoperative complications were found to be higher in

Table 5.5 Preoperative radiotherapy: effect of locoregional recurrence and survival* (University of Miami 1971–1975)

	No. of patients	Recurrence at primary site
Surgery alone	13	8/13 61%
Surgery with preoperative XRT	14	8/14 57%
XRT alone	17	13/17 76%

* Locoregional recurrence rates of "operable" squamous cell carcinoma of the upper aerodigestive tract in a prospective randomized trial with 2-year follow-up comparing treatment with surgery alone, irridiation alone, and preoperative irradiation of 4000 cGy given over 4 weeks (51).

the group that received preoperative radiotherapy ($p = 0.07$).

Conclusions

The consensus among most oncologists is that preoperative radiotherapy is effective in reducing local and regional recurrences of squamous cell carcinoma of the head and neck. However, a corresponding increase in survival with the use of combination therapy in this manner has not been generally noted due primarily to increased mortality from distant metastases and second primaries.

Because of these findings and the acknowledged increase in surgical complications that result from operating in an irradiated field, a shift away from the use of preoperative irradiation to its use postoperatively developed in the 1970s (52, 51). It was felt by some investigators that preoperative irradiation does not deliver a sufficiently strong attack on the tumor and therefore allows microscopic seeding of viable tumor cells to develop into clinically apparent distant metastases (53). The combination of prompt surgical removal of tumor, the ability to carefully control margins with frozen section, and the larger doses of irradiation that could be given postoperatively was expected to result in both improved local control and a lower metastatic rate which would be reflected in increased survival with radiotherapy given after surgery. For these reasons, and because of the decreased risk of operative complications, combination therapy in the 1970s came to be most commonly administered as postoperative radiation therapy for carcinoma of the head and neck.

Postoperative Radiation Therapy

The advantages in using radiation therapy postoperatively are more practical than theoretical. The identification of tumor extent using both intraoperative frozen section control and postoperative pathologic assessment of the resected specimen permits a more definitive evaluation of the tumor than can be obtained through preoperative studies. This additional information serves to improve radiation treatment planning (40). Both the clinical and pathological evaluation of tumor margins are more reliable prior to the administration of radiation therapy (54). In a retrospective study of combined therapy, Eisbach and Krause found local recurrence rates to be significantly higher in patients with hypopharyngeal carcinoma treated with preoperative radiotherapy than in those treated with surgery alone (55). They interpreted these data to suggest that preoperative irradiation had impaired the ability to determine adequate resection margins despite the use of frozen section control intraoperatively (55). The technical performance of an operation is easier in tissue that has not been altered by the fibrosis, fusion of planes, and increased vascularity that characterizes recently irradiated tissue. The problems with healing which are also associated with irradiation and include increased vulnerability to infection and fistula formation are markedly diminished by administering radiotherapy after the surgery rather than before.

A practical disadvantage to the use of postoperative radiotherapy lies in the delay that recovery from surgery may cause in the administration of the irradiation. Adequate wound healing usually requires from 3 to 4 weeks before beginning irradiation, and any delay in healing may further delay the start of radiation therapy.

As was true in the evaluation of preoperative radiotherapy, most information regarding the proper dosage and timing of postoperative radiotherapy has been derived from retrospective studies.

Time–Dose Factors

It is generally held that radiotherapy given after surgery requires a larger treatment volume and a higher dose to adequately cover the operated area than if it had been administered preoperatively (40). Local dissemination of the tumor by the surgical procedure and decreased oxygenation of tumor cells from scarring and surgical interruption of the blood supply are reasons given for increasing the radiation dose and field (22).

The Dose of Irradiation

Initial reports of the use of radiotherapy postoperatively generally described unstandardized techniques applied without protocol. An early report published in 1970 listed several ways in which postoperative radiotherapy was used, including administration to isolated areas of questionable margins, treating a "generous margin of a gross recurrence," and employing comprehensive irradiation to the whole neck on one or both sides (56). A more systematic approach to the delivery of postoperative radiotherapy followed as experience with its use accumulated.

Feldman and Fletcher described the evolution of their method of postoperative radiotherapy which developed during the treatment of 81 patients from 1955 to 1976 (7). They noted that although previous studies had shown from 4500 to 5000 cGy to be sufficient to eradicate more than 90% of expected occult deposits of tumor when given to a previously unoperated area, high recurrence rates were seen when this same dosage was used in treating persistent microscopic disease following surgery. Patterns of recurrence also suggested to them that the entire surgical area, all wound extensions, and all areas of the neck should be included in the irradiated field. They increased the dose to 6500–7000 cGy locally for specific situations which included positive resection margins.

On the basis of a retrospective review of 71 patients with head and neck carcinoma of advanced stage treated with postoperative radiotherapy, Marcus et al. from the University of Florida reported in 1979 that recurrence rates were reduced with an increased dose up to 7000 cGy (33). Although they note that it may be reasonable to treat with lower doses in order to decrease the risk of complications, they routinely treated the upper neck and primary site with 6500 cGy over 7 to 1½ weeks. Oral cavity and oropharyngeal tumors resected with positive margins are treated with 7000 cGy. They indicated that smaller doses could be employed in the lower neck since none of their patients developed recurrent tumor in this region when treated with 4000 cGy or more.

A similar association between an increased postoperative dose of irradiation and increased locoreg-

Table 5.6 Postoperative radiotherapy: time–dose factors effect of dosage on local recurrence rates*
(University of Nebraska College of Medicine 1979–1985)

Postoperative radiation dose (cGy)	No. of patients	No. of local recurrences	Recurrence rate	Surgical margins		
				Negative Microscopic	Positive	Gross
4000–5000	13	4/13	30%	10/13	3/13	0/13
6000	30	6/30	20%	19/30	8/30	3/30
6600	31	3/31	10%	22/31	7/31	2/31

* Recurrence rates of squamous cell carcinoma of the upper aerodigestive tract at the primary site as a function of dosage of postoperative radiotherapy. Doses of 4000–5000 cGy were employed from 1979 to 1981; 6000–6600 cGy were employed from 1981 to 1985 (57).

ional control was reported in a retrospective study of 76 patients from the University of Nebraska in 1987 (57). Patients receiving 6600 cGy showed a higher local control rate than those receiving 6000 cGy, who, in turn, showed a higher local control rate than those treated with 4000–5000 cGy. These investigators suggest that greater local control of stage III and IV cancers of the head and neck will be obtained with higher postoperative doses (6600 cGy delivered to the surgical bed (Table 5.6).

The Timing of Radiotherapy

It is generally felt that radiation therapy is best administered as soon as possible following surgery, with limitations imposed primarily by the speed with which wound healing occurs. Early treatment following surgery allows the delivery of radiation therapy to microscopic aggregates of residual tumor cells while they are small enough to be radiocurable. Several authors have reported that postoperative irradiation is not effective if it is administered after a recurrence has become grossly detectable (58, 56). Jesse and Lindberg noted that beginning radiation therapy within 3 to 4 weeks following surgery is important to the point that the extent of a surgical procedure should be kept to a minimum so that

wound healing will occur in time to allow early application of radiotherapy (22). A significant delay in treatment results in the delivery of irradiation to a wound after the initial period of healing is completed and when the vascularity has diminished with scarring, rendering the residual tumor cells hypoxic and therefore radioresistant.

Despite these theoretical reasons to begin radiation therapy as soon postoperatively as possible, the number of clinical studies which support this principle is small. Most of the data which address this issue come from retrospective reviews of patients treated at the Memorial Sloan–Kettering Cancer Center (52, 59). The largest study to date is an uncontrolled review of 114 patients with stage III and IV squamous cell carcinoma of the head and neck who were treated with combined therapy employing from 5000 to 6000 cGy postoperatively (59). Radiation therapy was begun once healing of the surgical wounds was judged to be adequate by the operating surgeon. Recurrence of disease in the head and neck was found to occur significantly more frequently when irradiation was delayed for more than 6 weeks after the operation, than when begun within 6 weeks (Table 5.7).

These findings have prompted others to begin radiation therapy within the first 6 weeks postopera-

Table 5.7 Postoperative radiotherapy: time–dose factors effect of timing on local recurrence rate* (Memorial Sloan-Kettering Cancer Center 1975–1980)

Interval from radical neck dissection to beginning XRT	No. of patients	Total	Recurrences in the neck	
			With single-level metastases	With multiple-level metastases
Less than 6 weeks	53	(1/53) 2%	(0/10) 0%	(1/43) 3%
More than 6 weeks	41	(9/41) 22%	(3/9) 33%	(9/32) 27%

* Recurrence rates in the neck of squamous cell carcinoma of the upper aerodigestive tract as a function of time from neck dissection to institution of radiotherapy. Megavoltage external from radiation therapy was directed to the primary site and both sides in dosage ranging from 5000 to 6000 cGy to the upper neck (52).

tively, despite the presence of an unhealed wound or fistula. Isaacs et al. reported treating 13 such patients without apparent complication from the irradiation (60).

Controlled Studies

As was true in the evaluation of preoperative radiotherapy, most information regarding the results of treatment with postoperative radiotherapy has been derived from retrospective studies. Although these studies are of value in assessing patient tolerance to different treatment regimes, the impact of postoperative radiotherapy on tumor recurrence and patient survival is best evaluated by protocols that randomize patients to a study and control group. Retrospective studies of postoperative radiotherapy may be even more susceptible to the development of erroneous conclusions than when radiotherapy is used preoperatively, since patients with the worst prognosis are generally selected for combined therapy. Three studies that have evaluated the use of postoperative radiotherapy in a prospective, controlled manner are presented.

Kokal WA, Neifeld JP, et al. (1988): City of Hope National Medical Center, Duarte California and Massey Cancer Center, Medical College of Virginia. From 1981 through 1984, 51 patients with stage III or IV squamous cell carcinomas of the oral cavity, larynx, and pharynx were randomized to treatment with either surgery alone or surgery with postoperative radiation therapy (61). Patients were treated with excision of the primary tumor coupled with an ipsilateral neck dissection. In that group randomized to receive combined therapy, irradiation was begun prior to the end of the sixth postoperative week and encompassed both the primary site, the ipsilateral neck, and the contralateral neck to a dose of 5000 cGy, given over 5 to 5.5 weeks. Although 5 patients who were randomized to receive postoperative irradiation were excluded from the study either

because they refused treatment or developed contralateral tumor prior to the onset of radiotherapy, the groups were otherwise similar with regard to primary site of disease, clinical stage, and incidence of histologically proven lymph node metastases. Locoregional recurrence rates and survival rates at 3 years were similar between the two groups (Table 5.**8**). A complication rate of 37% (7 of 19 patients) directly related to radiation therapy occurred in the combined therapy group, including severe mucositis, trismus, osteoradionecrosis of the mandible, and pharyngeal stricture. Because of the high complication rate attributed to irradiation and the failure to demonstrate benefit from its use in this study, the authors conclude that the routine use of postoperative radiation therapy should be reconsidered.

Vandenbrouck C, Sancho H et al. (1977): Gustave–Roussy Institute, Villejuif, France and Henri Becquerel Center, Rouen, France. Between 1967 and 1969, 177 patients with squamous cell carcinoma of the hypopharynx were evaluated in a study which compared pre- versus post-operative radiotherapy as treatment. In this prospective study, the two groups were similar as to site of the tumor, TNM status, and patient age. Preoperative radiotherapy was administered to 5500 cGy over a 5½-week period followed by surgery 2 weeks later. Postoperative irradiation was administered over a 6-week period beginning within 4 weeks of the surgery. In both groups the surgery consisted of a total laryngectomy with partial pharyngectomy and ipsilateral radical neck dissection.

The high number of postoperative deaths in the group receiving preoperative radiotherapy was found to be significant enough early in the study that the protocol was discontinued after only 49 of a planned 260 patients were treated. In those who received preoperative radiotherapy, carotid hemorrhage contributed to the high postoperative mortality rate of 31%. Five-year survival for the entire group of patients treated with preoperative irradiation was only 14% compared to 56% for those who received

Table 5.8   Postoperative radiotherapy: effect on locoregional recurrence and survival* (Medical College of Virginia and City of Hope National Medical Center 1981–1984)

	No. of patients	Total	Recurrence		
			Locoregional	Contralateral unoperated neck out	Distant mets only
Surgery only	27	(15/27) 55.5%	(6/27) 22.2%	(4/27) 14.8%	(4/27) 14.8%
Surgery with postop XRT	19	(7/19) 36.8%	(5/19) 26.3%	(1/19) 5.3%	(1/19) 5.3%
		$p = NS$	$p = NS$	$p = NS$	$p = NS$

* Locoregional recurrence and survival rates in a prospective randomized trial comparing surgery alone and surgery with 5000 cGy administered to the head an neck of patients with squamous cell carcinoma of the oral cavity, larynx, and pharynx (61).

Table 5.9   **Postoperative radiotherapy: effect on survival and complications** * (Gustave–Roussy Institute, Villejuif, France and Henri Becquerel Center, Rouen, France 1967–1969)

	No. of patients	5-year survival (randomized)	Carotid hemorrhage	No. of patients able to complete study	5-year survival of those who were able to complete therapy
Preoperative irradiation	25	14%	5	16	36%
Postoperative irradiation	24	56%	0	23	56%

* Survival and carotid hemorrhage rates in a prospective randomized trial comparing treatment of hypopharyngeal squamous cell carcinoma with laryngectomy and ipsilateral neck dissection with 5000 cGy to the tumor bed and neck administered either preoperatively or postoperatively (29).

radiotherapy postoperatively. A significant difference was also noted between the two groups as to both complications and quality of life, that favored the postoperative group. It has been suggested that the high complication may have resulted from the short interval of 2 weeks between completion of irradiation and surgical treatment (51). Locoregional recurrence rates were not evaluated in this study.

Snow JB, Gelber RD, et al. (1981); Kramer S, Gelber RD, Snow JB, et al. (1987): Radiation Therapy Oncology Group, Nineteen participating institutions. A large multi-institution prospective, randomized study comparing pre- and post-operative radiotherapy in patients treated for advanced carcinoma of the head and neck was begun in 1973, with patient accrual terminated in 1979 (62–67). In this study, 277 patients were stratified according to sex, site of primary, and T and N category and then randomized to combined treatment with either preoperative or postoperative irradiation. Forty-two patients in the preoperative group and 41 in the postoperative group failed to complete the treatment protocol. Preoperative irradiation was administered as 5000 cGy to the primary site as well as both sides of the neck over a 5-week period, and was followed by surgery from 4 to 8 weeks later. Postoperative radiotherapy consisted of 6000 cGy to the primary site and 5000 cGy to both sides of the neck over 5 weeks with an additional 1000 cGy to residual neoplasm in the neck. The postoperative irradiation was begun as soon as wound healing allowed which was always within 4 weeks of the surgical date. An additional group of patients with oral cavity and oral pharyngeal tumors were randomized to receive treatment with radiation therapy alone. This was administered as 5000 cGy to the primary site and both sides of the neck in 5 weeks plus 1500 cGy in 1½ weeks to a coned down field using an intersititial implant.

Overall there was no statistically significant difference in survival at any site with a median follow-up of 60 months (Table 5.**10** A). There was no signifi-

Table 5.**10**   **Postoperative radiotherapy: effect on recurrence rate and survival** * (Radiation Therapy Oncology Group (RTOG 73–03) 1973–1979)

A	No. of patients	Locoregional control	Overall survival
Preoperative irradiation	136	48%	33%
Postoperative irradiation	141	65%	38%
		p = 0.04	p = 0.10

B	4-year locoregional control			
	Oral cavity	Oropharynx	Supraglottic larynx	Hypopharynx
Preoperative irradiation	40%	47%	53%	50%
Postoperative irradiation	44%	61%	77%	61%

* Locoregional recurrence rates and overall survival in a prospective randomized trial comparing treatment of advanced, operable squamous cell carcinoma of the upper aerodigestive tract with either 5000 cGy preoperatively or 6000 cGy postoperatively (62).

cant difference in complication rate between the groups treated with either pre- or post-operative radiotherapy. Although the numbers were small, no significant difference was seen in recurrence or survival between treatment of oral cavity and oral pharyngeal tumors with either combined therapy or radical irradiation. A significant difference ($p = 0.04$) in favor of postoperative radiotherapy was seen for locoregional control rates in assessing all sites combined (Table 5.**10**). This improved locoregional control with postoperative radiotherapy resulted primarily from improved control of cancer of the supraglottic larynx, which was the largest group studied (Table 5.**10** B).

Conclusions

Despite the fact that the only prospective randomized trial designed to compare tumor recurrence with postoperative radiotherapy and tumor recurrence with surgery alone (Kokal et al.) showed no significant difference, many centers today utilize postoperative combined therapy in the hope of improving survival rates (61). It is generally assumed that because preoperative radiotherapy has been shown to decrease local recurrence rates and because radiotherapy gives similar rates of local control and survival when administered either preoperatively or postoperatively, that postoperative radiotherapy should improve local control over treatment with surgery alone (40, 68).

Strong support for the use of postoperative radiotherapy comes from retrospective studies. Vikram et al. reported results of treating 114 patients with stage III or IV squamous cell carcinoma of the upper aerodigestive tract between 1975 and 1980 with postoperative radiotherapy to a dose of 5000−6000 cGy over 5 to 6 weeks. When radiation was begun within 6 weeks of surgery, 2-year follow-up showed only one neck recurrence among 53 patients treated with positive nodes in the neck. This same cohort of patients showed similarly low recurrence rate at the primary site with the use of postoperative radiotherapy as described (69). Although one should be cautious about attaching too much significance to retrospective studies, additional support for the use of irradiation postoperatively rather than preoperatively comes from a study performed at the University of Illinois in which consecutive series of patients are compared (70).

Sixty patients treated with postoperative radiotherapy between 1975 and 1979 were compared to 92 patients treated with preoperative radiotherapy between 1963 and 1974. Those patients receiving preoperative radiotherapy had been enrolled in a prospective randomized study to compare low-dose preoperative radiotherapy given as 2000 cGy over 5 days followed immediately by surgery with high-dose radiotherapy given as 5000 cGy over 5 weeks followed by surgery from 3 to 6 weeks later. The results from this treatment was compared to the postoperative radiotherapy administered as 6000−6500 cGy over 6½ to 7 weeks with contralateral neck nodes and supraclavicular areas treated to from 4500 to 5000 cGy. Although survival rates were similar among the three treatment groups, the incidence of complications following treatment with postoperative radiotherapy was significantly lower than when treatment was given with either high- or low-dose radiotherapy preoperatively. This difference in complication rate occured as a function of immediate complications which included fistula formation and wound dehiscence. The incidence of the delayed complications of esophageal stenosis, stomal stenosis, osteomyelitis of the mandible, and carotid rupture were similar between the three treatment groups (70).

As a result of these considerations, most institutions currently employ radiotherapy postoperatively when treating head and neck cancer with combined therapy. Recent reports of local control rates following combined therapy with high dose postoperative irradiation have improved to the point that Shah proposes that neck recurrence rates may fall to negligible levels if radiotherapy is begun within 6 weeks of surgery in every case (68). Although improved local–regional control is associated with improved survival in most areas of the body, the use of combined therapy in the treatment of squamous cell carcinoma of the head and neck appears to the unique in improving local control without improving survival. As a result, further modifications in the application of combination therapy as well as additional treatment modalities need to be investigated.

Intraoperative Radiotherapy

The technique of administering radiotherapy intraoperatively has recently gained interest in several centers in the United States after its introduction in Japan in the 1960s (71). A significant advantage to the use of radiation at the time of surgery includes the ability to administer large single doses of radiation directly to the area involved with tumor. The capacity to use large doses is facilitated by direct shielding of sensitive structures and movement of skin and other soft tissue structures out of the radiation field. Disadvantages to the use of intraoperative radiotherapy include the difficult logistics in administering radiotherapy to an anesthetized patient with an open wound requiring sterile technique. The coordination of effort between the surgeons, anesthesiologists, and radiation therapists is also difficult and expensive.

Despite these drawbacks, initial experience with this technique is promising. Garrett et al. in 1986 reported on the use of intraoperative doses of from 1500 to 2000 cGy to achieve a 1-year control rate of 65% in treating fixed neck disease (72). These results parallel those of conventional combination therapy, with success obtained in controlling positive or close surgical margins, but not residual gross disease. Although prospective randomized studies evaluating intraoperative radiotherapy have not yet been reported, initial successes with its use warrant further investigation.

Sandwich Therapy

Sandwich therapy refers to the administration of radiation before and after surgery (36). This treatment method permits the delivery of higher total doses of irradiation either pre- or post-operatively, and was in commonly used in Europe in the early and mid part of the 1900s.

In addition to the application of external beam irradiation by the external technique, methods of using sandwich therapy employing interstitial radiation therapy are possible (73). External radiation may be used to precede surgical excision at which time radioactive implants may be placed to increase the local delivery to the region of the tumor bed. Although the use of implants has recently regained popularity in the case of patients who are known to have residual disease following surgery, its use as a planned treatment in combination with preoperative irradiation is still not common today. The application of external irradiation by the "sandwich" technique may find benefit in special cases in which tissue tolerance for postoperative radiation is diminished by the surgical procedure. Gastric mucosa and small intestine have a reduced tolerance to radiation relative to other tissue normally present in the head and neck. Reconstruction of hypopharyngeal defects with gastric pull-ups or jejeunum-free flaps limits the amount of postoperative radiotherapy that may be delivered. Doses of irradiation to this tissue in excess of 5000 cGy are frequently associated with the complications of ulceration, stricture, and perforation (47). The administration of preoperative radiotherapy followed by a reduced dose of postoperative therapy may find some benefit in situations such as these.

A trial of sandwich therapy in an attempt to decrease the reported high incidence of stomal recurrence rate of 17% following emergency tracheostomy for airway obstruction due to laryngeal cancer was reported from the University of Cincinnatti in 1988 (74). These researchers treated 18 patients with laryngeal cancer with 2000 cGy in five fractions after emergency tracheostomy and performed a laryngectomy within 24 to 48 hours of completing radiotherapy. Although they demonstrated a stomal recurrence rate of 11%, an unac-

ceptably high local recurrence rate of 56% outside the stoma was noted despite the use of postoperative radiotherapy in 16 of these patients. They concluded that the short course of preoperative radiotherapy restricted the dose of postoperative radiotherapy that could be given, and that a moderate-to-high dose postoperative radiation should be adequate prophylaxis against stomal recurrence.

It is generally held that full treatment with either pre- or post-operative radiotherapy is preferable to partial treatment with both. As a result the sandwich technique of applying radiotherapy has not found general use.

Indications for Combined Therapy in the Treatment of Squamous Cell Carcinoma

Is Combined Therapy Worthwhile?

Despite over 30 years of experience in dual modality treatment of head and neck cancer, the reason for using combined therapy in the treatment of advanced disease has not changed—in a large number of cases, single modality therapy fails to control the disease. The question still remains: is combination therapy better than single modality therapy?

Most authors today recognize that local recurrence rates in the treatment of head and neck cancer are decreased when radiotherapy is added to the surgical treatment of higher staged squamous cell carcinomas. Although there are differences of opinion, it is generally recognized that 5-year survival is not increased when radiation therapy is used to supplement primary surgery at most sites in the head and neck.

A debate ensues as to whether it is worthwhile to treat with a second modality if all that is accomplished is to change the case of death from locoregional recurrence to either distant metastases or the development of a second primary (75). DeSanto et al. point out that changing the cause of death without improving survival may not be sufficient justification to employ radiotherapy, which may introduce its own morbidity (54, 76). Immune suppression from radiation exposure may adversely affect treated patients. Dental disease, muscositis, xerostomia, as well as osteoradionecrosis and chondroradionecrosis are well recognized complications of radiotherapy to the head and neck. Additionally, radiation is a carcinogen that may affect growth centers when administered to younger patients. The additional cost of radiotherapy is another argument for using it with reserve.

Despite these arguments against supplementing surgical treatment with radiotherapy, the prevailing opinion among head and neck oncologists today is that the coupling of radiotherapy with surgery is worthwhile even if a decrease in locoregional recurrence is the only objective. Most oncologists feel that death from local recurrence is worse than that from distant metastases and, when local disease is controlled, the quality of life is improved (6, 75). Despite this general consensus, differences still exist among oncologists as to what characteristics of a tumor predict that an increased chance of local control can be realized by adding a second treatment modality.

Indications for Use of Combined Therapy

When megavoltage first became available in the 1950s, it was initially used postoperatively to treat either disease known to be present at a margin of resection or a gross recurrence (56). Initial success in treating patients with positive margins stimulated its use in other situations known to be associated with a high recurrence rate such as the findings on histopathology of close margins or perineural involvemnt. Later, in the 1960s when it became apparent that there was a correlation between the presence of metastatic tumor in the neck dissection specimen and subsequent recurrence in the neck, postoperative radiotherapy came to be used commonly based on the pathologists report of disease in the neck specimen (7).

Snow et al. found the histologic characteristics of metastases to neck nodes to be far more meaningful than the preoperative clinical evaluation in predicting prognosis (77, 78). A recurrence rate of 21% in the neck was determined in a study of 327 patients who were treated with a radical neck dissection with histologic evidence of lymph node metastases. Preoperative clinical evaluation was found to have prognostic significance only if lymph node fixation was noted. In contrast, the histologic parameters of extranodal spread, increasing number of lymph nodes with metastasis, and assignment of a poorly differentiated grade were all indicators of a high risk of tumor recurrence in the neck (78). Characteristics of a tumor metastatic to the neck that indicate a high likelihood of recurrence following surgery are used to help determine the need for postoperative radiotherapy. Most cancer treatment centers today will employ postoperative irradiation if the neck disease shows extracapsular spread of tumor in cervical lymph nodes, multiple metastatic lymph nodes, or extension of tumor into the soft tissues of the neck (34, 79, 76).

Characteristics of a tumor at a primary site that indicate either a high chance of local recurrence or regional metastasis will also prompt the addition of postoperative radiotherapy. Most tumors staged as T3 or T4 are treated with combined therapy (80). Depending on the histopathologic assessment of the resection confirming the extent of the tumor, postoperative radiotherapy may then either be held or

implemented. Vascular or nerve invasion are other indicators that some oncologists use to identify an aggressive tumor that should be treated with adjuvant radiotherapy (68). The finding of bone invasion or an endophytic rather than exophytic appearance are additional aggressive characteristics of a tumor that may prompt the use of postoperative radiotherapy (68).

In the 1960s the most common reason for treating with postoperative radiotherapy was incomplete excision of a tumor as indicated either by the postoperative finding of positive microscopic margins or the intraoperative observation that gross tumor was left behind. Although the concept central to the use of combined therapy is that tumor not eradicated by sugery may be eradicated by adjuvant radiotherapy, gross residual tumor has been found to respond poorly to postoperative irradiation. Reexcision to obtain a margin of normal tissue about the tumor offers the best chance for cure in the treatment of incompletely excised tumors. If gross residual tumor remains after surgery that cannot be comletely excised because of its involvement of vital structures; postoperative radiotherapy to treat macroscopic residual tumor must be considered palliative rather than curative.

The concept underlying the use of postoperative radiotherapy is that this second treatment modality will eradicate subclinical disease left behind after surgery in a significant number of cases. As a result, the primary indication for the addition of postoperative radiotherapy occurs when there is thought to be a significant risk of subclinical disease remaining after surgery. The indications for using combined therapy that are listed above are merely characteristics of tumors that have been statistically associated with a high incidence of recurrence following surgery. The use of irradiation as the sole modality to treat residual microscopic tumor as indicated by positive margins is controversial and will be discussed in the next section.

Controversial Areas

Tumor at Resection Margins

Controversy exists not only in how to best use the skills of the pathologist to assess tumor involvement of surgical margins, but also how to deal with positive margins.

Evaluation of Tumor Margins

Frozen section evaluation of surgical margins is relied upon by many surgeons to assess the adequacy of tumor excision intraoperatively. Although some surgeons permit the pathologist to sample tissue from the excised specimen intraoperatively, it is our preference to sample tissue from the patient for frozen section assessment after the tumor has been excised with a margin that is considered adequate by gross evaluation. By either of these techniques, the report of a positive margin will indicate to the surgeon either that the tumor is unresectable or that more tissue needs to be removed in order to adequately excise the tumor. Negative margins obtained intraoperatively are used by many surgeons as an indicator that the tumor has been adequately excised. With this information, the procedure may be terminated or a reconstructive procedure may be undertaken with an improved chance that it is being performed on a patient free of tumor.

Unfortunately, the intraoperative evaluation of resection margins is far from perfect. The recurrence rates reported following surgical excision with margins considered to be adequate by histopathologic assessment varies according to the tumor type, tumor location, and treatment administered (81). Looser reported that of 62 patients with head and neck cancer excised with positive margins, 44 recurred (71%) compared to 1713 tumors excised with negative margins, of which 31.7% recurred (82). The application of Moh's technique to ensure the adequacy of resection of mucosal malignancies of the head and neck offers an interesting method to improve upon this high rate of recurrence but may add significantly more time to procedures that are usually already lengthy (83–86).

Although we employ intraoperative frozen section control to evaluate resection margins for the excision of most mucosal tumors, occasionally the report of a positive margin is obtained several days postoperatively when a review of the permanent slides alters the interpretation of a margin determined to be negative intraoperatively. Additionally, the report of tumor involving bone adjacent to a margin may be delayed to a week or more after the surgery because of the time required in the decalcification of bone to allow its histopathologic assessment. The finding of positive margins postoperatively is even more common among surgeons who do not employ intraoperative frozen section evaluation of resection margins and rely on evaluation of the adequacy of the resection from review of permanent section slides obtained from the resected specimen. It is in these cases in which there is a strong indication that tumor persists in the surgical wound that debate ensues as to the value of postoperative radiation therapy versus reoperating to excise the residual tumor.

Although the development of a second primary tumor may present as a recurrence, the location and timing of tumor recurrences most commonly implicates that subclinical disease has been left behind following surgical resection (87, 88). It is therefore likely that the finding of a positive resection margin, in many cases, merely reflects a greater amount of residual subclinical tumor than persists following an apparently complete excision that recurs.

Treatment of Positive Tumor Margins

There is strong support from clinical studies indicating that gross disease persisting after surgery is not adequately treated by radiotherapy alone. There is also support from both laboratory animal studies and clinical data that postoperative radiotherapy may successfully prevent the local recurrence of subclinical tumor residual. Controversy exists regarding the capacity of radiotherapy to adquately treat residual disease that lies in between these two extremes: not grossly apparent, but sufficiently large to be recognized as a positive margin histologically.

A frequently cited article in support of the use of irradiation to treat incompletely resected tumors was published by Fletcher and Evers in 1970 (56). Of 19 patients who received radiotherapy because the surgical specimen did not reveal an adequate margin, 8 patients (40%) showed no evidence of recurrence. To assume that these 8 patients would have developed tumor recurrences without radiotherapy is not correct. A study by Bauer, Lesinski and Ogura published in 1975 which examined laryngeal specimens after hemilaryngectomy discovered 39 patients with positive margins defined as close, grossly involved or with intraepithelial microscopic invasion (82). Despite the fact that none of these patients received further treatment, only 7 (18%) recurrences developed. A similar study reported by Lee in 1973 noted that a local recurrence developed in only 27 of 54 patients (50%) without further treatment who were noted to have positive margins following resection of tumors from the oral cavity, oropharynx, hypopharynx, and larynx. A third study examining recurrence rates following surgical treatment with positive microscopic margins was reported by Looser et al. in 1978 (82). These investigators noted a 32% local recurrence rate when the margins were free of tumor that compared to a 71% local recurrence rate following excision characterized either by tumor within 0.5 cm of the margin, atypia and premalignant change at the margin, or in situ carcinoma at the margin. It is clear from these studies that, just as the microscopic finding that the resection margins are free of tumor does not guarantee against recurrence, the report of a positive margin following tumor resection does not mean that tumor recurrence will occur without further treatment.

Lee evaluated patients with head and neck tumors excised with positive margins who were subsequently treated with reexcision, radiation therapy or observation (81). Although the three groups were not comparable as to tumor stage, a 5-year determinate survival was noted of 100% for those treated with reexcision, 43% for those who received radiotherapy, and 28% for those who received no treatment. He concluded that where possible, reexcision should be attempted following the report of a positive margin.

Sadeghi et al. from a retrospective study of patients treated from 1956 to 1980 at UCLA and from 1974 to 1980 at Emory University offered more insight into the value of postoperative radiotherapy in the treatment of positive margins (89). They reported results of treatment of 104 patients with squamous cell carcinoma of the upper aerodigestive tract found to have positive margins following resection. Positive margins were identified by extension of cancer to within 0.5 cm of a margin with either carcinoma in situ or dysplasia. Based on the predisposition of the involved oncologist, the positive margins were either not treated or treated postoperatively with radiation ranging from 5000 to 6500 cGy. Despite the fact that the postoperative radiotherapy group was comprised of more patients with positive nodes (83% vs. 17%), T3 and T4 primary tumors (79% vs. 21%), and poorly differentiated carcinoma (76% vs. 33%), the 2-year NED survival rate was higher in those who received postoperative irradiation than in those who received no further treatment.

It is our practice to reoperate to excise additional tissue when radiologic assessment indicates microscopic residual tumor at the resection margin. If excessive morbidity would be introduced by reoperating, treatment with radiotherapy alone may be considered as a less effective, but potentially beneficial, adjunctive measure.

Can Use of Irradiation Alter the Surgical Plan?

Conversion of Unresectable to Resectable

An established principle of head and neck cancer surgery is that a planned surgical excision should not be diminished despite apparent tumor regression resulting from preoperative irradiation. This treatment philosophy derives from clinical experience which has shown that identification of tumor extension is unreliable by gross evaluation in tissue altered by irradiation (53, 90). As a result, it is important to record tumor size and location prior to treatment in order to direct the surgical excision appropriately. In addition to hand-drawn diagrams of the tumor, photographs, videorecordings, and radiographic studies may be used to record the extent of the tumor. Margins about mucosal lesions may also be recorded prior to irradiation by tattooing about the periphery of the tumor with India ink (91).

Histologic studies of tumor specimens resected following preoperative radiotherapy have also demonstrated that resection margins should not be diminished despite response to radiotherapy (28, 36, 46). Goldman et al. evaluated excised laryngeal specimens following combined therapy with preoperative radiotherapy and total laryngectomy (92). Thin coronal sectioning allowed close histologic inspection which showed that although a small percentage of larynges had no identifiable tumor cells, the majority of specimens contained small noncontiguous nests of tumor cells randomly distributed throughout the original tumor bed (46). These findings led the authors to conclude that irradiation does not cause a centripetal regression or tumor and therefore, "surgery can never be reduced in its extent" despite the use of preoperative irradiation (46).

Despite these findings, when complete surgical excision of a lesion is not possible, some current investigators suggest a trial of preoperative radiotherapy to "shrink" the tumor to change it from unresectable to resectable (40, 93, 94). Most investigators note that this treatment plan should be employed when there are no alternative options and with the knowledge that there is a high likelihood that either local recurrence or distant metastases will occur following treatment of tumors of this type (95–97).

The limits that define a tumor as unresectable vary from institution to institution but in general terms refer to involvement of a structure that the surgeon is unwilling to sacrifice. Involvement of the base of skull, vertebral artery, common carotid artery, internal carotid artery or deep musculature and spine are limits often used to define a tumor as unresectable (93, 96). Because of the dismal prognosis following traditional combined therapy of these lesions with external beam radiotherapy, new techniques such as intraoperative irradiation and brachytherapy with iodine-125 implant in the area of residual tumor are under investigation (98–101).

Organ Preservation

Although the use of surgery to treat recurrences following attempted cure with radiotherapy is a distortion of the classic interpretation of combination therapy, this treatment strategy is used by many oncologists and deserves further mention. This approach to advanced head and neck cancer is primarily used in place of planned combined therapy in an attempt to spare the patient loss of an important organ such as the base of tongue, palate, or larynx (88, 91, 103–104). Although most head and neck surgeons would agree that local recurrence rates and survival are improved when surgery is a part of the treatment plan for advanced head and neck cancers, the morbidity from resection of an important structure may be sufficient to justify use of a less successful but less invasive treatment such as irradiation alone. In these instances, a simple evaluation of recurrence rates and survival can not be used as the only consideration in determining treatment. It should be emphasized that irradiation does introduce its own morbidity which, depending on the dose and location, may be more extensive than that of radical surgery performed with a successful reconstruction (105–109).

When the patient is competent to make decisions, a partnership should exist between himself and the physician in which treatment is offered and accepted or rejected based on a discussion of alternative therapies. It is no longer reasonable to assume that the best and only treatment method is the one most likely to prolong the patients life (110). The difficult task—to maximize the patient's well being—must entail not only attention to the "quantity of life," but also the "quality of life" (111).

An ethical dilemma of this type develops frequently in therapeutic decision making for patients with advanced laryngeal and oropharyngeal tumors. Jesse and Sugarbaker in 1976 described a treatment plan whereby T3 lesions of the oropharynx were treated with a curative dose of irradiation, reserving resection for those in whom residual or recurrent cancer became manifest (88).

Consideration of the disability created by large surgical resections in the oropharynx and oral cavity and the lack of data demonstrating a clear advantage to the use of systematic combined therapy prompted the use of this treatment plan by these investigators and by others (104). Additional experience in the treatment of oral cavity and oropharyngeal lesions has failed to definitively clarify this issue. Kramer et al. in 1987 reported similar survival rates and complication rates among 129 patients randomized to two groups which received combined therapy with either pre- or post-operative radiotherapy and another group treated with definitive irradiation and surgical salvage (62). Although they did note improved locoregional control with surgery as part of the planned combined treatment, they acknowledged that the number of patients entered in the trial was not large enough to show significance differences between the three treatment groups.

Another hotly debated topic is the the treatment of T3 and T4 laryngeal carcinomas (38, 41). Harwood et al. at the University of Toronto have supported the use of primary irradiation with surgical salvage for many years for T3N0 and T4N0 laryngeal carcinomas (111, 112). This treatment policy evolved from the discovery that there was no difference in survival between patients with T3 or T4 tumors who were treated with high-dose preoperative irradiation whether surgery was performed electively from 6 to 8 weeks later, or performed later as salvage surgery (113, 114). Harwood et al. stress that salvage surgery is an essential part of this treatment plan because control rates following irradiation alone are inferior to surgery alone. They relate that overall control rates are similar between surgery alone and primary irradiation with surgical salvage when two-thirds of the irradiation failures are salvaged surgically (103).

DeSanto takes issue with this approach for advanced laryngeal cancers and stresses that "life is more important than a larynx and the first treatment should be the one most likely to get the patient well" (115). In dissecting Harwood's data and evaluating his own, DeSanto relates that significantly greater number of cures result from treatment of advanced laryngeal carcinomas with surgery as the primary modality than when it is reserved for salvage with irradiation as the initial treatment (103, 122, 114–116). With the primary radiation and surgical salvage approach, he presents the argument that some patients must die in order that others may preserve their larynx.

Although differences in surgical and irradiation techniques as well as regional differences in patient populations may explain the conflicting results seen by these two investigators, the standard of care at most locations today is to treat most advanced laryngeal cancers (T3 and T4) with total laryngectomy, reserving postoperative irradiation following pathologic evaluation of the surgical specimen. It should be reemphasized that this approach is individualized with the patient as an active participant in the decision-making process.

Interesting data from protocols designed to preserve the larynx that employ chemotherapy prior to irradiation are emerging that indicate potential benefit from this approach (117).

Until methods are developed that guarantee the cure of head and neck cancer, diversity will persist among treatment plans. Continued critical reappraisal of these treatment plans is necessary to improve patient care. Failure to significantly improve upon survival statistics over the past three decades has made it apparent that new methods are needed in the treatment of advanced head and neck cancer (118, 119). It is important that these methods be introduced in a systematic fashion that permits an unbiased appreciation of their value relative to traditional treatment.

References

1. Bowing HH, Fricke RE. Preoperative radium treatment of rectal carincoma. Am J Roentgenol 1935; 34:766–9.
2. May EA. Surgical and roentgen treatment of carcinoma of the rectum. Am J Roentgenol 1924; 11:246–51.
3. Westermark N. The result of the combined surgical and radiological treatment of cancer mammae at Radium Hemmet 1921–1923. Acta Radiol vol. XI fasc 1. 1930; 30:IV(59):1–30.
4. Forssell, G. Radiotherapy of malignant tumors in Sweden. Br J Radiol, 1930; 3:198–234.
5. Fletcher GH. The evolution of the basic concepts underlying the practice of radiotherapy from 1949 to 1977. Radiology 1978; 127:3–19.

6. Fletcher GH. Combination of irradiation and surgery. In: Fletcher G, ed. Textbook of radiotherapy 3rd ed. Philadelphia: Lea and Febiger; 1980:219−24.

7. Feldman M, Fletcher GH. Analysis of the parameters relating to failures above the clavicles in patients treated by postoperative irradiation for squamous cell carcinomas of the oral cavity or oropharynx. Int J Radiat. Oncol Biol Phys 1982; 8:27−30.

8. Agostino D, Nickson J. Properative X-ray therapy in a simulated colon carcinoma in the rat. Radiology 1960; 74:816−19.

9. Inch WR, McCredie JA. Effect of a small dose of X-radiation on local recurrence of tumors in rats and mice. Cancer 1963; 16:595−8.

10. Strong EW, Henschke WK, Nickson JJ, Frazell EL, Tollefsen R, and Hilaris BS. Preoperative X-ray therapy as an adjunct to radical neck dissection. Cancer 1966; 19:1509−16.

11. Powers WE, Ogura JH. Preperative irradiation in head and neck cancer surgery. Arch Otolaryngol 1965; 81:153−60.

12. Rolander TL, Everts EC, Shumrick DA. Carcinoma of the tonsil: A planned combined therapy approach. Laryngoscope 1971; 81:1199−207.

13. Moss WT, Brand WN, Battifora H. Combinations of radiotherapy and surgery. In: Moss, et al., eds. Radiation oncology rationale. St Louis: CV Mosby, 1979:37−51.

14. Hewitt HB, Blake ER. The growth of transplanted murien tumors in pre-irradiated sites. Br J Cancer. 1968; 22:808−24.

15. Vermund et al. Effects or roentgen irradiation on the tumor bed. Radiat Res 1956; 5:354−64.

16. Sumners WC, et al. X-irradiation of the tumor bed. Radiology 1964; 82:691−703.

17. Hoye RC, Smith RR. The effectiveness of small amounts of preoperative irradiation in preventing the growth of tumor cells disseminated at surgery. Cancer 1961; 14:284−95.

18. Read J. The effect of ionizing radiants on the broad bean root. Br J Radiol 1952; 25:89.

19. Sapareto SA. The radiobiology of head and neck cancer. In: Jacobs JR, et al., eds. Head and neck cancer: scientific perspectives in management and strategies for cure. New York: Elsevier, 1987:248−66.

20. Fletcher GH. Clinical dose−response curves of human malignant epithelial tumors. Br J Radiol 1973; 46:1−12.

21. Brady LW, Davis LW. Treatment of head and neck cancer by radiation therapy. Semin Oncol 15(1). From Department of Radiation Oncology and Nuclear Medicine, Hahnemann University, Philadelphia and Department of Radiation Therapy, Albert Einstein College of Medicine, Bronx, New York, February, 1988:29−38.

22. Jesse RH, Lindberg RD. The efficacy of combining radiation therapy with a surgical procedure in patients with cervical metastasis from squamous cancer of the oropharynx and hypopharynx. Cancer 1975; 35:1163−66.

23. Clifford P. Combined modality therapy in head and neck cancer. In: Chambers RG, et al., eds. Cancer of the head and neck—Proceedings of an International Symposium, Montreux, Switzerland, April 2−4, 1975. Amsterdam, Oxford: Excerpta Medica; New York: Elsevier, 67−72.

24. Coutard H. Roentgen therapy of epitheliomas of the tonsillar region, hypopharynx and larynx from 1920 to 1926. Am J Roentgenol 1932; 28:313.

25. Ketcham AS, Hoye RC, Chretien PB, Brace KC. Irradiation twenty-four hours preopertively. Am J Surg 1969; 118:691−97.

26. Henschke U, et al. Value of preoperative X-ray therapy as an adjunct to radical neck dissection. Radiology 1966; 86:450−3.

27. Strong MS, Vaughan CW, et al. A randomized trial of preoperative radiotherapy in cancer of the orpharynx and hypopharynx. Am J Surg 1978; 136:494−500.

28. Goldman J, et al. High dosage pre-operative radiation and surgery from carcinoma of the larynx and laryngopharynx—a 14 year program. Laryngoscope 1972; 5:1869−82.

29. Vanderbrouck C, Sancho H, LeFur R, Richard JM, Cachin Y. Results of a randomized clinical trial of preoperative irradiation versus postoperative in treatment of tumors of the hypopharynx. Cancer 1977; 39:1445−9.

30. Smits RG, Krause CJ, McCabe BF. Complications associated with combined therapy of oral and pharyngeal neoplasms. Ann Otol, 1972; 81:496−500.

31. Fletcher G. Elective irradiation of subclinical disease in cancers of the head and neck. Cancer 1972; 29:1450−4.

32. Committee for Radiation Oncology Studies. Control of local and regional subclinical disease by radiation therapy. Cancer 1976; 37:2123−8.

33. Marcus RB, Million RR, Cassissi NJ. Postoperative irradiation for squamous cell carcincomas of the head and neck: Analysis of time−dose factors related tocontrol above the clavicles. Int J Radiat Oncol Biol Phys 1979; 5:1943−9.

34. Perez CA, Powers WE. Studies on optimal dose of preoperative irradiation and time for surgery in the cure of a mouse lymphosarcoma. Radiology 1967; 89:116−22.

35. Moore C, Mullins F, Scott RM. Preoperative irradiation in cancer of the head and neck. Am J Surg 1972; 24:555−8.

36. Goldman JF, et al. Combined radiation and surgical therapy for cancer of the larynx and laryngopharynx—II Laryngoscope 1964; 74:1111−34.

37. Buschke F, Galante M. Radical preoperative roentgen therapy in primarily inoperable advanced cancers of the head and neck. Radiology 1959; 73:845−8.

38. Karim ABMF, Kralendonk JH, et al. Radiation therapy for advanced (T3T4N0−N3M0) laryngeal carcinoma: the need for a change of strategy: a radiotherapeutic viewpoint. Int J Radiat Oncol Biol Phys 1987; 13:1625−33.

39. Harwood AR, Hawkins NV, et al. Management of advanced glottic cancer. Int J Radat Oncol Biol Phys 1979; 5:899−904.

40. Million RR, Cassisi NJ. General priciples for treatment of cancers in the head and neck: combining surgery and radiation therapy. In: Million RR, Cassisi NJ, eds. Management of head and neck cancer: a multidisciplinary approach. Philadelphia: JB Lippincott, 1984:91−5.

41. Terhaard CHJ, Wiggenraad RG, Hordijk GR, Ravasz LA. Regression after 50 cGy as a secletion for therapy in advanced laryngeal cancer. Int J Radiat Oncol Biol Phys 1988; 15:591−7.

42. Karim ABMF, Snow GB, et al. Dose−response in radiotherapy for glottic carcinomna. Cancer 1978; 5:1728−32.

43. Suit HD. Predictors in radiation response. In: Karcher KH, Kogelnik HD, Szepesi T, eds. Progress in radio-oncology III. New York: Raven Press, 1987:5−13.

44. Parsons JT. Time, dose, volume relationship in radiation therapy. In: Million RR, Cassisi NJ, eds. Management of head and neck cancer: a multidisciplinary approach. Philadelphia: JB Lippincott, 1984:137−72.

45. Mantyla M, Kertekangas AE, Valevaava RA, Nordman EM. Tumor regression during radiation treatment as a guide to prognosis. Br J Radiol 1979; 652:972−7.

46. Goldman JL. High dosage preoperative radiation and surgery for carcinoma of the larynx and laryngopharynx. Ann Otol 1972; 81:488−95.

47. Henk JM. Biological basis of pre- and postoperative radiotherapy. In: Bloom, et al., eds. Head and neck oncology. New York: Raven Press, 1986:447−50.

48. Strong EW. Preoperative radiation and radical neck dissection. Surg Clin North Am 1979; 43:271−6.

49. Terz JJ, King ER, Lawrence W. Preoperative irradiation for head and neck cancer: Results of a prospective study. Surgery 1981; 4:449−53.

50. Lawrence W, Terz JJ, Rogers C, King RE, Wolf JS, King ER. Preoperative irradiation for head and neck cancer: A prospective study. Cancer 1974; 33:318−23.

51. Hintz B, Komanduri C, Chandler JR, Sudarsanam A, Garciga C. Randomized study of control for the primary tumor and survival using preoperative radiation, radiation alone, or surgery alone in head and neck carcinomas. J Surg Oncol 1979; 12(I):75−85.

52. Vikram B, Strong EW, Shah J, Spiro RH. Elective postoperative radiation therapy in stages III and IV epidermoid carcinoma of the head and neck. Am J Surg 1980; 140:580−4.

53. Schuller DE, et al. Symposium: Adjuvant cancer therapy of head and neck tumors: increased survival with surgery alone vs. combined therapy. Laryngoscope 1979; 89:582−94.

54. DeSanto LW, Holt JJ, Beahrs OH, O'Fallon WM. Neck dissection: Is it worthwhile? Laryngoscope 1982; 92:502−9.

55. Eisbach KJ, Krause CJ. Carcinoma of the pyriform sinus: a comparison of treatment modalities. Laryngoscope 1977; 87:1904−10.

56. Fletcher, GH, Evers WT. Radiotherapeutic management of surgical recurrences and postoperative residuals in tumors of the head and neck. Radiology 1970; 95:185−8.

57. Kumar PP, Good RR, Epstein BE. Relationship of dose to local control in advanced stage III and IV head and neck cancer treated by surgery and postoperative radiotherapy. Am J Clin Oncol 1987; 10(3):240−2.

58. Lindberg RD, Jesse RH, Fletcher GH. Radiotherapy—Before or after surgery? In: Neoplasia of the head and neck. Chicago: Chicago Year Book Medical Publishers, 1974:46−58.

59. Vikram B, Strong EW, Shah JP, Spiro R. Failure in the neck following multimodality treatment for advanced head and neck cancer. Head Neck Surg 1984; 6:724−9.

60. Isaacs JH, Thompson WB, Cassisi NJ, Million R. Postoperative radiation of open head and neck wounds. Laryngoscope 1987; 97:267−70.

61. Kokal WA, Neifeld JP, Eisert D, et al. Postoperative radiation as adjuvant treatment for carcinoma of the oral cavity, larynx and pharynx: Preliminary report of a prospective randomized trial. J Surg Oncol 1988; 38:71−6.

62. Kramer S, Gelber RD, Snow JB, et al. Combined radiation therapy and surgery in the management of advanced head and neck cancer: Final report of study 73−03 of the radiation therapy oncology group. Head Neck Surg 1987; 10:19−27.

63. Marcial VA, Gelber R, Kramer S, Snow JB, Davis L, Vallecillo LA. Does preoperative irradiation increase the rate of surgical complications in carcinoma of the head and neck? Cancer 1982; 49:1297−301.

64. Snow JB, et al. Evaluation of randomized preoperative and postoperative radiation therapy for supraglottic carincoma. Ann Otol 1978; 87:686−91.

65. Snow JB, Gelber RD, Kramer S, Davis LW, Marcial VA, Lowry LD. Randomized preoperative and postoperative radiation therapy for patients with carcinoma of the head and neck: A preliminary report. Laryngoscope 1980; 90:930−45.

66. Snow JB, Gelber R, Kramer S, Davis LW, Marcial VA, Lowry LD. Comparison of preoperative and postoperative radiation therapy for patients with carcinoma of the head and neck. Acta Otolaryngol (Stockh) 1981; 91:611−26.

67. Marcial VA, Gelber R, et al. Does preoperative irradiation increase the rate of surgical complications in carcinoma of the head and neck? Cancer 1982; 49:1297−301.

68. Shah JP. Preoperative or postoperative radiotherapy? A Surgeons View. In: Shah JP, Blume HJG, Hanham IWF, eds. Head and neck oncology. New York: Raven Press, 1986:51−7.

69. Vikram B, Strong EW, Shah JP, Spiro R. Failure at the primary site following multimodality treatment in advanced head and neck cancer. Head Neck Surg 1984; 6:720−3.

70. Mantravadi RVP, Skolnik EM, Applebaum EL. Complications of postoperative and preoperative radiation therapy in head and neck cancer. Arch Otolaryngol 1981; 107:690−3.

71. Abe M, Takahashi M. Intraoperative radiotherapy: the Japanese experience. Int J Radiat Oncol Biol Phys 1981; 7:863−8.

72. Garrett P, Pugh N, Ross D, Hamaker R, Singer M. Intraoperative radiation therapy for advanced or recurrent head and neck cancer. Int J Radiat Oncol Biol Phys 1987; 13:785−8.

73. MacComb W, Fletcher GH. Planned combination of surgery and radiation in treatment of advanced primary head and neck cancer. Am J Roentgenol, Radium Ther Nucl Med 1957; 77(3):397−414.

74. Breneman JC, Bradshaw A, Gluckman J, Aron BS. Prevention of stomal recurrence in patients requiring emergency tracheostomy for advanced laryngeal and pharyngeal tumors. Cancer 1988; 2:802−5.

75. Collins SL. Controversy in management of cancer of the neck. In: Thawley SE, Panje WR, eds. Comprehensive management of head and neck tumors. Philadelphia: WB Saunders, 1987: chap 56, 1386−43.

76. DeSanto LW. Controversy in The Management of Laryngeal Tumors—Surgical Perspective. In: Thawley SE, Panje WR, eds. Comprehensive management of head and neck tumors .Philadelphia: WB Saunders, 1987:1029−39.

77. Snow GB, Balm A, Arendse J, et al. Prognostic factors in neck node metastasis. In: Larson DL, Ballantyne AJ, Guillamondegui OM, eds. Cancer in the neck—evaluation and treatment. New York: Macmillan, 1986:53−63.

78. Snow GB, Annyas AA, Van Slooten EA, et al. Prognostic factors of neck node metastasis. Clin Otolaryngol 1982; 7:185−92.

79. Moss WT, Cox ID, eds. Radiation oncology: rationale, techniques, results. In: Radiation oncology. 3rd ed. St Louis: CV Mosby, 1989.

80. Fletcher GH, Jessee RH. The place of irradiation in the management of the primary lesion in head and neck cancers. Cancer 1977; 39:862−7.

81. Fletcher GH. The place of irradiation in the management of head and neck cancers. Semin Oncol 1977; 4(4):375−85.

82. Looser, KG, Shah JP, Strong EW. The significance of "positive" margins in surgically resected epidermoid carcinomas. Head Neck Surg 1978; 1:107−11.

83. Baker SR, Swanson NA. Complete microscopic controlled surgery for head and neck cancer. Head Neck Surg 1984; 6:914−20.

84. Davidson TM, Haghighi P, et al. Mohs for head and neck mucosal cancer: Report on 111 patients. Laryngoscope 1988; 98:1078−83.

85. Davidson TM, Nahum AM, et al. Microscopic controlled excisions for epidermoid carcinoma of the head and neck. Otolaryngol Head Neck Surg 1981; 89:244−51.

86. Davidson TM, Nahum AM, et al. The biology of head and neck cancer detection and control by parallel histologic section. Arch Otolaryngol 1984; 110:193−6.

87. Slaughter DP, Southwick HW, Smejkal W. "Field cancerization" in oral stratified squmoaus epithelium. Cancer 1953; 6:963−8.

88. Jesse R, Sugarbaker E. Squamous cell carcinoma of the oropharynx: Why we fail. Otolaryngol Head Neck Surg 1976; 132:435−8.

89. Sadeghi A, Kuisk H, Tran LM, Mackintosh, Mclaren JR, Parker GR. The role of radiation therapy in squamous cell carcinoma of the upper aerodigestive tract with positive surgical margins. Am J Clin Oncol 1986; 9(6):500−3.

90. Wang Z, Million R, Mendenhall W, Parsons J, Cassisi N. Treatment with preoperative irradiation and surgery of squamous cell carcinoma of the head and neck. Cancer 1989; 64:32−8.

91. Perez C, Purdy J, Breaux S, Ogura J, Von Essen S. Carcinoma of the tonsillar fossa—A nonrandomized comparison of preoperative radiation and surgery or irradiation alone: Long-term results. Cancer 1982; 50:2314−22.

92. Goldman JF, et al. Histopathology of larynges and radical neck specimens in a combined radiation and surgical program for advanced carcinoma of the larynx and laryngopharynx. Ann Otol 1966; 75:313−35.

93. Byers R, Ballantyne M. Selection criteria for modified neck dissection with postoperative irradiation for N3 staged cervical metastasis. In: Chretien P, Johns M, Shedd D, Strong E, Ward P, eds. Head and neck cancer, vol 1. Proceedings of the International Conference. Philadelphia: BC Decker, 1985:157−9.

94. Goldman J, Bloom B, Zak F, Friedman W, Gunsberg M, Silverstone S. Serial microscopic studies of radical neck dissections. Arch Otolaryngol 1969; 89:620−8.

95. Santos V, Strong S, Vaughan C, DiTroia J. Role of surgery in head and neck cancer with fixed nodes. Arch Otolaryngol 1975; 101:645−8.

96. Kennedy JT, Drause C, Loevy S. The importance of tumor attachment to the carotid artery. Arch Otolaryngol 1977; 103:70−3.

97. Krause C. Management of the N3 neck–Introduction. In: Chretien P, Johns M, Shedd D, Strong E, Ward P, eds. Head and neck cancer, vol 1. Proceedings of the International Conference. Philadelphia: BC Decker, 1985:156−7.

98. Stafford N, Dearnaley D. Treatment of "inoperable" neck nodes using surgical clearance and postoperative interstitial irradiation. Br J Surg 1988; 75:62.

99. Goffinet D, Paryani S, Fee W. Management of patients with N3 cervical lymphadenophathy and/or carotid artery involvement. In: Chretien P, Johns M, Shedd D, Strong E, Ward P, eds. Head and neck cancer, vol I. Proceedings of the International Conference. Philadelphia: BC Decker, 1985:159−62.

100. Hamaker R, Singer M, Pugh N, Ross D, Garrett P. Management of the N3 neck: intraoperative radiation. In: Chretien P, Johns M, Shedd D, Strong E, Ward P, eds. Head and neck cancer, vol 1. Proceedings of the International Conference. Philadelphia: BC Decker, 1985:162−6.

101. Gunderson L, Cohen A, Dosoretz D, et al. Residual unresectable, or recurrent colorectal cancer: External beam irradiation and intraoperative electron beam boost +/− resection. Int J Radiat Oncol Biol Phys 1983; 9:1597−606.

102. Horton D, Tran L, Greenberg P, Selch M, Parker R. Primary radiation therapy in the treatment of squamous cell carcinoma of the soft palate. Cancer 1989; 63:2442−5.

103. Harwood A, Hawkins N, Beale F, Rider W, Bryce D. Management of advanced glottic cancer: A 10 year review of the Toronto experience. Int J Radiat Oncol Biol Phys 1979; 5:899−904.

104. Hanham I, Mould R. Role of surgery in patients with tongue cancer treated by radiotherapy: A radiotherapist's view. In: Bloom H, Hanham I, Shaw H, eds. Head and neck oncology. New York: Raven Press, 1986:59−63.

105. Beumer J, Curtis T, Harrison R. Radiation therapy of the oral cavity: Sequelae and management, Part 1. Head Neck Surg 1979; 1:301−12.

106. Beumer J, Curtis T, Harrison R. Radiation therapy of the oral cavity: Sequelae and management, Part 2. Head Neck Surg 1979; 1:392−408.

107. Metson R, Freehling D, Wang C. Surgical complications following twice-a-day versus once-a-day radiation therapy. Laryngoscope 1988; 98:30−35.

108. Marchetta F, Sako K, Maxwell W. Complications after radical head and neck surgery performed through previously irradiated tissues. Am J Surg 1967; 114:835−8.

109. Raymond C. Childhood cancers' improved survival rates can exact a price in late effects of therapy. JAMA 1988; 260:3400−5.

110. Veatch RM. The patient as partner: The ethics of working with head and neck cancer patients. In: Fee W, Goepfert H, Johns M, Strong E, Ward P, eds. Head and Neck Cancer, vol 2. Toronto: BC Decker, 1990:10−16.

111. McNeil B, Weichselbaum R, Pauker S. Speech and survival—tradeoffs between quality and quantity of life in laryngeal cancer. New Eng J Med 1981; 05:982−7.

112. Harwood A, Bryce D, Rider W. Management of T3 glottic cancer. Arch Otolaryngol 1980; 106:697.

113. Bryce D, Rider W. Pree-operative irradiation in the treatment of advanced laryngeal carcinoma. Laryngoscope 1971; 81:1481−90.

114. Rider B. Evolution in management of laryngeal cancer at the University of Toronto. J Otolaryngol 1982; 11:3.

115. DeSanto LW. Controversy in the management of laryngeal tumors: surgical perspective. In: Thawley SE, Panje WR, eds. Comprehensive management of head and neck tumors. Philadelphia: WB Saunders, 1987:1029−39.

116. DeSanto L, Magrina C. Stage III supraglottic cancer. In: Fee W, Goepfert H, Johns M, Strong E, Ward P, eds. Head and neck cancer vol 2. Proceedings of the International Conference. Toronto: BC Decker, 1990:126−30.

117. Wolf G, Hong W, Fisher S, et al. Laryngeal preservation with induction chemotherapy (CT) and radiation therapy in advanced laryngeal cancer: Preliminary results of VASCP #268. Abstract, in Otolaryngol Head Neck Surg 1989; 101:153.

118. Wolf G, Al-Sarraf M, Crissman J, Forastiere A, et al. Head and neck oncology reserach—A Summary of the Second International Head and Neck Oncology Research Conference. Head and Neck Surgery (suppl II): 1988; 590−596.

119. Snow GB. Surgical management—The next decade. In: Fee W, Goepfert H, Johns M, Stong E, Ward P, eds. Head and neck cancer, vol 2. Proceedings of the International Conference. Toronto: BC Decker, 1990:17−23.

6 Multimodal Chemotherapy

Induction Chemotherapy

B. W. Morrison, J. R. Clark

Introduction

In analyzing adjunctive treatments for cancers of the head and neck, and in particular squamous cell carcinomas of the head and neck (SCCHN), one must first define the present obstacles to cure. Local invasion and regional lymph node metastases remain the principal causes of patient morbidity and mortality due to SCCHN as up to 60% of patients with advanced disease develop local–regional recurrences after conventional surgery or radiotherapy (1–4). Distant metastasis is a less frequent cause of mortality as only 15 to 25% of patients relapse at distant sites. There is a suggestion, however, that as local–regional control has improved metastatic disease has become an increasing problem (5–7). Therefore, in the attempt to improve the survival of patients with locally advanced SCCHN, efforts should be focused primarily at increasing local–regional control and facilitating reductions in local treatment, and secondarily at eliminating micrometastatic disease. There are reasons to believe that induction chemotherapy as an adjunctive treatment to surgery or radiotherapy can achieve both these goals.

The objective of this chapter is to review the theoretic and experimental evidence for the use of induction (neoadjuvant, up-front, primary, or protoadjuvant) chemotherapy in the multidisciplinary treatment of patients with advanced SCCHN. By definition, induction chemotherapy refers to the use of chemotherapy as initial treatment prior to definitive surgery or radiotherapy for patients with potentially curable, M0, disease. Promising results with induction chemotherapy have been reported in the management of several human tumors including non-small cell lung cancer (8, 9), osteogenic sarcoma (10–12), locally advanced breast cancer (13–16), and transitional cell carcinoma of the bladder (17–19). As with SCCHN, these tumors typically present management problems related to locally aggressive disease with a propensity for relapse at local or distant sites despite relatively morbid surgery or radiotherapy. The practical utility of induction chemotherapy for these and other malignancies will only be determined by appropriately designed prospective, randomized trials that compare standard treatment with and without induction therapy.

For the present, the use of investigational therapies in the management of these tumors is justified on clinical grounds. That induction chemotherapy is an appropriate investigative approach which may be more effective than adjuvant chemotherapy after surgery or radiotherapy, or concurrent chemotherapy and radiation, is based on numerous preclinical and clinical studies. The evidence supporting the use of chemotherapy as induction treatment is reviewed, and we will consider the impact of timing (early versus late) in the delivery of systemic treatment and the influence of dose intensity and drug delivery on treatment outcome.

The Rationale for Induction Chemotherapy

The Impact of Time in the Delivery of Systemic Chemotherapy

The most compelling theory in support of induction chemotherapy comes from the spontaneous mutation model of Goldie and Coldman (20, 21). This mathematical model assumes that drug-resistant tumor cells arise spontaneously at a defined rate per cell division. From this model one can predict that the fraction of drug-resistant cells increases with increasing tumor size. The probability that a given tumor will be free of resistant cells, and thus "curable" by chemotherapy, decreases as the tumor grows. Moreover, this model suggests that as little as a 2 log increase in cell number (from 4 to 7 tumor doublings) may decrease the probability that a tumor is free of resistant cells from 95 to 5%).

These data suggest that if chemotherapy is to be used in an attempt to increase survival it should be used as early as possible in order to minimize the risk that a tumor will develop spontaneous, or de novo, drug resistance. The use of chemotherapy as induction treatment, the earliest possible use of chemotherapy, is supported by this model. However, the direct application of this model to the clinic is difficult. Although it predicts that there is a critical point in the life of a tumor when a drug-resistant population develops, one cannot ascertain when this will occur. In many instances, drug resistance may already have occurred by the time the patient first presents (22). Conversely, residual disease may not become resistant to potentially curative adjuvant chemotherapy until months after surgery or radiotherapy. In these instances, the importance of timing in the delivery of chemotherapy may be insignificant. Where drug resistance develops prior to presentation, chemotherapy as curative therapy will be ineffective. When drug resistance is delayed, chemotherapy may be uniformly effective.

Perhaps the greatest limitation of the Goldie–Coldman model is that it does not consider the relative impact of multidisciplinary treatment. This model is most easily applied to situations involving drug therapy for micrometastatic disease. The relative impact of a small population of drug-resistant tumor cells within local–regional disease may be negligible if those cells can be removed with subsequent surgery or radiotherapy.

The Goldie–Coldman model can also be used to argue in favor of initial surgical resection. The original model (20) assumed that all cells in a given tumor have stem cell capacity and predicts that any method of decreasing tumor burden will decrease the likelihood that a given tumor will become drug resistant. For example, a surgical resection of all gross disease can result in at least a 2 to 3 log reduction in tumor mass. If one assumes that the tumor is free of resistant cells at presentation and that drug delivery is not jeopardized by surgery, then an immediate 2 to 3 log kill with surgery would be preferable to a similar degree of cytoreduction with chemotherapy that may take from 8 to 12 weeks to develop. In this example, the emergence of drug-resistant cells would be delayed by initial surgery.

A modification of the original model (21) removes the assumption of a uniform stem-cell capacity within tumors and assumes that a defined proportion of tumor cells do not replicate and eventually die. This model predicts that large, slow-growing tumors with a substantial subpopulation of dying cells are more likely to develop drug-resistant cells than faster growing tumors. This would imply that large, slow-growing lesions that typify SCCHN have a high likelihood of giving rise to resistant populations and should be removed as soon as possible to prevent dissemination of resistant cells.

In conclusion, the mathematical models of tumor cell growth and spontaneous resistance argue both for and against induction chemotherapy. Appropriately designed small animal studies are required to validate these mathematical predictions and define the potential advantage of induction chemotherapy. While many small animal studies have evaluated adjuvant chemotherapy, relatively few have specifically addressed the use of induction chemotherapy.

Van Putten and colleagues (23, 24) have evaluated induction versus adjuvant cyclophosphamide in the treatment of three transplantable tumors. In these studies, local treatment was surgical amputation and the therapeutic endpoints were survival and the control of distant metastases. With mammary carcinoma 2661, preoperative chemotherapy cured 20% of mice, whereas no survivors were seen with postoperative treatment. With Lewis lung carcinoma, the use of cyclophosphamide before amputation resulted in fewer cures and a shorter time to relapse when compared with postoperative adjuvant therapy. With osteosarcoma C22LR, the use of induction or adjuvant cyclophosphamide resulted in an increased cure rate that was independent of the time of drug administration.

Similar studies have been conducted by Fisher and colleagues (25). After subcutaneous injection of C3H/HeJ mouse mammary carcinoma cells into the hind legs of mice, these investigators studied the effect of cyclophosphamide administered either 5 days prior to, at the time of, or 3 or 7 days after removal of the tumor by limb amputation. In this study, all approaches lead to increased survival but the best survival was seen in animals given chemotherapy 5 days preoperatively.

Thus, the combined experience of Van Putten and Fisher argues both for and against induction therapy. It would appear that the relative value of induction or adjuvant chemotherapy in murine systems is heavily dependant on the biology of the specific tumor under evaluation. However provocative, these data provide limited information about the relative effects of induction and adjuvant chemotherapy on macroscopic disease and local–regional recurrence. The latter endpoints are extremely relevant to the treatment of patients with SCCHN and have not been formally evaluated in animal models.

Given the paucity of preclinical data that specifically address induction chemotherapy, one must look to the experience with adjuvant chemotherapy for implications regarding the impact of timing in the delivery of systemic chemotherapy. The seminal work in this area has been performed at the Southern Research Institute by Schabel, Griswold, and their colleagues (26–31). In multiple different murine models of subcutaneously transplanted tumors treated with surgery and adjuvant chemotherapy, they demonstrated that the length of time between tumor implantation and either surgical resection or adjuvant chemotherapy was critical to the prevention or elimination of micrometastatic disease. In these studies chemotherapy was maximally effective when delivered soon after surgery.

Numerous investigations have cited these results in their arguments for induction chemotherapy. It is frequently assumed that if the early use of chemotherapy is critical to the success of adjuvant therapy, then preoperative chemotherapy would yield even better results. That this assumption is naive is suggested by studies that reveal that micrometastases are uniquely sensitive to chemotherapy in the immediate postoperative period. There is evidence that the growth rate of micrometastases may be increased, and the proportion of cells in the G0 or resting phase of the cell cycle may be decreased, for a limited time after surgical removal of the primary tumor (25, 32−35). Given that dividing cells are relatively sensitive to chemotherapy, resection of the primary tumor may be a critical factor in demonstrating the importance of the timing in the delivery of adjuvant chemotherapy. Given this effect, extrapolation of the results of Schabel and Griswold to the setting of induction chemotherapy may not be possible.

Clinical studies have also addressed the importance of timing in the delivery of systemic chemotherapy. Retrospectively analyzed data from the early experience with dactinomycin in the treatment of a Wilms tumor suggested that delays in the use of chemotherapy for even a few days after surgery might be prejudicial to outcome (36). The initiation of systemic therapy within hours of resection has become standard practice. Additional data comes from a Scandinavian trial of postoperative cyclophosphamide in the adjuvant treatment of breast cancer (37, 38). In this randomized, multi-institutional study the administration of adjuvant therapy after mastectomy was associated with a significant improvement in survival in all but one participating hospital. At the latter institution, the administration of chemotherapy was delayed for several weeks while postoperative radiotherapy was given. All other institutions had given chemotherapy prior to radiotherapy and had documented a benefit with adjuvant treatment. A multifactorial analysis suggested that the delay in delivery of chemotherapy accounted for this difference.

Other studies have not been able to confirm these observations. The M. D. Anderson Hospital performed a retrospective analysis of 460 breast cancer patients treated with adjuvant therapy. Groups in which the delay between mastectomy and chemotherapy varied between less than 10 weeks to more than 18 weeks had similar disease-free and overall survivals (39). However, the shortest postmastectomy interval evaluated in the M. D. Anderson study was 10 weeks, while in the Scandinavian study, chemotherapy began within 4 weeks of surgery. In the M. D. Andersen study, chemotherapy may have been administered too late in the postoperative period to discern an impact of time to adjuvant chemotherapy on outcome.

This issue was additionally addressed in two cooperative group studies. The Southwest Oncology Group performed a similar retrospective analysis evaluating the relationship between the time interval from mastectomy to adjuvant chemotherapy and patient outcome (40). They found that an interval of less than 14 days yielded the same disease-free survival as a delay of from 29 to 42 days. The Eastern Cooperative Oncology Group similarly found no difference in the survival rate of patients who began chemotherapy within 3 weeks or more than 3 weeks after surgery (41).

The importance of timing in the delivery of systemic chemotherapy has been most specifically evaluated in a recently published trial by the Ludwig Breast Cancer Study Group (42). In their prospective trial of adjuvant chemotherapy, women with node positive disease were randomized to receive either one course of adjuvant cyclophosphamide, methotrexate, and 5-fluorouracil (CMF) within 36 hours of mastectomy, or identical perioperative treatment plus six additional courses of CMF, or six courses of CMF beginning 25 to 32 days after surgery. For the two groups receiving multiple courses of adjuvant CMF, disease-free and overall survival were not significantly different. Survival for these patients, however, was superior to that recorded in the group that received a single perioperative course of CMF. This trial clearly demonstrated that postponing the initiation of adjuvant chemotherapy for 4 weeks does not jeopardize its efficacy and is consistent with the majority of the previously cited retrospective studies. However provocative the Ludwig Group results are, they still do not adequately evaluate the relative impact of perioperative therapy given the absence of controls receiving either no CMF, or only a single course of CMF from 25 to 32 days after surgery. The relative importance of multiple courses of CMF therapy may have outweighed a relative sensitivity to chemotherapy in the perioperative period.

The issue of timing in the delivery of adjuvant chemotherapy remains unsettled and additional trials are warranted. Two ongoing prospective randomized trials are of note. In premenopausal patients with newly diagnosed, high-risk operable breast cancer, Ragaz is conducting a randomized evaluation of six cycles of adjuvant CMF either with or without an additional cycle delivered approximately 1 week prior to mastectomy (43). At the Dana−Farber Cancer Institute, women with node positive breast cancer who have had lumpectomy and axillary dissection are being randomized either to postoperative radiotherapy followed by chemotherapy or to postoperative adjuvant chemotherapy followed by radiation. By trial design there will be a delay of from 6 to 8 weeks in the initiation of adjuvant chemotherapy between treatment groups. Results from these trials are eagerly awaited.

The Impact of Dose Intensity and Drug Delivery on Response to Chemotherapy

It is an axiom of modern medical oncology that a relationship exists between the dose intensity of administered chemotherapy (i. e., the cumulative dose of chemotherapy administered over time) and tumor response, and that maximally tolerated doses should be administered whenever possible (44). This concept must be considered in the treatment of patients with SCCHN for it is generally felt that these patients tolerate chemotherapy less well than those receiving similar therapies for other cancers. The latter impression has been attributed to the relatively poor performance status and multitude of concurrent medical problems that are common to patients with SCCHN. While the relative tolerance of induction or adjuvant chemotherapy for SCCHN has not been formally evaluated by randomized trial, studies of patients receiving both induction and adjuvant therapy have clearly demonstrated an improved tolerance of induction treatment (45, 46). These results, as well as those of studies evaluating only adjuvant chemotherapy for SCCHN, have led to the common belief that radiotherapy, and to a lesser extent surgery, reduce the intensity of chemotherapy administered after local–regional treatment. The dose intensity and potential antitumor activity of induction chemotherapy may be superior to that which can be achieved with adjuvant treatment.

The final argument in favor of induction therapy over adjuvant chemotherapy concerns the influence of drug delivery on response to chemotherapy. There is evidence that surgery and radiotherapy compromise tumor vascularity and subsequent drug delivery to residual disease within the field of treatment (47, 48). Such changes would be expected to diminish the effect of adjuvant chemotherapy on residual disease. Induction therapy administered through a minimally perturbed vascular supply may be more active against local disease.

The relative contribution of induction or adjuvant chemotherapy to local–regional control of disease has not been adequately evaluated in the treatment of any human tumor. For some tumors, both induction and adjuvant chemotherapy appear to increase local control of disease. In nonrandomized studies of patients with locally advanced breast cancer, the use

of induction therapy has been associated with enhanced local control of disease and allowed many patients to avoid mastectomy (13–16). However, in randomized trials of patients with stage II breast cancer, adjuvant chemotherapy or hormonal therapy can decrease the rate of local recurrence after either mastectomy or local excision and radiotherapy (49–51). Whether induction chemotherapy would be superior in this regard is unknown, but clearly the issues of vascular supply, drug delivery to residual disease, and local–regional control after surgery and radiotherapy for breast cancer or other malignancies such as SCCHN is neither simple nor settled.

The Potential Advantages of Induction Chemotherapy for SCCHN

Thus far this discussion has reviewed concepts and data that support the ability of induction chemotherapy to increase the cure rate of human tumors. As noted, experimental evidence advocating induction over adjuvant chemotherapy is suboptimal and additional preclinical and clinical studies are warranted. Nonetheless, even if induction chemotherapy does not significantly improve survival over that achieved with adjuvant therapy, there may still be important advantages to its use. The potential advantages of induction chemotherapy for the patient with advanced SCCHN are noted in Table 6.1.

The most obvious benefit of induction therapy is for the patient with a locally advanced or unresectable primary tumor, or a fixed neck lesion. Even a partial response to induction chemotherapy may enhance local–regional control and facilitate eventual resection with the same or decreased morbidity. Moreover, induction therapy may identify a subset of patients who after a good response to chemotherapy may receive less extensive surgery or radiation therapy without sacrificing local–regional control. Of course the classic rationale for induction therapy is not to replace or reduce surgery or radiotherapy but to add to standard treatment with the intent of improving local–regional control and survival.

Another advantage of induction chemotherapy is that it provides an in vivo assay system for the efficacy of chemotherapy. Response data gathered in trials of induction chemotherapy may be of considerable value in the development of curative chemotherapy. Experimental studies indicate a high degree of correlation between the responsiveness of macroscopic and micrometastatic disease to a given chemotherapy (52, 53). Knowledge of an individual's response to induction chemotherapy may be used to select the type of adjuvant chemotherapy that would benefit those at continued risk for relapse despite initial chemotherapy and optimal local treatment. The successful use of both induction and adjuvant chemotherapy for solid tumors was pioneered by

Table 6.1 Potential advantages of induction chemotherapy

- To promote regression of primary and nodal disease, and enhance local–regional control with subsequent surgery or radiotherapy

- To reduce the bulk of initially unresectable lesion, and facilitate eventual surgical resection

- To identify patients with responding lesion that can be effectively managed with single-modality surgery or radiotherapy

- To identify patients with responding tumors that many benefit from additional therapy after local–regional treatment

- To provide early systemic treatment for occult metastatic disease

Rosen and colleagues in their treatment of osteogenic sarcoma (53).

In addition, when surgical resection follows initial chemotherapy in vivo data on the biology of tumor regression are available. Comparative histopathologic analyses of the pretreatment biopsy and the resection specimen can provide valuable information regarding the influence of chemotherapy on tumor vascularity and stromal−tumor cell interactions. The opportunity to study morphological, cytokinetic, and immunological changes with chemotherapy also exists. Of practical importance is whether clinically observed tumor regression with chemotherapy results from a radial contraction of a tumor's margins with maintenance of initial tumor cell density, or from a decrease in tumor cell density without a change in initial tumor volume. Preliminary observations in SCCHN suggest that both patterns of tumor regression exist and may correlate with whether a clinically evident tumor is exophytic or infiltrative (54, 55). These data will have bearing on the extent of surgery or radiotherapy required after initial chemotherapy.

The Potential Disadvantages of Induction Chemotherapy for SCCHN

There are potential disadvantages to the use of induction chemotherapy. The most compelling fear is that the use of induction therapy will delay definitive treatment of primary and regional disease, compromise eventual local−regional treatment and contribute to dissemination of distant metastases (Table 6.2).

Several experimental animal models have addressed the latter concern and suggest that chemotherapy may promote metastatic spread of disease. These models have generally involved pretreatment of small animals with chemotherapy or radiotherapy prior to intravenous or subcutaneous inoculation with tumor cells. Such studies have demonstrated an increase in lung metastases in pretreated animals (56−59). By design, however, these models do not parallel the clinical situation in human cancer. The models of Moore and Dixon (60) and Poupon and

Table 6.2   **Potential disadvantages of induction chemotherapy**

- Causes a delay in local−regional treatment that may be associated with:
  - interval growth of tumor with compromise of subsequent surgery or radiotherapy
  - dissemination of distant metastases
- May select for drug or radioresistant tumor cells
- Increases the local toxicity of subsequent surgery or radiotherapy

colleagues (61) are of greater concern. In their studies, transplantable tumors were implanted subcutaneously and allowed to grow to a given size prior to treatment with radiotherapy and/or chemotherapy. Poupon and colleagues found that treatment with nitrosoureas led to an increase in lung metastases without a change in lymph node spread. Cyclophosphamide in their model decreased both local growth rate and systemic spread of tumor while methotrexate had no effect on either primary or systemic disease. Similarly, Moore and Dixon found that treatment of established tumors with cyclophosphamide and radiotherapy seemed to increase the metastatic potential of rat mammary carcinomas compared to either no treatment or to treatment with chemotherapy or radiation therapy alone. The explanation for these observations is not known but may be due to:

1. The immunosuppressive effect of the various treatments and the loss of immunosurveillance capabilities
2. Endothelial damage by chemotherapy at sites of potential metastatic spread that increases the likelihood that circulating tumor cells will adhere to endothelial cells and establish local growth, or
3. The mutagenic effects of chemotherapy and radiation with the consequent development of the metastatic phenotype (62)

Few clinical studies specifically address distant metastases after induction chemotherapy. One such trial is the recently completed Veterans Administration Cooperative Study on Operable Laryngeal Cancer. Results from this randomized trial of induction cisplatin and 5-fluorouracil reveal a significant decrease in distant relapse in patients receiving induction chemotherapy prior to local−regional treatment (63). It is likely that the risk of enhancing metastatic spread of disease with induction therapy is dependent on multiple interrelated factors that are evaluable only in properly designed clinical trials.

As previously mentioned, induction chemotherapy may jeopardize local−regional control by causing a delay in local−regional treatment. A few prospective, randomized trials of induction chemotherapy for patients with advanced SCCHN have noted an increase in local−regional failure after induction therapy (63, 64). However, the local−regional treatment delivered in these trials was not equivalent between treatment groups. Whether by design or conduct, fewer surgical resections were performed in patients treated with induction chemotherapy. Similar studies with more tightly regulated local−regional treatment have not reported such a difference (45, 65).

That induction therapy may cause detrimental delays in local−regional therapy is also suggested by results from three recently published randomized trials evaluating induction chemotherapy versus concurrent chemotherapy and radiotherapy (66–68). In these studies, disease-free survival, although not overall survival, was improved by concurrent chemotherapy and radiotherapy when compared to survival after a similar or identical regimen of induction chemotherapy followed by radiation therapy. The noted improvement in disease-free survival with concurrent treatment is support for the concept of dose intensity which predicts that a superior outcome will be achieved with the most concentrated course of treatment (44). A superior survival could also have been achieved with concurrent therapy due to a synergistic chemotherapy and radiation. However, additional interpretations of these data are possible. One might conclude that a delay in radiotherapy is detrimental in the face of ineffective induction chemotherapy.

A more recent concern regarding induction chemotherapy has to do with data documenting cross-resistance between chemotherapy and radiotherapy. Ozols and colleagues (69) have shown that ovarian cancer cell lines made resistant to cisplatin or melphalan can develop de novo resistance to radiation therapy. Moreover, these investigators implicated glutathione in this mechanism of resistance. Upon decreasing glutathione levels within these doubly resistant cell lines, sensitivity to both chemotherapy and radiation was restored.

There is supporting evidence for these observations from clinical studies of patients with SCCHN. A number of investigators have noted an association between a nonresponse to induction chemotherapy and a nonresponse to subsequent radiotherapy (70–74). The implications of these observations specifically for or against the use of induction chemotherapy are unclear. The radioresistance of lesions that fail to respond to induction chemotherapy may in large part be due to anatomical factors. Large, bulky, necrotic lesions are least likely to respond to either chemotherapy or radiotherapy. Regional hypoxia and a low growth fraction may contribute to the relative resistance of such lesions to chemotherapy or radiotherapy. The selective delivery of drugs to the well perfused peripheral portions of these lesions rather than to their necrotic core is certainly a contributing factor to drug resistance. The frequency of cross-resistance to chemotherapy and radiotherapy at the cellular or molecular level is unknown, but presumed to be rare. If in fact such cross-resistant cells make up even a small proportion of a presenting tumor, our present armamentarium of therapeutic modalities, however brilliantly orchestrated, may not be curative. Further research into the frequency of this problem in SCCHN is needed as are new tools to overcome these mechanisms of resistance.

It is clear that the potential advantages and disadvantages of induction chemotherapy have been inadequately evaluated. Additional preclinical and clinical studies addressing these issues are indicated. Nevertheless, clinical trials of induction chemotherapy for patients with advanced SCCHN have proceeded with both promising and controversial results.

Clinical Studies of Induction Chemotherapy for SCCHN

Several recent publications (75–77) have reviewed the phase I–II trials of induction single agent and combination chemotherapy for SCCHN. This chapter will outline the historical development of induction chemotherapy for SCCHN, summate the phase I–II and phase III experiences with induction combination chemotherapy, and relate strategies for continued clinical investigation.

Single-agent Trials of Induction Chemotherapy for SCCHN

The experience with induction chemotherapy for patients with SCCHN began in the early 1960s when several trials studied sequential single-agent chemotherapy and radiotherapy. The earliest trials were uncontrolled, employing methotrexate or other antimetabolites in a variety of doses and schedules before radiotherapy (78–81). Subsequent trials utilized bleomycin or cisplatin (82–86). Several of these studies suggested that induction chemotherapy improved local–regional control and survival for patients with advanced inoperable disease. To date, however, four prospective, randomized trials of single-agent induction chemotherapy have been published and none have reported a difference in disease-free or overall survival (87–90).

In these studies, the impact of chemotherapy was limited by the use of a single agent for only 2 to 4 weeks prior to local–regional treatment. Nonetheless, they demonstrated that induction chemotherapy causes only a slight increase in the incidence and severity of radiation-associated mucositis and no increase in subsequent surgical complications. These findings laid the foundation for initiating trials of induction combination chemotherapy and for the use of induction chemotherapy as preoperative therapy in patients with more limited disease.

Phase I–II Trials of Induction Combination Chemotherapy

Phase I–II trials of induction combination chemotherapy for patients with advanced SCCHN began in the late 1970s and continue as an area of active clinical investigation. Despite variations in design and conduct, the scientific objectives of these studies have always been to maximize the rate of complete response to chemotherapy, to identify prognostic factors for favorable treatment outcome, and to define the extent of surgery or radiotherapy required for optimal local–regional control after chemotherapy. The degree to which these objectives have been met can be summarized:

1. Induction chemotherapy causes significant tumor regression in 70–90% and complete clinical regression of tumor in 20–50% of patients prior to local–regional treatment (46, 91–95)
2. Tumor regression continues and response rates increase through at least three cycles of treatment (96, 97)
3. Of patients who achieve a complete clinical response to induction chemotherapy, 30–70% will be found to have had a complete pathologic regression of tumor after re-biopsy of the primary tumor site or upon analysis of a definitive surgical resection (92, 98–101)
4. Local–regional control of tumor and survival is highest in patients who achieve a complete response to initial chemotherapy (46, 92, 96, 100, 102, 103)
5. Single-modality surgery or radiotherapy may produce adequate local–regional control of tumor in selected patients who have a complete response to initial chemotherapy (92, 98)
6. An initially unresectable lesion may become resectable after a response to chemotherapy, however, whether such a resection enhances local–regional control beyond that achieved with chemotherapy and radiotherapy remains uncertain (103, 104)
7. Initial tumor extent whether defined by overall stage, T stage, N stage, or resectability predicts for response to chemotherapy and survival (94, 96, 97, 101, 105)
8. In some studies, a response to chemotherapy and survival have been associated with primary tumor site in the oral cavity (105, 106), oropharynx (106), or nasopharynx (46, 72), but others have not documented an influence of primary site on treatment outcome that was independent of tumor stage (107)
9. A poor performance status may not predict for response to chemotherapy, but does adversely influence survival (46, 105), perhaps due to reductions in the local–regional treatment delivered to this group of patients
10. When all patients are considered, the degree of squamous differentiation does not predict for response to induction chemotherapy or survival (102, 105, 108)
11. However, when only patients who achieve a complete clinical response to chemotherapy are considered, those with poorly differentiated tumors (108) or pathologically persistent disease

in the definitive resection specimen (99) may incur a greater risk for relapse despite surgery or radiotherapy; and
12. Induction chemotherapy does not significantly increase the toxicity of subsequent surgery or radiotherapy (93, 101, 103, 109)

Given these results, trials of induction chemotherapy for patients with initially inoperable or unresectable disease are increasingly rare. Conversely, trials of induction chemotherapy for patients with resectable and operable disease are relatively common, and many offer radiotherapy alone in a systematic fashion to those who achieve a complete response to chemotherapy. The majority of such patients will do well, but efforts are being made to identify those at high risk for relapse despite a complete response. As mentioned, preliminary results suggest that patients who achieve a complete clinical response, but had poorly differentiated lesions (108) or pathologically persistent disease (99), have an increased risk for relapse. The latter result, however, has been challenged (97). Once identified, high-risk patients with a favorable response to induction chemotherapy may be ideal candidates for alternative treatment strategies (e. g., radiation implants, adjuvant chemotherapy, concurrent chemotherapy, and radiotherapy, differentiation therapy with cis-retinoic acid or β-carotene, etc.).

The phase I–II experience with induction combination chemotherapy for patients with advanced SCCHN has answered many of the questions relevant to the proper use of chemotherapy in this setting, and has identified numerous variables important to the design, conduct, and interpretation of randomized trials. Unfortunately, a primary objective of the phase II experience with induction chemotherapy has not been achieved. At present, relatively little data exist to suggest what is the optimal regimen of induction therapy for SCCHN. While the combination of cisplatin and infusion 5-fluorouracil is generally accepted as the current "standard" for investigative studies, three studies cast doubt on the absolute superiority of this regimen.

Two trials have compared the activity of cisplatin and infusion 5-fluorouracil to other cisplatin-based regimens as induction therapy for patients with previously untreated SCCHN. Clark and colleagues at the Dana–Farber have performed a prospective, randomized phase II trial of two induction regimens (97). Preliminary results from the first 106 patients randomized to receive either cisplatin with infusion 5-fluorouracil or cisplatin with infusion bleomycin and mid-cycle methotrexate with leucovorin rescue did not indicate a significant difference in the rates of complete or overall response to chemotherapy. In a second study, Cognetti and colleagues compared their historical experience with either two cycles of induction CABO or three cycles of induction CF for patients with previously untreated SCCHN (105). In this report, the rate of complete response to chemotherapy was 15% in the 123 patients treated with CABO and 32% in the 25 patients treated with CF. This difference was not significant in multivariate analysis.

The relative activity of cisplatin and 5-fluorouracil has also been evaluated in patients with recurrent or metastatic SCCHN. In this setting, Clavel and associates within the EORTC randomized patients to receive either cisplatin, methotrexate, bleomycin, and vincristine (CABO), or cisplatin and infusion 5-fluorouracil (CF), or single-agent cisplatin (110). Preliminary results of this study indicate that CABO and CF result in similar rates of response, and that both regimens are superior to single-agent cisplatin in response.

The latter three trials compared cisplatin and infusion 5-fluorouracil to alternative cisplatin-based regimens. Although the power of these studies to detect small differences in tumor response is limited, they suggest that when the extent of disease and duration of treatment are controlled, the activity of present regimens of combination chemotherapy containing cisplatin is comparable. Continued progress in the development of induction chemotherapy will require the creation of increasingly active induction regimens. Accepting the premise that only a complete response to induction chemotherapy will convey a survival benefit to treated patients, phase I–II trials of induction chemotherapy for patients with advanced SCCHN continue in an attempt to develop combinations with enhanced antitumor activity. Such studies generally incorporate at least one of several strategies that may increase the rate of complete response to chemotherapy (Table 6.**3**).

Representative examples of this effort are numerous. The Southwest Oncology Group (SWOG) has organized a trial that will determine the activity of up to six cycles of induction cisplatin and infusion 5-fluorouracil prior to local–regional therapy (SWOG

Study 8810). Although preliminary results from the Dana–Farber (97) suggest that macroscopic regression of tumor and response rates do not change after three cycles of therapy, this finding requires confirmation. Moreover, these results do not consider the potential impact of additional (i. e., more than three) cycles of therapy on the treatment of microscopic disease located at the margin of surgery or radiotherapy or at distant sites, or its impact on overall survival.

The effect of prolonged courses of induction chemotherapy on response and survival can only be evaluated in well designed clinical trials. However, given the toxicity associated with present regimens of induction therapy, patient tolerance may be a limiting factor in determining the intensity and duration of chemotherapy prior to surgery or radiotherapy. Recognizing this fact, studies that evaluate new cytotoxic agents, drug analogues, or novel routes of drug administration are important for the identification of therapies with potentially increased antitumor activity or decreased toxicity compared to existing therapies. In this light, recent trials of carboplatin, a cisplatin analogue, and continuous infusion cisplatin are significant. In murine tumor models as well as clinical trials, carboplatin has been shown to possess similar antitumor activity, increased myelosuppression and thrombocytopenia, but decreased emetic potential, nephrotoxicity, neuro- and oto-toxicity when compared to the parent compound. To date, several studies of carboplatin with infusion 5-fluorouracil have been conducted in patients with either recurrent or metastatic SCCHN (111, 112), or previously untreated disease (113). This combination is active, but likely not more so than the combination of cisplatin and 5-fluorouracil. Nonetheless, carboplatin and 5-fluorouracil are extremely well tolerated and their use may facilitate the development of treatment programs that require multiple courses of chemotherapy.

The administration of cisplatin by prolonged (5-day) continuous intravenous infusion may be similarly advantageous as several studies have documented activity comparable to bolus cisplatin, but decreased gastrointestinal toxicity and improved patient tolerance with this means of drug delivery (114–119). Moreover, in a comparative study, Forastierre et al. (120) documented a pharmacologic advantage for infusion cisplatin over equivalent total doses of bolus therapy that warrants further clinical evaluation. Trials evaluating 5-day continuous infusions of cisplatin and 5-fluorouracil in patients with previously untreated SCCHN are in progress.

Some of the most interesting recent trials of combination chemotherapy for patients with SCCHN are those which have attempted to increase the intensity of treatment delivered through the use of high-dose chemotherapy, modifiers of cytotoxic drug activity,

Table 6.3   Strategies to increase the rate of CR to induction therapy

- The administration of additional (e.g., > 3) courses of induction chemotherapy

- The use of new cytotoxic agents, drug analogues, or novel routes of drug administration that result in increased antitumor activity or decreased toxicity

- The administration of increasingly intense treatment regimens that utilize:
  - high-dose chemotherapy,
  - modifiers of cytotoxic drug activity, or
  - additional cytotoxic agents (e.g., methotrexate, bleomycin, vindesine)

or the administration of additional cytotoxic agents (e. g., methotrexate, bleomycin) with cisplatin and 5-fluorouracil. Kish and associates evaluated bolus cisplatin at doses up to $200\,mg/m^2$ with infusion 5-fluorouracil (121). In this study of 11 patients with recurrent or metastatic SCCHN, 5 complete and 5 partial responses were recorded. The authors concluded that high-dose cisplatin and 5-fluorouracil resulted in increased myelosuppression but unchanged antitumor activity when compared to past experiences with regimens using conventional doses of these agents. Given the small number of patients in this study, however, the significance of the latter conclusion can be questioned. The activity of high-dose cisplatin, and its analogue carboplatin, deserves continued evaluation in patients with advanced SCCHN.

The modulating effect of calcium leucovorin on the activity of 5-fluorouracil is also under study in patients with advanced SCCHN. In patients with recurrent or metastatic disease, Vokes et al. (122) were the first to define a schedule of bolus cisplatin and infusion 5-fluorouracil with high-dose oral calcium leucovorin. In this phase I study, the antitumor activity of cisplatin, 5-fluorouracil, and leucovorin was not quantified. Clark and associates at the Dana–Farber are evaluating a related combination of 5-day continuous infusion cisplatin, 5-fluorouracil, and high-dose intravenous leucovorin as induction therapy in patients with untreated, advanced disease. Preliminary results indicate moderate or severe mucositis in 91% of 46 treated patients, but complete responses have been recorded in 65% (123). Similar results with cisplatin, 5-fluorouracil, and leucovorin have been reported by Loeffler and colleagues (124). In their study, a complete response to induction therapy was recorded in 23 of 45 (51%) patients with advanced SCCHN. Given the wealth of laboratory and clinical data that document the modulating effect of leucovorin on 5-fluorouracil (125), this combination warrants continued study.

The activity of induction regimens containing cytotoxic agents in addition to or alternating with cisplatin and 5-fluorouracil is also being evaluated. Ensley and colleagues are developing five-course programs of two alternating regimens: cisplatin with infusion 5-fluorouracil, and sequential methotrexate with 5-fluorouracil and leucovorin. In a completed study of 46 patients with unresectable disease, a complete response rate of 46% was achieved prior to surgery or radiotherapy (126). This alternating regimen was recently modified and preliminary results note that 11 of 17 patients with T4N3 disease developed a complete clinical response to induction treatment (127).

By design, the latter regimens of Clark, Loeffler, and Ensley for patients with previously untreated SCCHN are more intense than the parent regimen of cisplatin with infusion 5-fluorouracil. Although toxic, these regimens appear extremely active and ongoing evaluation in properly controlled studies may confirm their superiority to conventional cisplatin and 5-fluorouracil.

The use of extremely intense regimens of chemotherapy for patients with SCCHN remains poorly studied in comparison to treatment schemes for patients with other tumor types. A concept that has been applied to the treatment of several human tumors is the model of tumor growth proposed by Norton and Simon (128, 129). These authors have emphasized that the dose of chemotherapy required to eradicate clinical disease may be insufficient to eradicate microscopic disease. They note that after the attainment of complete clinical response, high-dose therapy of a relatively brief duration may be preferable to prolonged low-dose therapy in decreasing rates of recurrence (128). They have advocated intensification of therapy as tumors shrink. The application of this concept has yielded promising results in acute myelogenous leukemia (130) and non-Hodgkin's lymphoma (131). For patients with head and neck cancer a comparable approach might include conventional chemotherapy until a complete clinical response is acheived, then high-dose chemotherapy (e. g., with carboplatin regimens) followed by autologous bone marrow transplantation. Such treatment goes beyond traditional induction therapy and would not be tolerated by the majority of patients with advanced SCCHN. However, for selected patients with probable systemic disease, such as in young adults with advanced nasopharyngeal carcinomas or esthesioneuroblastomas, intensive drug therapy may hold special promise. For example, at the University of Virginia, 8 patients with recurrent Stage C esthesioneuroblastomas have been treated with high-dose chemotherapy and autologous bone marrow transplantation, and 4 have had durable complete remissions (132).

It should be evident that there are multiple means by which investigators in the treatment of patients with advanced SCCHN can and are attempting to increase the activity of chemotherapy for this disease. Through phase I–II analyses, considerable progress has been made in defining at least moderately active regimens of induction therapy. By intent, these studies have not attempted to identify induction chemotherapy as a standard treatment for patients with advanced SCCHN; they have nonetheless provided invaluable insight into the design, implementation, and interpretation of randomized, phase III trials of induction therapy.

Table 6.4 Randomized trials of induction combination chemotherapy for advanced SCCHN

Author	Induction regimen Drugs, schedule, and duration	No. of patients	Response Complete (CR)	Response Total (CR + PR)	Local treatment Surgery/RT	Local treatment RT alone	Local treatment Salvage surgery	Survival (2 year)* DFS	Survival (2 year)* OS
Stell et al. (135)	Bleomycin 60 mg iv infusion, d 1; Vincristine 1.5 mg/m² iv, d 1; Methotrexate 225 mg/m² iv, d 1; 5-Fluorouracil 350 mg/m² iv, d 1; Folinic Acid 15 mg po q 6 h × 4; Hydroxyurea 3 g/m² po, d 15; 6-Mercaptopurine 150 mg/m² po, d 15; Cytoxan 500 mg/m² iv, d 15; Duration: 28 days (1 cycle)	Control group: 39 patients	Not applicable		—	39(100%)	11(28%)	NA	55%
		Induction group: 47 patients	Not reported		—	46 (98%)	6(13%)	NA	22%
								No significant difference	
Head and Neck Contracts Program (45)	Cisplatin 100 mg/m² iv, d 1; Bleomycin 15 mg/m² iv, d 3; Bleomycin 15 mg/m²/d, iv-ci, d 3–7; Duration: 21 days (1 cycle)	Control group: 152 patients	Not applicable		144(95%)	?	—	55%	60%
		Induction group: 291 patients	3%	34%	270(93%)	?	—	60%	58%
								No difference	
Kun et al. (133)	Bleomycin 30 mg/day iv-ci, d 1–4; Cytoxan 200 mg/day iv, d 1–5; Methotrexate 30 mg/m² iv, d 1 and 5; 5-Fluorouracil 400 mg/m² iv, d 1–5; Duration: 42 days (2 cycles)	Control group: 40 patients	Not applicable		22(55%)	18 (45%)	—	64%[+]	43%[+]
		Induction group: 43 patients	5%	67%	14(33%)	28 (65%)	—	59%[+]	31%[+]
								No difference	
Schuller et al. (65)	Cisplatin 50 mg/m² iv, d 1; Methotrexate 40 mg/m² iv, d 1; Bleomycin 15 mg/m² iv, d 1 and 8; Vincristine 2 mg iv, d 1; Duration: 63 days (3 cycles)	Control group: 76 patients	Not applicable		70(92%)	?	—	44%[#]	55%
		Induction group: 32 patients	18%	70%	61(74%)	?	—	30%[#]	40%
								No difference	
Toohill et al. (134)	Cisplatin 100 mg/m² iv, d 1; 5-Fluorouracil 1 g/m²/d iv-ci, d 1–5; Duration: 63 days (3 cycles)	Control group: 33 patients	Not applicable		Not reported			70%[+]	67%[+]
		Induction group: 27 patients	19%	85%	Not reported			70%[+]	53%[+]
								No difference	

Table 6.4 (cont.)

Author	Induction regimen: Drugs, schedule, and duration	No. of patients	Response Complete (CR)	Response Total (CR + PR)	Local treatment Surgery/RT	Local treatment RT alone	Local treatment Salvage surgery	Survival (2 year)* DFS	Survival (2 year)* OS
Martin et al (137)	Bleomycin 10 mg/m²/d iv-ci, d 1–5; Methotrexate 120 mg/m² iv, d 2; Folinic acid rescue; 5-Fluorouracil 600 mg/m² iv, d 2; Cisplatin 120 mg/m² iv, d 4; Duration: 63 days (3 cycles)	Control group: 53 patients; Induction group: 54 patients	Not applicable; 6%	48%		Not reported; Not reported		42%; 39%; No difference	NA; NA
Carugati et al. (138)	Arm B1: Cisplatin 100 mg/m² iv, d 1 and 15; Bleomycin 20 mg/m² iv, d 1, 8, 15 and 22; or Arm B2: Cisplatin 100 mg/m² iv, d 4 and 19; Bleomycin 20 mg/m² iv, d 1, 8, 15 and 22; Methotrexate 50 mg/m² iv, d 1 and 15; Duration: 28 days (1 cycle)	Control group: 38 patients; Induction groups: B1: 43 patients; B2: 39 patients	Not applicable; NA; NA	44%; 59%		Not reported; Not reported		25%§; 33%§; No difference	18%§; 38%§
VA Coop (63)	Cisplatin 100 mg/m² iv, d 1; 5-Fluorouracil 1 g/m²/d iv-ci, d 1–5; Duration: 63 days (3 cycles)	Control group: 166 patients; Induction group: 166 patients	Not applicable; NA	NA	100%; 18%	–; 64%	–; 17%	72%; 63%; No difference	63%+; 63%+
Martin et al. (136)	Cisplatin 100 mg/m² iv, d 1; 5-Fluorouracil 1 g/m²/d iv-ci, d 1–5; Duration: 63 days (3 cycles)	Control group: 37 patients; Induction group: 38 patients	Not applicable; 46%	68%		Not reported; Not reported		NA; NA; No difference	NA; NA

* Estimate of 2-year survival determined from published actuarial graph unless otherwise noted.
+ Published 2-year survival by actuarial estimate.
# Two-year actuarial estimate of failure-free survival.
§ Five-year survival by actuarial estimate.

Abbreviations: CR, complete response; DFS, disease-free survival; NA, not available; OS, overall survival; PR, partial response; RT, radiotherapy; d, day; iv, intravenous; po, per os; iv-ci, intravenous continuous infusion.

Modified from Table 1 of reference (76).

Phase III Trials of Induction Combination Chemotherapy

Collectively, the single-institution and pilot experience with induction chemotherapy for patients with advanced SCCHN is encouraging and strongly suggests a role for chemotherapy in the multidisciplinary treatment of patients with this disease. However, the true value of induction chemotherapy can only be determined by prospective, randomized controlled trials. To date, results from nine such trials have been published (Table 6.**4**) as either completed manuscripts (45, 63, 65, 133–136) or meeting abstracts (137, 138). These results have supported many of the observations noted in phase II studies of induction chemotherapy including the dependence response to chemotherapy on stage of disease at presentation (45), and the absence of an increase in toxicity with surgery or radiotherapy after chemotherapy (45, 65, 133). Given that these studies contained a control group of patients treated with conventional surgery or radiotherapy alone, they have the potential to address the most pressing questions regarding induction chemotherapy:

1. What is the quality of life or survival of patients who receive induction chemotherapy compared to patients who receive similar local–regional treatment without chemotherapy?
2. What is the relative quality of life and survival of patients who are treated with induction chemotherapy prior to modified (more conservative) local–regional therapies compared to patients who receive unmodified surgery or radiotherapy without chemotherapy?

The first question has been addressed in all nine randomized trials of induction combination chemotherapy. To date, none of these studies have reported an improved survival after induction therapy (Table 6.**4**). However, these studies cannot be considered definitive assessments of induction chemotherapy due to limitations created by suboptimal patient accrual, the use of relatively inactive regimens of induction therapy or improperly controlled local–regional treatment.

As considered by Andersen and Kalish in Chapter 4, an "ideal" randomized study of induction chemotherapy for advanced SCCHN should be limited to the analysis of patients whose disease is restricted to one specific site and to a relatively narrow spectrum of TN stages. For example, such a trial might include only patients with operable laryngeal or perhaps tonsilar carcinomas. The extremely heterogeneous population of patients with advanced "unresectable" primary lesions or "fixed" neck disease would not be included. Under optimal conditions, over 200 patients must be randomized in a given study for a 20% difference in 2-year actuarial survival to be declared "significant" (assuming a 2-year actuarial survival of 50% for control patients, 80% power, and an alpha-level ≤ 0.05 in a 2-sided test). Suboptimal study conditions with a heterogeneous patient population, limited follow-up evaluation, a difference in observed survival of less than 20%, etc., will either decrease the power of a given study or increase the minimum number of patients that must be randomized in order to declare a "significant" difference in survival when one in truth exists. In addition, local–regional treatment options of surgery and radiotherapy, or radiotherapy alone must be strictly controlled and equivalent in all arms of therapy if chemotherapy is to be evaluated as an independent variable.

With these considerations in mind, it is clear that these nine randomized trials of induction combination chemotherapy for SCCHN were destined to yield "no significant difference in survival." Eight trials registered patients with multiple primary tumor sites and at least four trials (133–136) evaluated mixed groups of patients with "resectable" and "unresectable" disease prior to treatment. Despite these shortcomings, only two trials (45, 63) evaluated more than 75 patients per treatment arm. In addition, the majority of these trials have not reported whether surgery or radiotherapy were limited in patients treated with chemotherapy, and whether such limitations may have compromised their survival. Only five studies provide information regarding the local–regional treatment delivered to the control and experimental groups, and in four of these studies (63, 65, 133, 135), significant differences exist which may favor the control group. Kun et al. (133) did consider the impact of local–regional treatment on survival in his randomized trial of patients with "resectable" and "unresectable" disease. In this study, the type of local–regional treatment delivered (preoperative radiotherapy and surgery versus radiotherapy alone) was significantly associated with survival in both treatment groups. These data reveal the difficulties encountered in managing and interpreting studies that treat a mixed population of patients with different primary tumor sites, TN stages, and degrees of "resectability."

Even an "ideal" trial of induction chemotherapy will fail if the induction regimen is inactive. Recent studies indicate that a complete response rate of 20–54% can be expected in patients treated with three or more cycles of cisplatin-based combination chemotherapy prior to surgery and/or radiotherapy. Remarkably, the highest rate of complete response achieved in five of six randomized trials which reported this rate was only 19%. The Head and Neck Contracts Program (HNCP) (45) utilized low doses of cisplatin and only one cycle of induction chemotherapy, and reported a complete response rate of 3%. Kun et al. (133) administered either one or two cycles of an induction regimen without cisplatin, noted a complete response rate of 5% and did not report the percent of patients only receiving one course of treatment. Toohill and colleagues (134) used up to three cycles of cisplatin with infusion 5-fluorouracil, but reported a complete response rate of only 19%. This result was unexpected and remains in contrast to complete response rates of 46% and 54% achieved with the identical induction regimen at other institutions (93, 136). Institutional differences in the volume of disease treated and the intensity of drug administration may account for much of this difference. Schuller and colleagues (65) treated 82 patients with "resectable" advanced SCCHN using a 21-day, three-cycle regimen that contained less than maximal doses of cisplatin and recorded a complete response rate of 18%. Martin et al. (137) administered three cycles of full-dose cisplatin prior to local–regional treatment but noted a remarkably low complete response rate of 4%. Evaluation of this result is limited by its publication in abstract form. At present, it is not clear how many patients actually received three cycles of therapy, and it is uncertain whether the utilization of cisplatin on day 4 rather than on day 1 of treatment may have lessened the activity of this regimen.

One randomized prospective trial, the Veterans Administration Cooperative Study Project (VACSP No. 268), approximates the ideal in design and conduct (63). This recently completed study randomized patients with advanced, but resectable laryngeal carcinoma to receive either two courses of induction cisplatin and infusion 5-fluorouracil over 6 weeks or immediate laryngectomy and postoperative radiotherapy (Fig. 6.1). Patients who responded to two cycles of chemotherapy received a third cycle and then radiotherapy alone. In the latter group, laryngectomy is deferred until persistent or recurrent disease was documented despite radiotherapy. Patients who did not respond to induction chemotherapy received surgery and radiotherapy.

The first published report of the VACSP note that 332 patients with laryngeal cancer had been randomized either to laryngectomy and postoperative radiotherapy (166 patients) or to induction chemo-

therapy and perhaps radiotherapy alone (166 patients). While the overall rate of complete response was not mentioned, the report indicates that a complete clinical response was achieved at the primary site in 49% of patients completing three courses of chemotherapy. Complete pathologic regression of tumor has been documented at the primary site in 64% of 103 responding patients who were biopsied after chemotherapy. Of biopsied patients who had achieved a complete clinical response at the primary site, 88% were confirmed as having had a complete pathological response. Of 166 patients assigned to induction therapy, 107 (64%) had preservation of the larynx, and 59 (36%) underwent laryngectomy either before radiation (30 nonresponders to chemotherapy) or after radiation (29 patients with recurrent or persistent disease). To date, there is no significant difference in disease-free or overall survival between the two arms of this study. A significant difference in sites of failure has been noted, however, with fewer distant metastases and more local–regional relapses in those treated with chemotherapy.

That survival in the VACSP was not significantly improved by induction therapy is discouraging. It must be recalled, however, that this study was designed principally to demonstrate the ability of induction therapy to identify patients with a favorable response to chemotherapy that could be effectively managed with radiotherapy alone. Local–regional therapy was not equivalent between treatment groups and the impact of chemotherapy on overall survival could not be evaluated as an independent variable. The extent to which induction chemotherapy impacted on local–regional disease in the VACSP remains unclear given that this study did not contain a control group of patients treated with radiotherapy alone.

The success of the VACSP is found in its demonstration that induction chemotherapy and radiotherapy can be offered as an alternative to surgery and radiotherapy for selected patients with operable laryngeal cancers. Moreover, this study confirmed a significant effect of induction chemotherapy on dis-

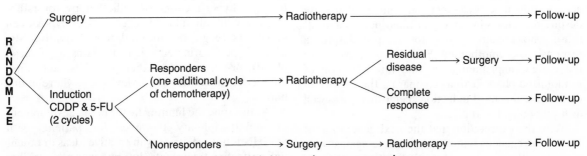

Fig. 6.1   **VA Cooperative Study: treatment of operable laryngeal squamous carcinoma**

tant metastases. Given that at least 17% (29/166) of patients required laryngectomy after chemotherapy and radiation, one wonders whether or not local–regional control and survival might have been improved if radiotherapy alone had not been offered to all patients with complete or partial response to chemotherapy.

In summary, of the two questions posed at the beginning of this section, only the second has been answered in the affirmative by randomized trial. Properly utilized, induction chemotherapy and radiotherapy can be offered to selected patients with advanced SCCHN with the expectation of improved quality of life and at least similar survival compared to results with surgery and radiotherapy. Confirmation of an improved survival with induction chemotherapy awaits the development of drug regimens with greater activity than cisplatin and infusion 5-fluorouracil, and the organization of randomized trials that are similar to the VACSP in their treatment of a large number of patients with limited heterogeneity of disease, but different in their use of comparable local–regional treatments.

Future Directions for Induction Chemotherapy

Despite over 25 years of active clinical investigation, a role for induction chemotherapy in the routine management of patients with advanced SCCHN has not been defined. As mentioned, continued progress in the development of this modality will require additional preclinical and clinical studies. Small animal models must clarify the influence of tumor type on the incidence of distant relapse after induction or adjuvant chemotherapy. More important to the situation with SCCHN, animal models must be developed that can evaluate the relative impact of induction or adjuvant chemotherapy on local–regional control of disease.

Phase I–II clinical studies of patients with previously untreated, M0 SCCHN must continue to develop induction regimens with potential antitumor activity that is greater than cisplatin and infusion 5-fluorouracil. Concurrent with this effort, phase II studies of induction chemotherapy must identify prognostic factors for response to chemotherapy, and define two subsets of patients: (1) those who can achieve adequate local–regional control of disease despite reductions in surgery or radiotherapy and (2) those who remain at risk for relapse despite a response to chemotherapy. Such data are crucial to the design, implementation, and interpretation of randomized phase II trials comparing the activity of different regimens of induction chemotherapy as well as future phase III studies.

With the expectation that the next generation of induction regimens will be more active against normal as well as malignant epithelial tissues, efforts must be made to broaden the therapeutic ratio for chemotherapy and limit normal tissue toxicity. At present, mucositis and myelosuppression are the principle toxicities that limit the delivery of induction chemotherapy. Recombinant human granulocyte colony stimulating factor (rhG–CSF), a myeloid growth factor, was serendipitously found to limit chemotherapy-associated mucositis (139) and may be useful in this regard.

Forthcoming prospective, randomized phase III trials of induction chemotherapy must determine the relative impact of the newer regimens of induction chemotherapy on overall survival, disease-free survival, quality of life, and financial cost of treatment. Such trials must have greater respect for biostatistical concerns than previous phase III studies. Considering the provocative results from the VACSP, it will be increasingly difficult to implement studies of induction chemotherapy that do not consider radiotherapy alone as local–regional treatment after chemotherapy. Treatment arms of phase III trials that evaluate quality of life as a principle objective (e. g., the VACSP) need not have comparable local–regional therapies and can offer radiotherapy alone to selected patients treated with induction chemotherapy and combined surgery and radiotherapy to control patients. Conversely, treatment arms of phase III studies that seek to document an improved survival with induction chemotherapy must have comparable local–regional therapies and should consider radiotherapy alone for both the experimental and control groups of patients. In studies of the latter design, surgery would be reserved for salvage patients with recurrent or persistent disease.

In the absence of a randomized phase III trial documenting a survival benefit with induction chemotherapy, clinicians cannot employ this modality as a standard treatment for patients with advanced SCCHN. Nonetheless, the preclinical and clinical foundation for the multidisciplinary treatment of many tumors, including SCCHN, with chemotherapy remains sound. Clinical investigators must continue their studies of induction chemotherapy as they must continue their analyses of other promising treatments for patients with SCCHN including concurrent chemotherapy and radiotherapy, adjuvant chemotherapy, intra-arterial chemotherapy, hyperfractionated radiotherapy, or radiotherapy with radiation sensitizers such as hypoxic cell sensitizers (e. g., the misonidazole derivative SR-2508), perfluorinated hydrocarbons (artificial blood), or regional hyperthermia. These and other adjunctive modalities are reviewed elsewhere in this book.

At this time the limiting factor in the development of multidisciplinary therapies for patients with SCCHN is not a deficiency in creative ideas or potentially effective treatments, but rather the availability of patients for clinical studies. The failure to consider patients for investigative treatment due to inappropriate pessimism, or false optimism with the injudicious use of "off-protocol" therapy must be discouraged. The probability that properly administered chemotherapy can improve the natural history of SCCHN is high.

References

1. Million RR, Cassisi NJ. Management of head and neck cancer, a multidisciplinary approach. Philadelphia: JB Lippincott, 1984.
2. Merino OR, Lindberg RD, Fletcher GH. An analysis of distant metastases from squamous cell carcinoma of the upper respiratory and digestive tracts. Cancer 1977; 40:145−51.
3. Snow JBJ, Gelber RD, Kramer S, et al. Randomized preoperative and postoperative radiation therapy for patients with carcinoma of the head and neck: preliminary report. Laryngoscope 1980; 90:930−45.
4. Vikram B, Strong EW, Shah JP, Spiro R. Failure at distant sites following multimodality treatment for advanced head and neck cancer. Head Neck Surg 1984; 6:730−3.
5. Jesse RH, Lindberg RD. The efficacy of combining radiation with a surgical procedure in patients with cervical metastasis from squamous cell cancer of the oropharynx and hypopharynx. Cancer 1975; 35:1163−6.
6. Carpenter RJ, DeSanto LW, Devine KD, et al. Cancer of the hypopharynx. Arch Otolaryngol 1976; 102:716−21.
7. Schuller DE, McGuirt WF, Krause CJ, et al. Symposium: Adjuvant cancer therapy of head and neck tumors. Increased survival with surgery alone vs. combined therapy. Laryngoscope 1979; 89:1735−8.
8. Skarin A, Jochelson M, Sheldon T, et al. Neoadjuvant chemotherapy in marginally resectable stage III M0 non-small cell lung cancer: Long-term follow-up in 41 patients. J Surg Oncol 1989; 40:266−74.
9. Dillman RO, Seagren SL, Probert K, et al. A randomized trial of induction chemotherapy plus high-dose radiation versus radiation alone in stage III non-small-cell lung cancer. New Engl J Med 1990; 323:940−5.
10. Eckardt JJ, Eilber FR, Grant TT, et al. Management of stage IIB osteogenic sarcoma: experience at the University of California, Los Angeles. Cancer Treat Symp 1985; 3:117−30.
11. Rosen G, Nirenberg A. Neoadjuvant chemotherapy for osteogenic sarcoma: a five-year follow-up (T-10) and preliminary report of new studies (T-12). In: Wagener DJ, Blijham GH, Smeets, JBE, Wils A, eds. Primary chemotherapy in cancer medicine. New York: Alan R Liss, 1985:39−51.
12. Winkler K, Beron G, Kotz RS, et al. Neo-adjuvant chemotherapy for osteogenic sarcoma: results of a cooperative German−Austrian study. J Clin Oncol 1984; 2:617−24.
13. Loprinzi CL, Carbone PP, Tormey DC, et al. Aggressive combined modality therapy for advanced local−regional breast carcinoma. J Clin Oncol 1984; 2:157−63.
14. Zylerberg B, Salat-Baroux J, Ravina JH, et al. Initial chemotherapy in infiltrating cancer in the breast. Cancer 1982; 49:1537−43.
15. Sherry MM, Johnson DH, Page DL, et al. Inflammatory carcinoma of the breast: Clinical review and summary of the Vanderbilt experience with multimodality therapy. Am J Med 1985; 79:355−64.
16. Hortobagyi GN, Ames FC, Buzdar AU, et al. Management of stage III primary breast cancer with primary chemotherapy, surgery and radiation therapy. Cancer 1988; 62:2507−16.
17. Ragavan D. First-line cisplatinum for invasive clinically nonmetastatic bladder cancer. In: Garnick MB, ed. Genitourinary cancer. New York: Churchill Livingstone, 1985: 193−207.
18. Ragavan D. Pre-emptive (neo-adjuvant) intravenous chemotherapy for invasive bladder cancer. Br J Urol 1988; 61:1−8.
19. Scher HI, Yagoda A, Steinberg CN, et al. Neo-adjuvant M-VAC for transitional cell carcinoma of the urothelium (abstr #417). Proc Am Soc Clin Oncol 1986; 5:108.
20. Goldie J, Coldman A. A mathematical model for relating the drug sensitivity of tumors to their spontaneous mutation rate. Cancer Treat Rep 1979; 63:1727−33.
21. Goldie J, Coldman A. Quantitative model for multiple levels of drug resistance in clinical tumors. Cancer Treat Rep 1983; 67:923−31.
22. DeVita V. The relationship between tumor mass and resistance to chemotherapy. Cancer 1983; 51:1209.
23. Van Putten L. Optimal timing of adjuvant chemotherapy in mouse modes. In: Wagener D, Blijham G, Smeets J, Wils R, eds. Primary chemotherapy in cancer medicine. New York: Alan R Liss, 1985:15−21.
24. Mulder JH, de Ruiter J, Edelstein MB et al. Model studies in adjuvant chemotherapy. Cancer Treat Rep 1983; 67:45.
25. Fisher D, Gunduz N, Saffer EA. Influence of the interval between primary tumor removal and chemotherapy on kinetics and growth of metastases. Cancer Res 1983; 43:1488−92.
26. Griswold DPJ. The potential for murine tumor models in surgical adjuvant chemotherapy. Cancer Chemother Rep 1975; 5:187−204.
27. Griswold DRJ, Corbett TH. Breast tumor modeling for prognosis and treatment. In: St Arneault G, Band P, Israel L, eds. Recent results in cancer research. Berlin: Springer, 1976:42−58.
28. Mayo JG, Laster WRJ, Andrews CM et al. Success and failure in the treatment of solid tumors. III. "Cure" of metastatic Lewis lung carcinoma with methyl-CCNU (NSC-95441) and surgery−chemotherapy. Cancer Chemother Rep 1972; 56:183−95.
29. Schabel FJ. Concepts for treatment of micrometastases developed in murine systems. Am J Roentgenol 1976; 126:500−11.
30. Schabel FJ. Surgical adjuvant chemotherapy of metastatic murine tumors. Cancer 1977; 40:558−68.
31. Schabel FJ. Recent studies with surgical adjuvant chemotherapy or immunotherapy of metastatic solid tumors of mice. In: Tones S, Salmon S, eds. Adjuvant therapy of cancer II. Orlando: Grune & Stratton, 1979:3−17.
32. Schabel FMJ. The use of tumor growth kinetics in planning "curative" chemotherapy of advanced solid tumors. Cancer Res. 1969; 29:2384−9.
33. Simpson-Herren L, Sanford AH, Holmquist JP. Effects of surgery on the cell kinetics of residual tumor. Cancer Treat Rep 1976; 60:1749−60.
34. Gunduz N, Fisher B, Saffer EA. Effect of surgical removal on the growth and kinetics of residual tumor. Cancer Res 1979; 39:3861−5.
35. Lange PH, Hekmat K, Bosl G, et al. Accelerated growth of testicular cancer after cytoreductive surgery. Cancer 1980; 45:1498−506.
36. Burgert EO, Glidewell O. Dactinomycin in Wilms' tumor. JAMA 1967; 199:464−68.
37. Nissen-Meyer R, Kjellgren K, Malmio K, et al. Surgical adjuvant chemotherapy: Results with one short course with cyclophosphamide after mastectomy for breast cancer. Cancer 1978; 41:2088−98.
38. Nissen-Meyer R, Host H, Kjellgren K, et al. Scandinavian trials with a short postoperative course versus a 12-cycle course. Recent Results Cancer Res 1984; 96:48−54.
39. Buzdar AU, Smith TL, Powell KD, et al. Effect of timing of initiation of adjuvant chemotherapy on disease-free survival in breast cancer. Breast Cancer Res Treat 1982; 2:163−9.
40. Glucksberg H, Rivkin SE, Rasmussen S, et al. Combination chemotherapy (CMFVP) versus 1-phenylalanine mustard (L-PAM) for operable breast cancer with positive axillary nodes: a Southwest Oncology Group Study. Cancer 1982; 50:423−34.
41. Taylor SG, Kalish LA, Olson JE, et al. Adjuvant CMFP versus CMFP plus tamoxiphen versus observation alone in post-menopausal, node-positive breast cancer patients: three-year results of an Eastern Cooperative Group study. J Clin Oncol 1985; 3:144−54.
42. Ludwig Breast Cancer Study Group: Combination adjuvant chemotherapy for node-positive breast cancer. N. Engl J Med 1988; 319:677−83.

43. Ragaz R. Emerging modalities for adjuvant therapy of breast cancer: Neoadjuvant chemotherapy. NCI Monogr 1986; 1:145−52.

44. Hrynuik WM. The importance of dose intensity in outcome of chemotherapy. In: DeVita VT Jr, Hellman S, Rosenberg SA, eds. Important advances in oncology. Philadelphia: JB Lippincott, 1988;121−41.

45. Head and Neck Contracts Program. Adjuvant chemotherapy for advanced head and neck squamous carcinoma. Final report of the Head and Neck Contracts Program. Cancer 1987; 60:301−11.

46. Ervin TJ, Clark JR, Weichselbaum RR, et al. An analysis of induction and adjuvant chemotherapy in the multidisciplinary treatment of squamous-cell carcinoma of the head and neck. J Clin Oncol 1987; 5:10−20.

47. Rheinhold, HS, Buisman GH, Radiosensitivity of capillary endothelium. Br J Radiol 1973; 46:54−7.

48. Rubin P, Casarett GW. Clinical radiation pathology. Philadelphia: WB Saunders, 1968.

49. Rubens RD, Knight RK, Fentmen IS, et al. Controlled trial of adjuvant chemotherapy with melphalan for breast cancer. Lancet 1983; 1:839−43.

50. Ludwig Breast Cancer Study Group. Randomized trial of chemo-endocrine therapy, endocrine therapy, and mastectomy alone in post-menopausal patients with operable breast cancer and axillary node metastases. Lancet 1984; 1:1256−60.

51. Bonnadona G, Valagrussa P, Rossi A, et al. Ten year experience with CMF-based adjuvant chemotherapy in resectable breast cancer. Breast Cancer Res Treat 1985; 5:95−115.

52. Benjamin RS, Chawla SP, Murray JA, et al. Response to preoperative chemotherapy of osteosarcoma improves disease-free survival and the chances of limb salvage (abstr). Proc Am Assoc Cancer Res 1985; 26:174.

53. Rosen G, Caparros B, Huvos AG, et al. Preoperative chemotherapy for osteogenic sarcoma: selection of postoperative adjuvant chemotherapy based on the response of the primary tumor to preoperative chemotherapy. Cancer 1982; 49:1221−30.

54. Crisman JD, Liu WY, Gluckman LJ, et al. Prognostic value of histopathologic parameters in squamous cell carcinoma of the oropharynx. Cancer 1984; 54:2995−3001.

55. Boheim K, Spoendlin H. The effect of chemotherapy in relation to pathohistologic tumor grading in head and neck cancer. Arch Otorhinolaryngol 1984; 238:197−204.

56. Milas L, Malenica B, Allergretti N. Enhancement of artificial pulmonary metastasis in mice caused by cyclophosphamide. Cancer Immunol Immunother 1979; 6:191.

57. Steel GG, Adams K. Enhancement by cytotoxic agents of artificial pulmonary metastasis. Br J Cancer 1977; 36:653.

58. Carmel RJ, Brown JM. The effect of cyclophosphamide and other drugs on the incidence of pulmonary metastases in mice. Cancer Res 1977; 37:145.

59. Van Putten LM, Kram LKJ, Van Dierendonck HH, et al. Enhancement by drugs of metastatic lung nodule formation after intravenous tumor cell injection. Int J Cancer 1975; 15:588−959.

60. Moore JV, Dixon B. Metastasis of a transplantable mammary tumor in rats treated with cyclophosphamide and or radiation. Br J Cancer 1977; 36:221.

61. Poupon LM, Pauwels C, Jasmin C, et al. An implicit pulmonary metastasis of rat rhabdomyosarcoma in response to nitrosourea treatment. Cancer Treat Rep 1984; 68:749−58.

62. Kerbel RS, Davis AJS. Facilitation of tumor progression by cancer therapy. Lancet 1982; 2:997.

63. Department of Veterans Affairs Laryngeal Cancer Study Group. Induction chemotherapy plus radiation compared with surgery plus radiation in patients with advanced laryngeal cancer. New Engl J Med 1991; 24:1685−90.

64. Toohill RJ, Duncavage JA, Grossman TW, et al. The effects of delay in standard treatment due to induction chemotherapy in two randomized prospective studies. Laryngoscope 1987; 97:407−11.

65. Schuller DE, Metch B, Stein DW, et al. Preoperative chemotherapy in advanced resectable head and neck cancer− Final report of the Southwest Oncology Group. Laryngoscope 1988; 98:1205−11.

66. Adelstein DJ, Sharan VM, Earle AS, et al. A prospective randomized trial of simultaneous vs. sequential chemoradiotherapy for squamous head and neck cancer (abstr #648). Proc Am Soc Clin Oncol 1989; 8:167.

67. SECOG. A randomized trial of combined multidrug chemotherapy and radiotherapy in advanced squamous cell carcinoma of the head and neck. Eur J Surg Oncol 1986; 12:289−95.

68. Merlano M, Rosso R, Sertoli MR, et al. Sequential versus alternating chemotherapy and radiotherapy in stage III−IV squamous cell carcinoma of the head and neck: a phase III study. J Clin Oncol 1988; 6:627−32.

69. Ozols RF, Masuda H, Hamilton TC. Keynote address: Mechanisms of cross-resistance between radiation and antineoplastic drugs. NCI Monogr 1988:6:159.

70. Ensley JF, Jacobs JR, Weaver A, et al. Correlation between response to cisplatinum–combination chemotherapy and subsequent radiotherapy in previously untreated patients with advanced squamous cell cancers of the head and neck. Cancer 1984; 54:811−14.

71. Hong WK, O'Donohue GM, Sheetz S, et al. Sequential response patterns in head and neck cancer: potential impact of treatment in advanced laryngeal cancer. In: Wagener DJT, Blijham GH, Smeets JBE, eds. Primary chemotherapy in cancer medicine. New York: Alan R Liss, 1985:191−7.

72. Hill BT, Price LA, MacRae K. Importance of primary site in assessing chemotherapy response and 7-year survival data in advanced squamous-cell carcinomas of the head and neck treated with initial combination chemotherapy without cisplatin. J Clin Oncol 1986; 4:1340−7.

73. Browman GP, Levine MN, Russell R, et al. Survival results from a phase III study of simultaneous versus 1-hour sequential methotrexate-5-fluorouracil chemotherapy in head and neck cancer. Head Neck Surg 1986; 8:146−52.

74. Glick JH, Marcial V, Richter M, et al. The adjuvant treatment of inoperable stage III and IV epidermoid carcinoma of the head and neck with platinum and bleomycin infusions prior to definitive radiotherapy. Cancer 1980; 46:1919−24.

75. Urba SG, Forastiere AA. Systemic therapy of head and neck cancer: most effective agents, areas of promise. Oncology 1989; 3:79−88.

76. Clark JR, Frei E III. Chemotherapy for head and neck cancer: progress and controversy in the management of patients with M0 disease. Semin Oncol 1989; 16(suppl 6):44−57.

77. Choksi AJ, Dimery IW, Hong WK. Adjuvant chemotherapy of head and neck cancer: the past, the present, and the future. Semin Oncol 1988; 15(suppl 3):45−59.

78. Condit PT, Ridings GR, Coin JW, et al. Methotrexate and radiation in the treatment of patients with cancer. Cancer Res 1964; 24:1524−33.

79. Friedman M, DeNarvaes FN, Daly JF. Treatment of squamous cell carcinoma of the head and neck with combined methotrexate and irradiation. Cancer 1970; 26:711−21.

80. Tarpley JL, Chretien PB, Alexander JC, et al. High dose methotrexate as a preoperative adjuvant in the treatment of epidermoid carcinoma of the head and neck. Am J Surg 1975; 130:481−6.

81. Ervin TJ, Kirkwood J, Weichselbaum RR, et al. Improved survival for patients with advanced carcinoma of the head and neck treated with methotrexate–leucovorin prior to definitive radiotherapy of surgery. Laryngoscope 1981; 7:1181−90.

82. Popkin JD, Hong WK, Bromer RH, et al. Induction bleomycin infusion in head and neck cancer. Am J Clin Oncol 1984; 7:199−204.

83. Jacobs C, Bertino JR, Goffinet DR, et al. 24-Hour infusion of cis-platinum in head and neck cancers. Cancer 1984; 42:2135−40.

84. Wittes R, Heller K, Randolf V, et al. Cis-diammineplatinum (II)-based chemotherapy as initial treatment of advanced head and neck cancer. Cancer Treat Rep 1979; 63:1533−8.

85. Schaefer SD, Middleton R, Reisch J, et al. Cis-platinum induction chemotherapy in the multi-modality initial treatment of advanced stage IV carcinoma of the head and neck. Cancer 1983; 51:2168−74.

86. Gad-El-Mawla N, Abul-Ela M, Mansour MA, et al. Preoperative adjuvant chemotherapy in relatively advanced head and neck cancer. Am J Clin Oncol 1984; 7:195−8.

87. Taylor SG, Applebaum E, Showel JL, et al. A randomized trial of adjuvant chemotherapy in head and neck cancer. J Clin Oncol 1985; 3:672−9.

88. von Essen CF, Joseph LBM, Simon GT, et al. Sequential chemotherapy and radiation therapy of buccal mucosal carcinoma in South India. Am J Roentgenol 1968; 102:530−40.

89. Knowlton AH, Percarpio B, Bobrow S, et al. Methotrexate and radiation therapy in the treatment of advanced head and neck tumors. Radiology 1975; 116:709−12.

90. Frazekas JT, Sommer C, Kramer S. Adjuvant intravenous methotrexate of definitive radiotherapy alone for advanced cancers of the oral cavity, oropharynx, supraglottic larynx or hypopharynx. Int J Radiat Oncol Biol Phys 1980; 6:533−41.

91. Peppard SB, Al-Sarraf M, Powers WE, Loh JK, Weaver AW. Combination of cis-platinum, oncovin, and bleomycin prior to surgery and/or radiotherapy in advanced untreated epidermoid cancer of the head and neck. Laryngoscope 1980; 90:1273−80.

92. Jacobs C, Goffinet DR, Goffinet L, Kohler M, Fee WE. Chemotherapy as a substitute for surgery in the treatment advanced resectable head and neck cancer. A report from the Northern California Oncology Group. Cancer 1987; 60:1178−83.

93. Weaver A, Fleming S, Ensley J, et al. Superior clinical response and survival rates with initial bolus of cisplatin and 120 hour infusion of 5-fluorouracil before definitive therapy for locally advanced head and neck cancer. Am J Surg 1984; 148:525−9.

94. Amrein PC, Weitzman SA. Treatment of squamous-cell carcinoma of the head and neck with cisplatin and 5-fluorouracil. J Clin Oncol 1985; 3:1632−9.

95. Spaulding MB, Kahn A, De Los Santos R, Kloth D, Lore JMJ. Adjuvant chemotherapy in advanced head and neck cancer. Am J Surg 1982; 144:432−6.

96. Rooney M, Kish J, Jacobs J, et al. Improved complete response rate and survival in advanced head and neck cancer after three-course induction therapy with 120-hour 5-FU infusion and cisplatin. Cancer 1985; 55:1123−8.

97. Clark JR, Fallon BG, Dreyfuss AI, et al. Chemotherapeutic strategies in the multidisciplinary treatment of head and neck cancer. Semin Oncol 1988; 15(suppl 3):35−44.

98. Fallon BG, Clark JR, Norris CM, Jr, et al. Induction chemotherapy for advanced squamous cell carcinoma of the head and neck: an analysis of clinical and histopathologic correlates after a complete response to chemotherapy. In: Wolf GT, Carey TE, eds. Head and Neck Oncology Research, Amsterdam, Berkeley: Kugler and Ghedini, 1987:281−6.

99. Al-Kourainy K, Kish J, Ensley J, et al. Achievement of superior survival for histologically negative versus histologically positive clinically complete responders to cisplatin combination chemotherapy in patients with locally advanced head and neck cancer. Cancer 1987; 59:233−8.

100. Kies MS, Gordon LI, Hauck WW, et al. Analysis of complete responders after initial treatment with chemotherapy in head and neck cancer. Otolaryngol Head Neck Surg 1985; 93:199−205.

101. Norris CM, Jr, Clark JR, Frei E III, et al. Pathology of surgery after induction chemotherapy: An analysis of resectability and locoregional control. Laryngoscope 1986; 96:292−302.

102. Weichselbaum RR, Clark JR, Miller D, et al. Combined modality treatment of head and neck cancer with cisplatin, bleomycin, methotrexate–leucovorin chemotherapy. Cancer 1985; 55:2149−55.

103. Pennacchio JL, Hong WK, Shapshay S, et al. Combination of cis-platin and bleomycin prior to surgery and/or radiotherapy compared with radiotherapy alone for the treatment of advanced squamous cell carcinoma of the head and neck. Cancer 1982; 50:2795−801.

104. Clark J, Fallon B, Weichselbaum R, et al. The influence of resectability on response to induction chemotherapy and survival in advanced squamous cell carcinoma of the head and neck (abstr). Proc Am Soc Clin Oncol 1985; 4:139.

105. Cognetti FC, Pinnaro P, Ruggeri EM, et al. Prognostic factors for chemotherapy response and survival using combination chemotherapy as initial treatment of advanced head and neck squamous cell cancer. J Clin Oncol 1989; 7:829−37.

106. Spaulding MB, Vasquez J, Khan A, Sundquist N, Lore JM. A nontoxic adjuvant treatment for advanced head and neck cancer. Arch Otolaryngol 1983; 109:789−91.

107. Hong WK, Popkin J, Bromer R, et al. Adjuvant chemotherapy as initial treatment of advanced head and neck cancer: survival data at three years. In: Jones SE, Salmon SE, eds. Adjuvant therapy of cancer, vol IV. Philadelphia: Grune & Stratton, 1984:127−34.

108. Ensley JF, Kish JA, Weaver AA, et al. The correlation of specific variables of tumor differentiation with response rate and survival in patients with advanced head and neck cancer treated with induction chemotherapy. Cancer 1988; 63:1487−92.

109. Posner MR, Weichselbaum RR, Fitzgerald TJ, et al. Treatment complications after sequential combination chemotherapy and radiotherapy with or without surgery in previously untreated squamous cell carcinoma of the head and neck. Int J Radiat Oncol Biol Phys 1985; 11:1887−93.

110. Clavel M, Cappelaere P, De Mulder P, et al. Cisplatin, methotrexate, bleomycin, vincristine (CABO), versus cisplatin–fluorouracil (CF) versus cisplatin alone in recurrent and metatstic head and neck squamous cell carcinoma (abstr 212). Proceedings of the Second International Conference on Head Neck Cancer, Boston, 1988:101.

111. Forastiere AA, Natale RB, Takasugi BJ, et al. A phase I−II trial of carboplatin and 5-fluorouracil combination chemotherapy in advanced carcinoma of the head and neck. J Clin Oncol 1987; 5:190−6.

112. Oliver IN, Bishop JF, Woods R, et al. Carboplatin and continuous infusion 5-fluorouracil in advanced head and neck cancer (abstr). Proc Am Soc Clin Oncol 1987; 6:124.

113. Volling P. Carboplatin: the better platinum in head and neck cancer. Arch Otolaryngol Head Neck Surg 1989; 115:695−8.

114. Lokich J, Zipoli T, Green R. Infusional cisplatin plus cyclophosphamide in advanced ovarian cancer. Cancer 1986; 58:2389−92.

115. Salem P, Khalyl M, Jabboury K, et al. cis-Diaminedichloroplatinum (II) by 5-day continuous infusion. A new schedule with minimal toxicity. Cancer 1984; 53:837−40.

116. Salem P, Hall SW, Bemjamin RS, et al. Clinical phase I−II study of cis-dichlorodi-aminineplatinum (II) given by continuous i.v. infusion. Cancer Treat Rep 1978; 62:1553−5.

117. Posner MR, Skarin AT, Clark J, et al. Phase I study of continuous infusion cisplatin. Cancer Treat Rep 1986; 70:847−50.

118. Posner MR, Ferrari L, Belliveau JF, et al. A phase I trial of continuous infusion cisplatin. Cancer 1987; 59:15−18.

119. Lokich JJ. Phase I study of cis-dichlorodi-aminineplatinum (II) administered as a constant 5-day infusion. Cancer Treat Rep 1980; 64:905−8.

120. Forastiere AA, Belliveau JF, Goren PG, et al. Pharmacokinetic and toxicity evaluation of five-day continuous infusion versus intermittent bolus cis-di-aminedichloroplatinum (II) in head and neck cancer patients. Cancer Res 1988; 48:3869−74.

121. Kish JA, Ensley JF, Jacobs JR, Binns P, Al-Sarraf M. Evaluation of high-dose cisplatin and 5-FU infusion as initial therapy in advanced head and neck cancer. Am J Clin Oncol 1988; 11:553−7.

122. Vokes EE, Choi KE, Schilsky RL, et al. Cisplatin, fluorouracil, and high-dose leucovorin for recurrent or metastatic head and neck cancer. J Clin Oncol 1988; 6:618−26.

123. Clark J, Dreyfuss A, Busse P, et al. Continuous infusion cisplatin, 5-FU and high-dose leucovorin: an induction therapy for SCCHN with high rates of complete response and radiotherapy alone as primary site management. In: Salmon SE, ed. Adjuvant therapy of cancer, vol IV. Philadelphia: WB Saunders, 1990:71−81.

124. Loeffler TM, Lindemann J, Luckhaupt H, Rose KG, Hausamen TU. Chemotherapy of advanced and relapsed squamous cell cancer of the head and neck with split-dose cisplatinum, 5-fluoruracil and leucovorin. Adv Exp Med Biol 1988; 244:267−73.

125. Grem JL, Hoth DF, Hamilton JM, King SA, Leyland-Jones B. Overview of current status and future direction of clinical trials with 5-fluorouracil in combination with folinic acid. Cancer Treat Rep 1987; 71:1249–64.

126. Ensley J, Kish J, Tapazoglou E, et al. An intensive, five course, alternating combination chemotherapy induction regimen used in patients with advanced, unresectable head and neck cancer. J Clin Oncol 1988; 6:1147–53.

127. Ensley J, Kish J, Tapazoglou E, et al. Continued intensification of an alternating regimen in patients with advanced, untreated squamous cancers of the head and neck (abstr #598). Proc Am Soc Clin Oncol 1988; 7:154.

128. Norton L, Simon R. Tumor size, sensitivity to chemotherapy, and the design of treatment schedules. Cancer Treat Rep 1977; 61:1307–17.

129. Norton L, Simon R. The Norton–Simon hypothesis revisited. Cancer Treat Rep 1986; 70:163–9.

130. Mayer RJ. Current chemotherapeutic treatment approaches to the management of previously untreated adults with de novo acute myelogenous leukemia. Semin Oncol 1987; 14:384–6.

131. Takvorian T, Canellos GP, Ritz J, et al. Prolonged disease-free survival after autologous bone marrow transplantation in patients with non-Hodgkin's lymphoma with a poor prognosis. N Engl J Med 1987; 316:1499–505.

132. Stewart FM, Lazarus HM, Levine PA, et al. High-dose chemotherapy and autologous marrow transplantation for esthesioneuroblastoma and sinonasal undifferentiated carcinoma. Am J Clin Oncol 1989; 12:217–21.

133. Kun LE, Toohill RJ, Holoye PY, et al. A randomized study of adjuvant chemotherapy for cancer of the upper aerodigestive tract. Int J Radiat Oncol Biol Phys 1986; 12:173–8.

134. Toohill RJ, Anderson T, Byhardt RW, et al. Cisplatin and fluorouracil as neoadjuvant therapy in head and neck cancer. A preliminary report. Arch Otolaryngol Head Neck Surg 1987; 113:758–61.

135. Stell PM, Dalby JE, Strickland R, et al. Sequential chemotherapy and radiotherapy in advanced head and neck cancer. Clin Radiol 1983; 34:463–7.

136. Martin M, Hazen A, Vergnes L, et al. Randomized study of 5-fluorouracil and cisplatin as neoadjuvant therapy in head and neck cancer: a preliminary report. Int J Radiat Oncol Phys 1990; 19:973–5.

137. Martin M, Mazeron JJ, Brun B, et al. Neo-adjuvant polychemotherapy of head and neck cancer: results of a randomized study (abstr #590). Proc Am Soc Clin Oncol 1988; 7:152.

138. Carugati A, Pradier R, de la Torre A. Combination chemotherapy pre-radical treatment for head and neck squamous cell carcinoma (abstr #589). Proc Am Soc Clin Oncol 1988; 7:152.

139. Garbrilove JL, Jarubowski A, Scher H, et al. Effect of granulocyte colony-stimulating factor on neutropenia and associated morbidity due to chemotherapy for transitional-cell carcinoma of the urothelium. N Engl J Med 1988; 318:1414–22.

Adjuvant Chemotherapy for Advanced Squamous Cell Carcinoma of the Head and Neck

J. B. Vermorken

Introduction

Squamous cell carcinomas of the head and neck region form a heterogeneous group of diseases with different biologic behavior and have a variety of outcomes. Overall, only one-third of patients present with localized disease easily curable by surgery and radiotherapy. Five-year survival rates in these circumstances vary from 70–90% (1–4). These treatment methods, however, have not provided adequate tumor control in the majority of patients who present with advanced local and regional disease. Despite optimal local treatment, local tumor control remains a significant problem, with local or regional recurrence in up to 50% of cases. Distant metastases develop in 10–30% of patients and second primaries and other medical problems account for the remainder of deaths (2, 5–8). Five-year survival rates for patients with advanced, resectable tumors range from 10–60% (5, 6, 8, 9). Unfortunately, even though local control of cancer above the clavicles has clearly improved with modern surgical and radiotherapeutic techniques, this survival rate has remained more or less the same over the past two decades. This is partly due to a changing pattern of failure and partly to an ever increasing number of second primary tumors that appear in head and neck cancer patients as time elapses from the definitive treatment of their primary cancer (7, 8, 10–12). It seems therefore reasonable to assume that important improvements in the long-term survival of patients with resectable head and neck cancer will probably not result from further refinement of these local therapies. However, the use of adjunctive systemic therapies, the development of more sophisticated methods for prevention, early detection, and effective treatment of second primary tumors might have greater impact.

The role of chemotherapy in the management of patients with head and neck cancer has been reserved historically for patients with metastatic disease or those with locally recurrent disease after maximal surgery or radiotherapy. Although the use of chemotherapy may be beneficial in these circumstances in terms of palliation, a major impact on survival is not evident. During the past 10 years, tremendous interest has arisen in using chemotherapy as part of the initial treatment of patients with advanced squamous cell carcinoma of the head and neck. In this multidisciplinary approach, chemotherapy can be used before definitive local therapy (induction chemotherapy), concomitantly with radiotherapy (simultaneous chemoradiotherapy), or after local treatments (adjuvant chemotherapy per se). There are three theoretical mechanisms whereby chemotherapy may be effective in these circumstances: initial tumor shrinkage, sensitization to radiotherapy, and eradication of micrometastases. This chapter will focus on the potential role of adjuvant chemotherapy (including both the classical adjuvant chemotherapy and adjuvant chemotherapy after induction chemotherapy) within the multimodal approach of patients with locally advanced squamous cell carcinoma of the head and neck.

Incidence of Distant Metastases

In 1906, Crile quoted the work of Hutchings who stated that metastases below the clavicle were found at autopsy in only one per cent of 4500 patients with head and neck cancer (13).

Although this reference was never documented, for a long time it has had its influence on the general conception that the occurrence of distant metastases in head and neck cancer was a rare event. As late as 1928, Dorrance and McShane reported that no distant metastases were found at autopsy in 15 patients with head and neck cancer at the Philadelphia General Hospital (14).

This idea has changed in the 1930s (15) when autopsy data reported in the period 1930–1950 indicated an incidence of distant metastases varying from 20–40% depending on the site of the primary tumor (16–22). Reports from the period 1960–1987 mention an even higher incidence, of 40–57% (23–26). Kotwall et al. (26), in their retrospective review of all head and neck cancer patients who died at Roswell Park Memorial Institute from 1961 to 1985, found histologically confirmed distant metastases at one or more sites in 387 of the 832 patients autopsied (47%). This study is of interest as it includes patients who have been treated in an era when the shift toward multimodality treatment of the head and neck cancer patients had taken place. Contrary to these autopsy data are the reports on the incidence of distant metastases based on the clinical findings. Generally, the figures presented are of a lower order, 5–25% (8, 10, 27–31). A comparison of these clinical data with those of autopsy studies is difficult to make. The percentages mentioned in the clinical reports most probably underestimate the magnitude of the development of distant metastases, as many patients did not live long enough to allow metastases to be detected clinically. On the other hand, several autopsy studies may have resulted in a percentage which is too high due to the fact that in some of these series there may have been a bias towards cases with distant metastases. Nevertheless, whatever the exact figure there will be a significant number of patients with locally advanced head and neck cancer who will develop distant metastases. Whereas distant metastases in many previous studies were often preceded by failure above the clavicle, with the more effective locoregional treatment available nowadays, distant metastases have become a major cause of mortality in these patients (8, 29). Selection of patients who are at high risk of developing distant metastases is therefore essential.

Patients at High Risk of Developing Distant Metastases

In none of the autopsy studies in the literature has there been a predominant site with a high incidence of distant metastases, mainly because of the relatively small number of cancers at each primary site. However, Dennington et al. (25) suggested that the probability of distant metastases was relatively high in patients with tumors of the nasopharynx, base of the tongue, and hypopharynx and particularly in patients with poorly differentiated carcinomas of the nasopharynx such as the lymphoepitheliomas. Also in the study of Kotwall et al. (26) the hypopharynx and base of the tongue had the highest incidence of distant metastases at the time of death (60% and 53%, respectively). In several studies the stage of the disease at presentation had a major impact, concerning both T stage (T3 and T4 lesions having the highest probability) and N stage (N2 and N3 > N1 and N0) (10, 21, 25, 26, 28, 29). Kotwall et al. (26) found the highest incidence of distant metastases in patients with stage IV disease (55%).

Both the study of Berger et al. (28) and Merino et al. (10) indicated that the rate of distant metastases correlated more with the appearance of cervical node metastases than with the T stage. These last two studies in contrast to the study of Kotwall did not include autopsy data. Distant metastases were observed in 12.5% in patients with N0/N1 stage versus 30.3% in those with N2/N3 stage in the first study (28). Therefore, not only for local recurrence, but also for the development of distant metastases the status of the cervical lymph nodes continues to be the single most important prognostic factor (32).

Of a series of 331 patients who underwent 383 radical neck dissections between 1973 and 1983 at the Free University Hospital, in Amsterdam, 78 (23.5%) developed distant metastases. Minimum follow-up period for these patients was 2 years and only 1 patient was lost to follow-up. Those who were found to have histologically positive nodes had a significantly greater likelihood of subsequent distant metastases than those who had histologically negative neck specimens (32). However, a further refinement in determining prognosis could be made by applying histologic prognostic factors. Extracapsular spread (ECS) and the number of positive nodes in that respect are considered the two histologic factors that are of most prognostic significance (33–42). Considering these two parameters it was found that patients with four or more positive nodes and ECS had a greater than 60% likelihood of developing distant metastases. This was significantly worse than in patients with only one histologically positive node with ECS, stressing the importance of a thorough investigation of the specimen.

It is important to mention that in the latter study more than 80% of distant metastases manifested within 2 years after radical neck dissection, a phenomenon that has also been reported by others (10, 29).

Rationale for Adjuvant Chemotherapy

Since distant metastases seem to become a growing problem in the treatment of patients with locally advanced head and neck cancer (see above), and chemotherapy or combined modality treatments fail to cure patients after recurrence of disease, the need for adjuvant therapy has arisen. An important question for the basis of such a treatment is whether squamous cell carcinoma of the head and neck has to be considered as a locoregional disease or a systemic disease. Crile (43) stated in 1923 that: "The collar of lymphatics about the neck forms an almost impossible barrier through which cancer rarely penetrates and every portion of their barrier is readily accessible to the surgeon." In this "contiguous hypothesis" the lymph nodes function as a barrier and the nodes are the instigator of distant spread. Contrary to this hypothesis is the later developed "systemic hypothesis," as described by Fischer et al. for breast cancer (44−47), whereby the regional lymph nodes are considered ineffective as barriers to tumor cell spread. These lymph nodes have a greater biological than anatomic importance and the bloodstream is considered of great importance in tumor dissemination with the disease being considered systemic from its conception. This last hypothesis was based on both laboratory and clinical investigations (44−47).

The biological rationale which, during the early 1970s led to the design of adjuvant chemotherapy studies was derived from studies performed in experimental animal systems (48, 49), which showed an inverse relationship between tumor cell burden and curability with chemotherapy and moreover indicated that the efficacy of chemotherapy was dose-dependent and related to the presence of resistant cells. The increased sensitivity of subclinical tumors was believed to result from their high growth fraction, shorter cell cycle time, and therefore greater fractional cell kill for a given dose of drug (50). When the same tumors increase in size (ultimately going from subclinical to clinical) their growth fraction falls, cell cycle time lengthens, sensitivity to treatment becomes less, the probability of cure diminishes, and ultimately will be lost. Not only are these alterations in cell kinetics related to tumor volume, but also the observation that in some tumors removal of the primary tumor leads to an increase in the labeling index of metastases has contributed to the enthusiasm in applying adjuvant chemotherapy (51, 52). However, tumor volume itself is not as good a predictor of curability in the clinic as one would have expected on the basis of available cell kinetic data (53). Certain bulky tumors (e.g. Burkitt lymphoma) can be eradicated with drug combinations. Contrary to this, drug combinations as adjuvants to surgery or radiotherapy in tumors such as lung cancer and colon cancer (both frequently occurring),

are no more effective than the same treatment in patients with advanced disease.

A more important consideration is the relationship of tumor cell resistance to tumor bulk. As stressed by Goldie and Coldman (54, 55), the probability of a tumor population containing resistant cells is a function of the total number of cells present (see below). Therefore, subclinical tumors are more likely than metastatic tumors to be cured by a specific schedule or type of chemotherapy.

Tumor Heterogeneity and Primary Drug Resistance

Late in the 1970s treatment failure began to find a more plausible explanation through new concepts dealing with tumor heterogeneity (56, 57) and primary drug resistance (54, 55). Tumors were viewed as complex entities with diverse cell populations that were heterogeneous for a variety of biological characteristics and included clones with metastatic potential and variants showing drug resistance. The number of the cellular subpopulations and their properties were thought to be constantly changing, not just in relation to selection pressures but also as a consequence of interactions, between the subpopulations themselves. Interactions between clonal subpopulations have a significant effect on the rate at which new subpopulations with altered metastatic properties are created. Of particular interest was the finding that events that restricted subpopulation diversity generated new variants. In fact, the question was raised as to whether restriction of cellular diversity via therapeutic elimination of susceptible cellular subpopulation would not stimulate the rate of formation of new variant tumor cells from any surviving subpopulations. Successful therapy of multiple metastases, populated by tumor cells with different responses to antineoplastic agents, will require treatment regimens that are capable of circumventing such cellular heterogeneity. One approach that has been suggested is to reduce the time interval between successive treatments with different agents.

The aim of such an approach would be to kill not only those populations that survive the previous treatment before they can generate large numbers of new variants, but also to kill new variant subpopulations as soon as they emerge (57).

It was Goldie and Coldman (54, 55) who hypothesized that most mammalian cells start with intrinsic sensitivity to antineoplastic drugs but develop spontaneous resistance at variable rates (somatic mutation theory). Since resistant cells would increase in number by both direct growth and by further mutations to doubly resistant lines, or by conversion of other sensitive lines to resistant lines, the resultant number of resistant cell lines and the size of resistant population will be directly dependent on the size of the population. They developed a mathematical model relating curability to the time of appearance of single or doubly resistant cells. Assuming a natural mutation rate, the model predicts a variation in size of the resistant fraction in tumors of the same size and type depending upon the mutation rate and the point at which the mutation develops. Tumors in which loss of stem cell capacity occurs with high frequency, i.e. slow-growing tumors with a substantial subpopulation of dying cells (as may be the case in squamous cell head and neck cancer), will theoretically have a great phenotypic heterogeneity and have a high likelihood of developing resistant cells (58).

These data may all have implications for adjuvant studies in the clinic:

1. It gives an explanation as to why chemotherapy may not be much more effective in the adjuvant setting than in patients with clinically evident tumors even though growth characteristics of micrometastases appear to make them more vulnerable to chemotherapy.
2. Tumors will be curable by chemotherapy if no permanently resistant cell lines are present and chemotherapy is started before such cells develop.
3. The probability of cure diminishes rapidly with the appearance of a single resistant line if only one effective therapy is available or with the appearance of a doubly resistant line if two equally effective therapies are available.
4. Combination chemotherapy could be effective because it offers the possibility of eradication of cell lines resistant to one drug, or one drug combination program, by an alternative drug, or alternative drug combination program. In fact, Goldie et al. (59) suggested that, provided certain conditions are met, the use of alternating non-cross-resistant chemotherapy could be a more effective strategy to adopt.
5. It stresses the importance of giving the adjuvant chemotherapy as early as possible in the course of the patient's malignant disease.

The Impact of Time of Drug Treatment

The time to first drug treatment in adjuvant chemotherapy may be a crucial step. In many murine models of subcutaneously transplanted tumors treated with surgery and adjuvant chemotherapy Schabel, Griswold and colleagues demonstrated that the length of time between tumor implantation and either surgical resection or adjuvant chemotherapy was critical for the prevention or elimination of micrometastatic disease. In these studies chemotherapy had its maximal effect when given soon after

surgery (60–64). Similar observations have been reported by others (65). Taking this to the extreme, the earliest possible use of chemotherapy, i.e. before any local treatment is given, would be an attractive option. Thus an advantage in the clinical situation would be that utilizing chemotherapy as the initial treatment, the patient's tumor is allowed to serve as a biologic indicator of responsiveness, and it would prevent pointless use of ineffective chemotherapy after local therapies for those not responding initially. It would allow rapid change to another program, or quick implementation of the standard local treatment, without the need to further expose the patient to ineffective and toxic drugs. The potential advantages and disadvantages of this so-called induction chemotherapy in general, and for patients with squamous cell head and neck cancer in particular, have been discussed by Morrison and Clark (see Section on Induction Chemotherapy, first part of Chapter 6). Two studies on induction chemotherapy of interest may be mentioned here—both applied chemotherapy intra-arterially, one with methotrexate alone, the other a combination of bleomycin and vincristine (66, 67). Beneficial effects were only observed in oral cavity tumors. In the study reported by Arcangeli et al. (66) the 5-year survival was significantly improved only in stage II patients, indicating that this approach seemed to give the most favorable results in early stage lesions. Such an observation has also been reported in adjuvant trials in patients with breast cancer (68) and is of interest for future adjuvant trials in patients with squamous cell carcinoma of the head and neck.

The Choice of Chemotherapy and the Effect of Dosing

Dosages and schedules of chemotherapy in the adjuvant setting are derived from experiences with chemotherapy in patients who have failed definitive treatment or from those obtained in patients who have received no prior treatment.

From studies in patients with recurrent disease it can be concluded that the four most active single agents are cisplatin, methotrexate, 5-fluorouracil, and bleomycin (69). Over the past 10 to 15 years, numerous combinations of active drugs have been evaluated. In nonrandomized trials, the complete response rate seems to have improved by about 10%. However, the overall duration of response and survival were not found to have been improved, and toxicities with these regimens were generally higher than those observed with single-agent chemotherapy. Therefore, present areas of investigation include diminishing toxicity by using continuous infusion schedules of cisplatin (70), by replacing cisplatin with a less toxic platinum analogue in the combination (71, 72), or by adding agents to the combination that may provide rescue from cisplatin-induced toxic effects (73). On the other hand, studies testing biochemical and pharmacological principles are focusing on improving the complete response rates in these circumstances (74–76). In randomized trials, combination chemotherapy with cisplatin does indeed result in better response rates, in some also better complete response rates than in those that can be achieved with cisplatin or methotrexate alone (77–79). However, these higher response rates have not been translated into a better survival of the patients.

Similar conclusions have been made in induction chemotherapy studies. Recently published reviews on the role of induction chemotherapy indicate that at the present time the best results seem to be obtained with CB-like (cisplatin and bleomycin) or CBM-like (CB + methotrexate) programs or with the cisplatin/5-fluorouracil (CF) infusion regimens (69, 70, 80). Response rates with these regimens have been variable in the different studies (37–100%) as have the complete response rates (0–54%) depending on the different patient categories treated. In a direct comparison of the CBM regimen with CF regimen at the Dana–Farber institute these two types of regimens have thus far not been shown to be different in terms of response rates (81). The concept of dose intensity has a strong basis from experiments performed in animal models (82). The impact of dose intensity (the amount of drug delivered per unit time, expressed as $mg/m^2/week$, regardless of the schedule or route of administration) in the clinic has recently attracted much attention. A clear-cut relationship between dose intensity and response rate has been retrospectively demonstrated in advanced ovarian cancer, breast cancer, colon cancer, and in lymphomas (83). There is some evidence from small studies in patients with head and neck cancer that dose escalation (dose intensification) of cisplatin may increase therapeutic response. Forastière et al. (84), using cisplatin at a dose of $40 \, mg/m^2/day \times 5$ or $50 \, mg/m^2/day \times 4$, every 28 days, found a 73% overall response rate in 22 patients, which was nearly double the expected 30–40% reported in similar patients treated with standard doses of cisplatin. Very recently, in a feasibility study of 6-weekly administration of cisplatin at doses up to $80 \, mg/m^2/week$, 9 of 12 patients with locally far-advanced head and neck cancer did respond, suggesting that dose intensity may play a role (85, 86). For methotrexate, bleomycin, and 5-fluorouracil the impact of dose intensity is less clear although it has to be stressed that for each of these drugs there are indications on how to use them most optimally. Weekly or twice-weekly conventional dose administration of methotrexate may be more effective than loading doses once every 3 or 4 weeks or daily administration of small doses (87). For bleomycin

there exists the clinical impression that the drug's clinical activity and therapeutic index are greater when it is given by continuous infusion than when administered by intermittent bolus. Nowadays, there is also a suggestion that 5-fluorouracil when given by continuous infusion (and by doing so a much a higher total dose can be given) its activity in head and neck cancer patients seems to be higher (69, 87).

The implications of giving adequate dosages in the adjuvant setting are clear from adjuvant studies in breast cancer patients (88), but also from adjuvant trials in patients with colorectal cancer, a tumor type for which the chemotherapeutic armamentarium is rather restricted. In a recently published meta-analysis (89) the strongest effects on the odds (of death) ratio were obtained in trials in which 5-fluorouracil was given over an extended period of time (odds ratio, 0.83; 95% ci 0.70 to 0.98). In one of the trials included in this analysis (Grage et al.) where 5-fluorouracil was found to have a significant effect on the disease-free interval in patients with Dukes C colonic cancer and in those with rectal cancer, those patients who were treated to toxicity, in terms of leukopenia, had a significantly longer disease-free interval and appeared to survive longer than those in whom the drug did not result in leukopenia (90). It is therefore clear that the general tendency of giving reduced dosages in adjuvant trials to restrict toxicity, should be avoided, since dose reductions reduce the therapeutic potential of a given drug or drug combination. Unfortunately, however, the use of inadequate dosages or schedules has been the rule rather than the exception in adjuvant trials in patients with head and neck cancer due to poor tolerance of those undergoing this chemotherapy after local therapies, in particular radiotherapy, and as a result of this poor patient compliance. Moreover, in those trials where adjuvant chemotherapy was used after previous induction chemotherapy, patient refusal has been reported to be a major obstacle (91).

If we restrict ourselves to classical adjuvant chemotherapy, there are several advantages of this approach: (1) the immediate initiation of effective and generally accepted local treatments such as surgery and/or radiotherapy; (2) no further prolongation of preoperative stress on the nutritional status of the patients; (3) the absence of intercurrent hematologic and immunologic suppression, potentially present with induction chemotherapy before local treatment; (4) no possibility of interference with radiotherapy, both in terms of doses that could be delivered or its continuity; and (5) no interference with planned surgery in operable cases.

On the other hand some negative aspects have also to be mentioned: (1) the adjuvant population is not homogeneous, i.e. some patients do not need chemotherapy and will be cured by surgery alone, some may benefit in cases where their tumors are responsive to the given chemotherapy, while some others may not benefit because of resistance to it and will only experience toxicity. These considerations would support the use of chemotherapy before local therapies, as this allows the patient's tumor to serve as a biologic indicator of responsiveness, as mentioned earlier; (2) there may be delay in the treatment of micrometastases; and (3) the compromised circulatory conditions related to previous surgery or radiation may reduce the uptake of drugs of the original tumor-bearing areas.

The available literature on adjuvant chemotherapy in head and neck therefore can be separated in two categories: (1) studies on the use of classical adjuvant chemotherapy, i. e. without first giving induction chemotherapy; and (2) studies on the use of adjuvant chemotherapy after induction chemotherapy and local therapies.

Clinical Studies on Adjuvant Chemotherapy

The data on trials evaluating conventionial adjuvant chemotherapy after surgery or radiation therapy in patients with head and neck cancer are very scarce. Lately, it has received more attention in several reviews which stressed the fact that this approach may have potential merit (80, 92, 93). Distant metastases are a major cause of treatment failure in patients with nasopharyngeal carcinoma (NPC), especially in those presenting with bulky cervical metastases. Systemic chemotherapy has been tried in this disease to improve control of distant metastases and prolong survival, both in children and in adults (94–97). Trials evaluating the role of adjuvant chemotherapy in patients with NPC will be discussed separately.

Nonrandomized Trials of Adjuvant Chemotherapy

The use of methotrexate (MTX) in the adjuvant setting has been studied by several investigators (98–100). Kirkwood et al. (98) reported a nonrandomized study of 24 patients with T3, T4, or N3 disease who received high-dose methotrexate with leucovorin rescue (LR) before and after definitive surgery and/or radiotherapy. Although the disease-free survival appeared to be prolonged in responding patients, no statistical analysis or survival data were given in this pilot study. Arlen (99) used a sandwich procedure of radiotherapy, chemotherapy (MTX and LR) followed by maintenance chemotherapy (MTX 40 mg weekly) for 2 years. The impact of this maintenance therapy, was, however, not clear from this publication. Finally, Taylor et al. (100), based on their pilot experience with escalating dosages of methotrexate (240, 360, and 480 mg/m² on days 1, 5, and 9, respectively, each time with leucovorin

rescue) in a 2-week course prior to surgery and/or radiotherapy (101), used the same 2-week regimen both for induction and maintenance chemotherapy before and after surgery and radiotherapy. Maintenance chemotherapy was given every 3 months for 1 year. In this latter study, 50 patients with tumors from variable sites (stages II, III, and IV) were randomized for either receiving methotrexate alone or methotrexate with immunotherapy (BCG alone or autologous tumor cell vaccine plus BCG). Recurrence rates were 50% and 35% for both groups, respectively. Forty-four percent of the total series remained disease-free after a median follow-up of 18 months. The lack of a control arm without systemic therapy, however, precluded any meaningful conclusions from this study. Nevertheless, an important message from this study was the observation that stomatitis was a much more severe problem during the course given following surgery and especially radiation therapy, requiring a substantial reduction in methotrexate dosages. Eighty-seven percent of patients had oral ulcerations following radiation therapy but only 40% had similar reactions with the initial course. Moreover, after radiation therapy the stomatitis occurred earlier, often preventing dose escalation and limiting the number of cycles of methotrexate to two.

Several reports have appeared on the use of multiagent chemotherapy after definitive treatment. Huang et al. (102) administered a combination of bleomycin, methotrexate, vinblastine, and CCNU to 31 patients (8 with stage III, 12 with stage IV, and 11 with recurrent cancer) once every 6 weeks for a total of six courses after surgery and/or radiotherapy. Contrary to the earlier mentioned experience with methotrexate alone, patient compliance was excellent. Two patients received only five courses due to reluctance to submit to the last course of therapy and 1 patient received only four courses due to an intercurrent event. With a minimum follow-up of 14 months, only 5 (16%) of the 31 patients relapsed between 18 and 22 months, 4 died due to tumor, 6 died of tumor-unrelated causes, resulting in a 67.7% overall survival. These data were considered superior to those of a nonrandomized control group of 24 patients who did not receive adjuvant chemotherapy. In the latter group, after a shorter period of follow-up (minimum 5 months), 16 (67%) relapsed, 13 died due to tumor (54%), 2 died of tumor-unrelated causes, giving an overall survival of 38%.

Similar positive results were observed by Johnson et al. (103, 104) in a study, in which 50 patients with resectable squamous cell head and neck cancer (30 with stage III, 20 with stage IV), all with histologic evidence of extracapsular spread (ECS), received adjuvant chemotherapy after surgery and irradiation for 6 months. Chemotherapy in this study consisted of sequential methotrexate and 5-fluorouracil (and leucovorin rescue), which was administered weekly, with 1-week rest following every second course. A total of 771 doses were administered. Dose reduction was required seventy-two times. Therapy was stopped in only 1 patient (2%) because of toxicity and only 3 other patients (6%) refused to complete the chemotherapy. After a minimum follow-up of 20 months, 8 patients have died of tumor-unrelated causes and 14 patients have relapsed (8 locoregional, 6 distant initially). The adjusted 2-year disease-free survival was 67%. This compared favorably with the 36% disease-free survival for concurrent controls and the 38% survival for historical controls (all patients with ECS treated with surgery and radiotherapy alone).

Although there may be several advantages to induction chemotherapy, one of the disadvantages is that compliance to surgery after induction chemotherapy has been reported to be less than 70% (105). In a pilot study of the Radiation Therapy Oncology Group (RTOG) using three courses of induction chemotherapy with cisplatin and 5-fluorouracil before surgery and irradiation, only 27 (64%) of the 42 evaluable patients underwent the planned surgery (106). Of the 15 patients who did not undergo surgery, 10 refused, 3 were judged to be unresectable, and 2 were lost to follow-up. In particular, those who respond very well to the chemotherapy may be reluctant to undergo surgery. In fact, in the RTOG study 9 (56%) of the 16 clinical complete responders subsequently refused surgery. In a next study the RTOG studied the feasibility and efficacy of cisplatin and 5-fluorouracil combination chemotherapy postsurgery, but before radiotherapy (107). A total of 29 patients entered this study (21% stage III, 79% stage IV). In 6 patients, chemotherapy was not given for medical conditions or because of patient refusal. Of the 23 patients who started chemotherapy, 18 (78%) received all three courses. Two patients had either one or two courses of chemotherapy and then refused further therapy. Three other patients did not finish chemotherapy because of medical condition at that time. Of the 25 patients who started radiotherapy, 24 (96%) completed it. Overall, 15 (52%) finished the treatment sequence. The authors very truly therefore stated that "it seemed that regardless of the first treatment modality in patients with advanced disease, 60% to 80% full compliance can be expected with each subsequent therapy." With a minimum follow-up of 24 months, 62% of the patients were alive at 2 years. Although this approach seemed feasible, the real value of this sequence of treatments will become clear from the ongoing phase III trial, which is ongoing in the Head and Neck Cancer Intergroup, comparing this combined modality therapy to standard treatment of surgery and postoperative radiotherapy.

The role of adjuvant chemotherapy for advanced NPC in childhood was recently reviewed by Kim et al. (95). All the studies reviewed included small groups of children, who had received chemotherapy either only after radiation therapy or before and after radiation therapy. Considering the fact that distant metastases generally occur within 2 years, the reported relapse-free survival beyond this time of 75–86% in the different series of patients with stage III and IV disease suggest that adjuvant chemotherapy might be useful for advanced NPC in childhood. Chemotherapy regimens used in the different series included in all cases cyclophosphamide and doxorubicin and some in addition methotrexate or vincristine ± 5-fluorouracil. Two carefully controlled comparisons with historical data in mostly adult patients with NPC resulted in different outcomes (96, 97). Thirty-four previously untreated patients with advanced NPC treated with combination chemotherapy (cisplatin and noncisplatin based) and sequential radiotherapy had a more favorable outcome in terms of disease-free survival and median survival than the 69 patients treated with radiotherapy alone in the control group (96). In the second study, two courses of a combination of vincristine, bleomycin, methotrexate, and 5-fluorouracil (VBMF) given before radiotherapy seemed to have a negative influence on survival when compared with the historical control group in which patients were treated with radiotherapy alone ($p = 0.002$). This negative influence was not seen in the group of patients who received VBMF plus cisplatin before and after radiotherapy. However, the distant relapses in both combined modality groups occurred at significantly shorter times after diagnosis than in the historical control group treated with radiotherapy alone ($p = 0.0001$). It was thought that postponement of radiotherapy by chemotherapy might have accounted for this (97). These latter two studies illustrate the wide variety of results obtainable when historical controls are used for comparison.

Randomized Trials of Classical Adjuvant Chemotherapy

Only four randomized studies on adjuvant chemotherapy per se have been carried out in head and neck cancer patients, one of which included only patients with NPC (108–111).

Szpirglas et al. (108) randomized patients with tumors of the tongue and floor of the mouth, who were in remission after local therapies to no treatment, chemotherapy or immunotherapy. The chemotherapy arm consisted of methotrexate (400 mg per month by intravenous infusion) followed by 100 mg of leucovorin intramuscularly and bleomycin in two 15 mg doses intramuscularly per week. The total dose of bleomycin never exceeded 450 mg in 15 weeks of treatment. Methotrexate was administered for 2 years.

The immunotherapy consisted of subcutaneous or intramuscular injections of *Corynebacterium parvum* every week for 2 years. The 95 patients included in the study were stratified for stage and initial treatment before randomization. There was a suggestion that the adjuvant therapies did delay recurrence to some extent, but they did not significantly decrease the recurrence rate. Moreover, no statistically significant difference in overall survival was found between the three groups. However, subset analysis demonstrated a significant survival advantage ($p < 0.01$) for the chemotherapy group in patients with T1−T2, N0 disease, while there was no advantage for patients with more advanced disease (T3N0, T1−T2−T3N+).

A total of 287 patients with tumors of the oral cavity, oropharynx, hypopharynx, larynx or unknown origin, and invaded cervical lymph nodes plus extracapsular spread (ECS), found at radical neck dissection, entered a protocol of the GETTEC (Group d'Étude des Tumeurs de la Tête et du Cou) from January 1983 till December 1985. Patients were randomized to surgery followed by radiotherapy or the same procedure plus chemotherapy, which started from 7 to 8 weeks after the completion of radiotherapy. The chemotherapy consisted of three cycles of a combination of cisplatin, methotrexate, and bleomycin and this was followed by 5-monthly courses of methotrexate and bleomycin. The results of this study appeared only in abstract form and were presented at ECCO-IV, November 1987. The minimum follow-up at that time was 32 months (median 40 months). There were less locoregional recurrences in the chemotherapy arm (14% vs. 27%), but somewhat more patients presented with distant metastases (33% vs. 25%) in comparison with the control group. The disease-free survival of the two groups was not significantly different. The survival curves showed a difference, of borderline significance, in favor of the control group. This difference disappeared when adjustments were made for adverse histological factors, such as vascular invasion and the number of lymph nodes with capsular rupture (109). It has to be mentioned, that in this study toxicity was again substantial. In the chemotherapy arm, 16% never started, 83% completed at least three cycles, but only 53% completed all planned treatment. Most important toxicities included hematologic toxicity, renal toxicity, and mucositis.

Bitter reported on a study involving a small but tightly defined patient population, in which postoperative chemotherapy was compared with postoperative radiotherapy (110). The study included only oral T3N1 and T3N2 lesions. Chemotherapy consisted of a combination of vincristine, bleomycin, and methotrexate (VBM) given in a timed sequence

for four cycles after surgery. When 33 patients had entered, a significant difference was observed in favor of the chemotherapy arm, the reason why further entry was stopped. Projected life table analysis demonstrated superiority for the chemotherapy group with $p < 0.02$ for recurrence (68% vs. 24% recurrence-free) and $p = 0.05$ for survival (65% vs. 29%). The reliability remains uncertain with this small number of patients. Nevertheless, these remarkable data warrant further study of postoperative chemotherapy.

The last study was carried out by an Italian Cooperative Group (111) in patients with locoregional nasopharyngeal carcinoma (squamous or undifferentiated) who were considered in complete response at the end of curative radiotherapy. Also patients with at least a $\geq 75\%$ clinical regression of the primary lesion were included in the study. Furthermore, patients with partial response of neck metastases could be included after removal of the residual disease by neck dissection. A total of 229 patients were randomized to receive no further treatment or 6-monthly cycles of VCA (vincristine, cyclophosphamide, adriamycin). The two groups were well balanced for all important prognostic factors. Radiotherapy was delivered to the nasopharynx, the base of the skull, and bilateral cervical nodes using a split course technique over 10 weeks up to the dose of 60−70 Gy to involved sites and 50 Gy to negative nodes. Eighty percent of the patients started adjuvant chemotherapy within the established 65 days. In 20% of cases it was delayed due to postsurgical problems, patient errors, leucopenia after radiotherapy, or other causes. Chemotherapy was not administered to 13 of the 113 patients randomized for chemotherapy (10 refused, 3 had early tumor relapse). In only 6 patients VCA had to be stopped for severe toxicity. Treatment was administered in most patients at a dose level $\geq 85\%$ of each drug. Only about 10% of patients received $< 75\%$ of the scheduled dose. Analysis at 48 months did not show significant differences between the two treatment groups in terms of relapse–free survival (RT, 55.8%; RT + VCA, 57.7%) and overall survival (RT, 67.3%; RT + VCA, 58.5%). Also, the pattern of relapse was similar in the two arms, with distant metastases being the cause of treatment failure in about 50% of relapsing patients.

Randomized Trials of Induction plus Adjuvant Chemotherapy

Specific data on the eight randomized trials evaluating the potential usefulness of induction chemotherapy plus adjuvant chemotherapy are summarized in Table 6.**5**. Two of these trials applied chemotherapy with methotrexate alone (113, 114). In the other studies, combination chemotherapy was used,

Table 6.5 Randomized trials of induction plus adjuvant chemotherapy

Author	Treatment schedule	No. of patients per arm	Prior treatment % CT	% S	% RT	Resp. IC % CR	% PR	LTC %	% Recurrence	% DFS (yrs)	% OS (yrs)
Tejada (112)	MTX 50 mg/m²/wk CDDP 20 mg/m²/wk IC 4 courses MC ? courses	Control 26	100	?	?			?	69[+]	576 D[#]	?
		Adjuvant 12	100	?	?	1	65	?	58[+]	530 D[#] (NS)	?
Rentschler (113)	MTX 40 mg/m²/wk escalation 10 mg/m²/wk IC 4 courses MC 12 courses (4 pre RT, 8 post RT)	Control 27	–	96	100	–	–	100	33	58(4)[§]	48(4)[§]
		Adjuvant 28	100	96	100	4	68	100	32	66 (NS)	48 (NS)
Taylor (114)	MTX 60 mg/m²/6 h × 4, d 1 90 mg/m²/6 h × 4, d 5 120 mg/m²/6 h × 4, d 9 Leucovorine rescue IC 1 course MC 3 courses q 3 mo or 4 courses of DOX 40 mg/m² q 3 wk CDDP 40 mg/m² q 3 wk	Control 41	–	66	80	–	–	88	49	35(4)[§]	36(4)[§]
		Adjuvant 41	100	80	71	6	34	78 (NS)	37	42 (NS)	37 (NS)
Stell (115)	A BLM 60 mg iv, d 1 VCR 1.5 mg/m² iv, d 1 MTX 225 mg/m² iv, d 1 5FU 350 mg/m² iv, d 1 FA 15 mg po q 6 h × 4 (Hydrocortisone 500 mg × 2) 2-week interval B HU 3 g/m² po, d 1 6MP 150 mg/m² po, d 1 CTX 500 mg/m² iv, d 1 IC 1 course (A + B) MC A alternate B, q 3 wk × 12	Control 39	–	28*	100	–		?	NA	NA	56(2.5)
		Adjuvant 47	100	13*	98	–		?	NA	NA	22(2.5) (NS)
Kun (116) Holoye (117)	BLM 30 U/d × 4 CTX 200 mg/m²/d × 5 MTX 30 mg/m², d × 5 5FU 400 mg/m²/d × 5 IC 2 courses q 3 wk MC 2 courses (50% dose of BLM)	Control 40	–	55	100	–	–	75	43	64(2)	43(2)
		Adjuvant 43**	100	35	100	10	61	57 (NS)	50	59 (NS)	31 (NS)

Table 6.5 (cont.)

Author	Treatment schedule	No. of patients per arm	Prior treatment % CT	% S	% RT	Resp. IC % CR	% PR	LTC %	% Recurrence	% DFS (yrs)	% OS (yrs)
Stolwijk (118)	VLB 6 mg/m² iv, d 1 BLM 15 mg im, d 1 MTX 40 mg/m² iv, d 2 CTX 400 mg/m² iv, d 2 5FU 15 mg/kg iv, d 2 IC 2 courses q 2 wk MC 13 courses q (3 wk—3 mo)	Control 35	—	?	?	—	—	63	NA	NA	53(2.5)
		Adjuvant 33	100	?	?	—	21	54 (NS)	NA	NA	36(2.5) (NS)
Ervin (119) Clark (81)	A CDDP 20 mg/m²/d iv, d 1–5 BLM 10 U/m²/d ci, d 3–7 MTX 200 mg/m² iv, d 15, 22 Leucovorin oral rescue	Control 20	100	S a/o RT	100	Included only CR/PR		100	40	61(2)	NA
	B CDDP 20 mg/m²/d iv, d 1–3 BLM 10 U/m²/d ci, d 2–4 MTX 200 mg/m² iv, d 15, 22, 29, 36 Leucovorin oral rescue IC 2 courses (A) q 4 wk MC 3 courses (B) q 6 wk	Adjuvant 26	100	S a/o RT	100	Included only CR/PR		100	11	84 (NS)	NA
H and N Contracts Program (120)	A CDDP 100 mg/m² iv, d 1 BLM 15 mg/m² iv, d 3 BLM 15 mg/m² ci, d 3–7	Control 152	—	95	?	—	—	95	44	55(5)	35(5)
		Induction 140	100	96	?	3	34	96	44	49	37
	B CDDP 80 mg/m² iv, q 4 wk IC 1 course of A MC 6 courses of B	Adjuvant 151	100	87	?	3		87	39	64 (NS)	45 (NS)

Abbreviations: IC, induction chemotherapy; MC, maintenance chemotherapy; CT, chemotherapy; S, surgery; RT, radiotherapy; CR, complete response; PR, partial response; DFS, disease-free survival; OS, overall survival; LTC, local tumor clearance; MTX, methotrexate; CDDP, Cisplatin; BLM, Bleomycin; VCR, Vincristine; 5FU, 5-Fluorouracil; FA, folinic acid; HU, hydroxyurea; 6MP, 6-mercaptopurine; CTX, Cyclophosphamide; iv, intravenous; im intramuscular; ci, continuous infusion; po, per os; NA, not available; d, day; wk, week; mo, month; NS, not significant.

* Salvage surgery.

+ Follow-up 19–36 months.

Mean DFS.

§ Estimated from published curves.

** Postoperative chemotherapy was stopped during the study due to toxicity and poor compliance.

three including cisplatin in the combination (112, 119, 120) and three using a combination without cisplatin (115–118). Only the Head and Neck Contracts Program used cisplatin alone in the maintenance arm (120). Unfortunately, apart from this latter study, all other trials included only limited numbers of patients (< 50 patients per treatment arm). Moreover, they all included patients with tumors from different sites, resulting in even smaller numbers in each subgroup. Only the Head and Neck Contracts Program was large enough to allow subset analysis (121). All studies included patients with stages III and IV squamous cell carcinoma of the head and neck. Only three of them included also poor-risk patients with stage II tumors (114, 117, 120). This category, however, was represented in such low numbers that separate analysis could not be performed in any of these studies. Overall, the results of these eight studies do not indicate a positive influence of induction chemotherapy plus adjuvant chemotherapy on disease-free survival or overall survival. However, bearing in mind the limited sample size and the relatively large number of tumor sites included, this would hardly have been expected. In addition, some interesting data came forward from these trials, which are worth mentioning and may have had influence on the outcome.

Induction chemotherapy in most of these trials was not given in its optimal form, according to modern standards, taking into account both the regimen itself and the number of cycles given. Local treatments were given after 2 to 4 weeks of chemotherapy in six of the eight trials (112–115, 118, 120), and after 6 to 8 weeks of chemotherapy in two (117, 119). It is therefore not surprising that the complete response rates in six of the seven studies, in which this was reported, varied from 0% to 10%. The only exception is the study of the Dana–Farber Institute with a complete response rate of 26% after two cycles of CBM (119).

Local treatments in the different studies included surgery alone, radiotherapy alone, or a combination of both, mostly reflecting differences in tumor site, stage, pathology findings, and resectability. In some studies, maintenance chemotherapy was given only to patients who had local tumor clearance after local treatments (113, 119, 120). In others, it was also given to patients in whom this was not reached (114, 117, 118). Interestingly, in those latter studies the percentage of patients with local tumor clearance was always slightly higher in the control arm in comparison with the experimental arm.

Maintenance chemotherapy started from 2 to 8 weeks after the completion of local treatments in the different studies and was either identical to the induction chemotherapy (112–115, 118) or similar, but given with a reduced dose (or deletion) of one or more of the drugs (117, 119, 120). In one trial, maintenance chemotherapy changed completely during the course of the study due to the poor tolerance of the original regimen after radiation and surgery (114). In those studies in which induction chemotherapy was given for more than one cycle, the interval between courses of maintenance chemotherapy increased in four and was the same in two. In two studies it was clearly mentioned that maintenance chemotherapy was only given to patients who had shown an initial response to induction chemotherapy (117, 119).

In several studies, maintenance chemotherapy could not be given according to protocol due to toxicity or poor compliance. In three studies, methotrexate-induced stomatitis was much worse after radiation and surgery then when given before (112–114). In one study the investigators even abandoned postoperative chemotherapy during their study as result of the observed toxicities (117). Moreover, patient refusal occurred frequently (112, 114, 119, 120). Maintenance chemotherapy with doxorubicin and cisplatin was refused in 25% in the study reported by Taylor et al. (114). At the Dana–Farber Institute only 46 of the 73 patients eligible for randomization to adjuvant chemotherapy accepted this (119). Of the 26 patients who were ultimately randomized to receive adjuvant chemotherapy, 3 refused treatment after randomization, 3 received only one course of therapy, 10 received two courses and 10 patients received all three planned courses of treatment. Of the 151 patients randomized to receive maintenance chemotherapy in the Head and Neck Contracts Program, only 13 (9%) completed all six cycles. Forty-one patients (27%) completed at least three cycles. Sixty-seven patients (45%) never received any maintenance chemotherapy. The most common reasons for this were patient refusal (37%), cancer recurrence (33%), or death (16%). Lethal toxicity to chemotherapy used in these eight trials has been reported in three of the five trials, in which this was mentioned, and ranged from 1% to 3% (115, 118, 119). In the large Head and Neck Contracts Program, treatment-related deaths occurred in 6 patients (1%), not specifying whether this was related to the use of chemotherapy (120). Chemotherapy-related lethal toxicities which were reported in the five trials (with a total of 265 study patients receiving chemotherapy) included lung toxicity in 1 patient and septicemia in 2 (overall 1.1%).

Despite these critical remarks and the overall negative results, one should not overlook the promising observations that have been made in at least some of these trials. The randomized trial at the Dana–Farber Institute of adjuvant chemotherapy initially demonstrated that such treatment significantly improved failure-free survival by decreasing locoregional failures (119). This was predominantly due to benefit in the patients who had had a partial response to induction chemotherapy with CBM. In a later update, this study continued to show substantial differences in favor of adjuvant chemotherapy (84% vs. 61%, see Table 6.5), but these differences were no longer significant (81). A similar trend has been observed in the study reported by Rentschler et al. (113) and in two of the earlier mentioned randomized studies with classical adjuvant chemotherapy (108, 110). A second important observation was made in the Head and Neck Contracts Program (120). Maintenance chemotherapy with cisplatin alone caused significantly fewer distant relapses (9% vs. 19%, $p = 0.025$) and a trend towards improved survival (45% vs. 35% in the control group), despite the low compliance rate. Even more interesting is the recently published subset analysis (121). Of the 192 patients with oral cavity cancer in this study, those on the maintenance arm had a significantly improved 3-year disease-free survival (67%) compared to the standard arm (49%) or the induction arm (44%) (overall $p = 0.05$). When analyzing the data based on stage of disease, maintenance chemotherapy improved the relapse-free interval in patients with less extensive tumors (T1 and T2), but not in those with more bulky disease (T3 and T4). The same was true for the extent of nodal disease; maintenance chemotherapy significantly improved the disease-free survival in patients with N1 or N2 disease, but not in those with N3 disease. These observations led the authors to suggest with some degree of circumspection (because of the potential flaws in such a retrospective analysis) it is possible to conclude that adjuvant chemotherapy may be more effective in patients with less extensive disease.

Conclusions and Future Research Directions

The promising results with adjuvant chemotherapy obtained in the nonrandomized studies have not been confirmed in randomized trials when survival benefit was taken as an endpoint.

Therefore, the routine use of adjuvant chemotherapy in patients with squamous cell head and neck cancer cannot be advocated at the present time. However, considering the many imperfections of previous trials and the limited numbers of patients involved in most of them, only a dramatic impact of chemotherapy would have been possible to detect. As we now know, based on experiences with adjuvant chemotherapy in patients with breast cancer or colorectal cancer, such an expectation is unrealistic. Nevertheless, in this reviewer's opinion, there is sufficient evidence from previous trials, to suggest that when sufficiently large trials could be performed in a proper manner, the probability of detecting a positive influence of chemotherapy on the outcome of this disease is very high.

From several trials there is an indication that the chance of finding a beneficial effect of adjuvant chemotherapy on survival is highest in poor-risk patients with less bulky and resectable disease (66, 108, 120). Moreover, there is a suggestion from the same trials that oral cavity tumors are the most likely to benefit from adjuvant chemotherapy. Stell and Rawson (122) in their meta-analysis on twenty-three trials of adjuvant chemotherapy did not, however, find this. Their subgroup analysis for site did not, unfortunately, include all the trials mentioned above. Moreover, their analysis did not include a subgroup analysis based on stage. Their review, which included all types of adjuvant chemotherapy, i.e. induction, maintenance, and simultaneous chemoradiotherapy, did, however, reveal that locoregional failure rate decreased significantly with the use of chemotherapy, thus improving the quality of survival. In contrast, the failure rate for distant metastases was only slightly reduced. Nevertheless, the Head and Neck Contracts Program, being the largest study on maintenance chemotherapy, clearly showed a significantly lower metastatic rate in the experimental arm (120).

The negative phase III trial on adjuvant chemotherapy in patients with nasopharyngeal carcinoma was rather disappointing, especially as about 70% of the tumors were of the undifferentiated type, and only 9% of the patients refused adjuvant chemotherapy after randomization. Further studies with chemotherapy are necessary because distant metastases were the cause of treatment failure in about 50% of relapsing patients. The investigation of intensive high-dose chemotherapy with hematopoietic growth factors or even autologous bone marrow transplantation, especially in younger patients, warrant consideration.

Future studies on adjuvant chemotherapy in patients with squamous cell head and neck cancer should focus on a better selection of patients for this approach, and should take into account the heterogeneity of the disease with survival differences dependent on site and stage. Moreover, future studies should make use of more optimal chemotherapy regimens than have been used in the past. These concepts should be adequately tested in order to avoid the possibility that a potentially beneficial treatment is withheld from patients.

References

1. Krause CJ, Lee JG, McCabe BF. Carcinoma of the oral cavity: a comparison of therapeutic modalities. Arch Otolaryngol 1973; 97:354−8.
2. Fu KK, Eisenberg L, Dedo HH, Phillips TL. Results of integrated management of supraglottic carcinoma. Cancer 1977; 40:2874−81.
3. Perez CA, Purday JA, Breaux SA, et al. Carcinoma of the tonsillar fossa: nonrandomized comparison of preoperative radiation and surgery or irradiation alone. Long-term results. Cancer 1982; 50:2314−32.

4. Chacko DC, Hendrickson FR, Fisher A. Definitive irradiation of T1–T4N0 larynx cancer. Cancer 1983; 51:994–1000.
5. Snow JB, Kramer S, Marcial VA, et al. Evaluation of randomized preoperative and postoperative radiation therapy of supraglottic carcinoma. Ann Otol Rhinol Laryngol 1978; 87:686–91.
6. Arriagada R, Eschwege F, Cachin Y, Richard JM. The value of combining radiotherapy with surgery in the treatment of hypopharyngeal and laryngeal cancers. Cancer 1983; 51:1819–25.
7. Wagenfeld DJH, Harwood AR, Bryce DP, et al. Second primary respiratory tract malignancies in glottic carcinoma. Cancer 1980; 46:1883–6.
8. Vikram B. Changing patterns of failure in advanced head and neck cancer. Arch Otolaryngol 1984; 110:564–5.
9. Cachin Y, Eschwege F. Combination of radiotherapy and surgery in the treatment of head and neck cancers. Cancer Treat Rev 1975; 2:177–91.
10. Merino OR, Lindberg RD, Fletcher GH. An analysis of distant metastases from squamous cell carcinoma of the upper respiratory and digestive tracts. Cancer 1977; 40:145–51.
11. Goepfert H. Are we making any progress? Arch Otolaryngol 1983; 110:562–3.
12. De Vries N. Magnitude of the problem of second primary cancers in head and neck cancer patients. In: De Vries N, Gluckman JL, eds. Multiple primary tumors in the head and neck. Stuttgart: Georg Thieme, 1990.
13. Crile GW. Excision of carcinoma of the head and neck with special reference to the plan of dissection based on 132 operations. J Am Med Assoc 1906; 47:1780–6.
14. Dorrance GM, McShane JK. Cancer of the tongue and floor of mouth. Ann Surg 1928; 88:1007–21.
15. Willis RA. The spread of tumours in the human body. London: Churchill, 1933.
16. Burke EM. Metastases in squamous cell carcinoma. Am J Cancer 1979; 30:493–503.
17. Martin HE, Sugarbaker EL. Cancer of the floor of mouth. Surg Gynecol Obstet 1940; 71:347–59.
18. Martin HE, Munster H, Sugarbaker ED. Cancer of the tongue. Arch Surg 1940; 41:888–936.
19. Martin HE, MacComb WS, Blady JV. A report on cancer of the lip. Ann Surg 1941; 114:226–42.
20. Martin HE. Cancer of the gums. Am J Surg 1941; 54:765–806.
21. Braund RR, Martin HE. Distant metastasis in cancer of the upper respiratory and alimentary tracts. Surg Gynecol Obstet 1941; 73:63–71.
22. Peltier LF, Thomas LB, Barclay THC, Kremen AJ. The incidence of distant metastases among patients dying with head and neck cancer. Surgery 1951; 30:827–33.
23. Gowen GF, DeSuto-Nagy G. The incidence and sites of distant metastases in head and neck carcinoma. Surg Gynecol Obstet 1963; 116:603–7.
24. O'Brien PH, Carlson R, Steubner EA, Staley CT. Distant metastases in epidermoid cell carcinoma of the head and neck. Cancer 1971; 27:304–7.
25. Dennington MO, Carter DR, Meyers AD. Distant metastases in head and neck epidermoid carcinoma. Laryngoscope 1980; 90:196–201.
26. Kotwall C, Sako K, Razack MS, et al. Am J Surg 1987; 154:439–42.
27. Castigliano SG, Rominger CJ. Distant metastasis from carcinoma of the oral cavity. Am J Roentgenol 1954; 71:997–1006.
28. Berger DS, Fletcher GH. Distant metastases following local control of squamous-cell carcinoma of the nasopharynx, tonsillar fossa and base of the tongue. Radiology 1971; 100:141–3.
29. Probert JC, Thompson RW, Bagshaw MA. Patterns of spread of distant metastases in head and neck cancer. Cancer 1974; 33:127–33.
30. Amer MH, Al-Sarraf M, Vaitkevicius VK. Factors that effect response to chemotherapy and survival of patients with advanced head and neck cancer. Cancer 1979; 43:2202–6.
31. Papac RJ. Distant metastases from head and neck cancer. Cancer 1984; 53:342–5.
32. Snow GB, Balm AJM, Arendsen JW, et al. Prognostic factors in neck node metastasis. In: Larson DL, Ballantyne AJ, Guillamondequi OM, eds. Cancer in the neck. New York: Macmillan, 1986:53–63.
33. Bennet SH, Futrell JW, Roth JA, et al. Prognostic significance of histologic host response in cancer of the larynx and hypopharynx. Cancer 1971; 28:1255–65.
34. Noone RB, Bonner H, Raymond S, et al. Lymph node metastases in oral carcinoma: a correlation of histopathology with survival. Plast Reconstr Surg 1974; 53:158–66.
35. Shah JC, Cendon RA, Farr HW, Strong EW. Carcinoma of the oral cavity (factors affecting treatment failure at the primary site and neck). Am J Surg 1976; 132:504–7.
36. Sessions DG. Surgical pathology of cancer of the larynx and hypopharynx. Laryngoscope 1976; 86:814–39.
37. Kalnins IK, Leonard AG, Sako K, Razack MS, Shedd DP. Correlation between prognosis and degree of lymph node involvement in carcinoma of the oral cavity. Am J Surg 1977; 134:450–4.
38. Zoller M, Goodman ML, Cummings CW. Guidelines for prognosis in head and neck cancer with nodal metastasis. Laryngoscope 1978; 88:135–40.
39. Cachin Y, Sancho-Garnier H, Micheau Ch, Marandas P. Nodal metastasis from carcinomas of the oropharynx. Otolaryngol Clin North Am 1979; 12:145–54.
40. Johnson JT, Myers EN, Bedetti CN, et al. Cervical lymph node metastases. Arch Otolaryngol 1985; 111:534–7.
41. Snow GB, Annyas AA, Van Slooten EA, et al. Prognostic factors of neck node metastasis. Clin Otolaryngol 1982; 7:185–92.
42. Johnson JT, Barnes EL, Myers EN, et al. The extracapsular spread of tumors incervical node metastasis. Arch Otolaryngol 1981; 107:725–9.
43. Crile GW. Carcinoma of the jaws, tongue, cheek and lips. Surg Gynecol Obstet 1923; 2:159–84.
44. Fisher B, Redmond C, Fisher ER. The contribution of recent NSABP clinical trials of primary breast cancer therapy to an understanding of tumor biology. An overview of findings. Cancer 1980; 46:1009–25.
45. Fisher B, Fisher ER. The interrelationship of hematogenous and lymphatic tumor cell dissemination. Surg Gynecol Obstet 1966; 122:791–8.
46. Fisher B, Fisher ER. Transmigration of lymph nodes by tumor cells. Science 1966; 152:1397–8.
47. Fisher B, Saffer EA, Fisher ER. Studies concerning the regional lymph node in cancer. Cancer 1974; 33:271–9.
48. Schabel FM Jr. Concept for systemic treatment of micrometastases. Cancer 1975; 35:15–24.
49. Martin DS, Fugmann RA, Stolfi RL, Hayworth PE. Solid tumor animal model therapeutically predictive for human breast cancer. Cancer Chemother Rep 1975; 5:89–109.
50. Salmon SE. Kinetics of minimal residual disease. Recent Results Cancer Res 1979; 67:5–15.
51. Simpson-Herren L, Sanford AH, Holmquist JP. Effects of surgery on the cell kinetics of residual tumor. Cancer Treat Rep 1976; 60:1749–60.
52. Gunduz N, Fisher B, Saffer EA. Effect of surgical removal on the growth and kinetics of residual tumor. Cancer Res 1979; 39:3861–5.
53. DeVita VT Jr. The relationship between tumor mass and resistance to chemotherapy. Implication for surgical adjuvant treatment of cancer. Cancer 1983; 51:1209–20.
54. Goldie JH, Coldman AJ. A mathematical model for relating the drug sensitivity of tumors to their spontaneous mutation rate. Cancer Treat Rep 1979; 63:1727–33.
55. Goldie JH, Coldman AJ. The genetic origin of drug resistance in neoplasms: implications for systemic therapy. Cancer Res 1984; 44:3643–53.
56. Heppner GH. Tumor heterogeneity. Cancer Res 1984; 44:2259–65.
57. Fidler IJ, Poste G. The cellular heterogeneity of malignant neoplasms: implications for adjuvant chemotherapy. Semin Oncol 1985; 12:207–21.
58. Goldie JH, Coldman AJ. Quantitative model for multiple levels of drug resistance in clinical tumors. Cancer Treat Rep 1983; 67:923–31.

59. Goldie JH, Coldman AJ, Gudauskas GA. Rationale for the use of alternating non-cross-resistant chemotherapy. Cancer Treat Rep 1982; 66:439–49.

60. Griswold DP Jr. The potential for murine tumor models in surgical adjuvant chemotherapy. Cancer Chemother Rep 1975; 5:187–204.

61. Mayo JG, Laster WRJ, Andrews CM, et al. Success and failure in the treatment of solid tumors III. "Cure" of metastatic Lewis lung carcinoma with methyl-CCNU (NSC-95441) and surgery–chemotherapy. Cancer Chemother Rep 1972; 56:183–95.

62. Schabel FJ. Concepts for treatment of micrometastases developed in murine systems. Am J Roentgenol 1976; 126:500–11.

63. Schabel FJ. Surgical adjuvant chemotherapy of metastatic murine tumors. Cancer 1977; 40:558–68.

64. Schabel FJ. Recent studies with surgical adjuvant chemotherapy or immunotherapy of metastatic solid tumors of mice. In: Jones S, Salmon S, eds. Adjuvant therapy of cancer, vol II. Orlando: Grune & Stratton, 1979:3–17.

65. Mulder JH, de Ruiter J, Edelstein MB, et al. Model studies in adjuvant chemotherapy. Cancer Treat Rep 1983; 67:45–50.

66. Arcangeli G, Nervi C, Righini R, et al. Combined radiation and drugs: the effect of intra-arterial chemotherapy followed by radiotherapy in head and neck cancer. Radiother Oncol 1983; 1:101–7.

67. Richard J, Molinary R, Sancho-Garnier H, et al. A randomized trial comparing surgery preceded or not by intra-arterial chemotherapy in squamous cell carcinoma of the head and neck. Proceedings of the International Conference on Head and Neck Cancer, Baltimore, 1984 (abstr # 113).

68. Bonadonna G, Valagussa P. Adjuvant systemic therapy for resectable breast cancer. J Clin Oncol 1985; 3:259–75.

69. Al-Sarraf M. Head and neck cancer: Chemotherapy concepts. Semin Oncol 1988; 15:70–85.

70. Choksi AJ, Hong WK, Dimery IW, et al. Continuous cisplatin (24-hours) and 5-fluorouracil (120-hours) infusion in recurrent head and neck squamous cell carcinoma. Cancer 1988; 61:909–12.

71. Gonzales-Vela JL, Panasci L, Black M, et al. Combination chemotherapy with carboplatin and bleomycin for advanced and recurrent head and neck cancer: a phase II study. J Surg Oncol 1988; 39:215–6.

72. Olver IN, Dalley D, Woods R, et al. Carboplatin and continuous infusion 5-fluorouracil for advanced head and neck cancer. Eur J Cancer Clin Oncol 1989; 25:173–6.

73. Paredes J, Hong WK, Felder JB, et al. Prospective randomized trial of high-dose cisplatin and fluorouracil infusion with or without sodium diethyldithiocarbamate in recurrent and/or metastatic squamous cell carcinoma of the head and neck. J Clin Oncol 1988; 6:955–62.

74. Mackintosch JF, Coater AS, Tattersall MHN, et al. Chemotherapy of advanced head and neck cancer: updated results of a randomized trial of the order of administration of sequential methotrexate and 5-fluorouracil. Med Pediatr Oncol 1988; 16:304–7.

75. Browman GP, Levine MN, Goodyear MD, et al. Methotrexate/fluorouracil scheduling influences normal tissue toxicity but not antitumor effects in patients with squamous cell head and neck cancer: results from a randomized trial. J Clin Oncol 1988; 6:963–8.

76. Vokes EE, Choi KE, Schilsky RL, et al. Cisplatin, fluorouracil, and high-dose leucovorin for recurrent and/or metastatic head and neck cancer. J Clin Oncol 1988; 6:618–26.

77. Vogl SE, Schoenfeld DA, Kaplan BH, et al. A randomized prospective comparison of methotrexate with a combination of methotrexate, bleomycin, and cisplatin in head and neck cancer. Cancer 1985; 56:432–42.

78. Chauvergne J, Cappelaere P, Fargeot P, et al. Étude randomisee comparant la cisplatine seul ou associe dans le traitement palliatif de carcinomes des voies aerodigestives superieures. Analyse d'une serie de 209 patients. Bull Cancer (Paris) 1988; 75:9–22.

79. Clavel M, Cappelaere P, Cognetti F, et al. Comparison between C (cisplatin) alone and two cisplatin-containing mul-

tiple drug regimens: CABO (cisplatin, methotrexate, bleomycine, oncovin) and CF (cisplatin-FU) in advanced head and neck carcinomas. Report on a randomized EORTC trial 24842 including 380 patients. Cancer Chemother Pharmacol (suppl) 23:C73. Abstr # 292 (S).

80. Choski AJ, Dimery IW, Hong WK. Adjuvant chemotherapy of head and neck cancer. The past, the present and the future. Semin Oncol 1988; 15:45–59.

81. Clark JR, Fallon BG, Dreyfuss AJ, et al. Chemotherapeutic strategies in the multidisciplinary treatment of head and neck cancer. Semin Oncol 1988; 15:35–44.

82. Schabel FM Jr, Griswold DP Jr, Corbett TH, et al. Testing therapeutic hypotheses in mice and man: observations on the therapeutic activity against advanced solid tumors in mice treated with anticancer drugs that have demonstrated or potential clinical utility for treatment of advanced solid tumors of man. In: DeVita VT, Busch H, eds. Methods in cancer research. New York: Academic Press, 1979:3–51.

83. De Vita VT Jr. Principles of chemotherapy. In: DeVita VT, Hellman S, Rosenberg SA, eds. Cancer: Principles and practice of oncology. Philadelphia: JB Lippincott, 1989:276–300.

84. Forastiere AA, Takasugi BJ, Baker SR, et al. High-dose cisplatin in advanced head and neck cancer. Cancer Chemother Pharmacol 1987; 19:155–8.

85. Planting AST, Van der Burg MEL, Stoter G, Verweij J. Phase I/II study of a short course of weekly high-dose cisplatin in advanced solid tumors. Sixth International Symposium on Platinum and Other Metal Coordination Compounds in Cancer Chemotherapy, San Diego, 1991:123 (abstr).

86. Verweij J. Personal communication.

87. Million RR, Cassisi NJ, Clark JR. Cancer of the head and neck. In: DeVita VT, Hellman S, Rosenberg SA, eds. Cancer: Principles and practice of oncology. Philadelphia: JB Lippincott, 1989:488–590.

88. Bonadonna G, Valagussa P. Dose–response effect of adjuvant chemotherapy in breast cancer. N Eng J Med 1981; 304:10–15.

89. Buyse M, Zeleniuch-Jacquotta A, Chalmers ThC. Adjuvant therapy of colorectal cancer. JAMA 1988; 259:3571–8.

90. Grage TB, Hill GJ, Cornell GN, et al. Adjuvant chemotherapy in large-bowel cancer: demonstration of effectiveness of single agent chemotherapy in a prospectively controlled, randomized trial. Recent Results Cancer Res 1978; 68:222–30.

91. Taylor SG IV. Integration of chemotherapy into the combined modality therapy of head and neck squamous cancer. Int J Radiat Oncol Biol Phys 1987; 13:779–83.

92. Vermorken JB. Combination of chemotherapy and radiotherapy. In: Veronesi U, Molinari R, Banfi A, Santoro CEA, eds. I tumori della testa e del collo. Ambrosiana: Milan, 1990:87–93.

93. Taylor SG IV. Head and neck cancer. In: Pinedo HM, Chabner BA, Longo DL, eds. Cancer chemotherapy and biological response modifiers, annual XI. Amsterdam: Elsevier, 1990:416–31.

94. Gasparini M, Lombardi F, Rottoli L, et al. Combined radiotherapy and chemotherapy in stage T3 and T4 nasopharyngeal carcinoma in children. J Clin Oncol 1988; 6:491–4.

95. Kim TH, McLaren J, Alvarado CS, et al. Adjuvant chemotherapy for advanced nasopharyngeal carcinoma in childhood. Cancer 1989; 63:1922–6.

96. Dimery IW, Legha SS, Peters LJ, et al. Adjuvant chemotherapy for advanced nasopharyngeal carcinoma. Cancer 1987; 60:943–9.

97. Teo P, Ho JHC, Choy D, et al. Adjunctive chemotherapy to radical radiation therapy in the treatment of advanced nasopharyngeal carcinoma. Int J Radiat Oncol Biol Phys 1987; 13:679–85.

98. Kirkwood JM, Miller D, Weichselbaum R, et al. Symposium: Adjuvant cancer therapy of head and neck tumors. Predefinitive and postdefinitive chemotherapy for locally advanced squamous carcinoma of the head and neck. Laryngoscope 1979; 89:573–81.

99. Arlen M. Epidermoid carcinoma of head and neck. NY State J Med 1979; Aug.:1384–8.

100. Taylor SG, Sisson GA, Bytell DE. Adjuvant chemoimmunotherapy of head and neck cancer. In: Bonadonna G, Mathé G, Salmon SE, eds. Adjuvant therapies and markers of postsurgical minimal residual disease, vol II. Adjuvant therapies of the various primary tumors. Recent Results Cancer Res 68. Berlin: Springer, 1979:297–308.

101. Taylor SG, Bytell DE, Sisson GA. Methotrexate (M) with leucovorin (L) as an adjuvant to surgery (S) and radiotherapy (R) in locally advanced squamous carcinoma in the head and neck. Proc Am Assoc Cancer Res and Am Soc Clin Oncol (abstr # C-320) 1977:346.

102. Huang AT, Cole TB, Fishburn R, et al. Adjuvant chemotherapy after surgery and radiation for stage III and IV head and neck cancer. Ann Surg 1984; 200:195–9.

103. Johnson JT, Myers EN, Srodes CH, et al. Maintenance chemotherapy for high-risk patients. A preliminary report. Arch Otolaryngol 1985; 111:727–9.

104. Johnson JT, Myers EN, Schramm VL, et al. Adjuvant chemotherapy for high-risk squamous cell carcinoma of the head and neck. J Clin Oncol 1987;5:456–8.

105. Al-Sarraf M. Chemotherapy strategies on squamous cell carcinoma of the head and neck. CRC Crit Rev Oncol Hematol 1984; 1:323–55.

106. Jacobs JR, Pajak ThF, Kinzie J, et al. Induction chemotherapy in advanced head and neck cancer. Arch Otolaryngol Head Neck Surg 1987; 113:193–7.

107. Jacobs JR, Pajak TF, Al-Sarraf M, et al. Chemotherapy following surgery for head and neck cancer. Am J Clin Oncol 1989; 12:185–9.

108. Szpirglas H, Chastang CL, Bertrand JCh. Adjuvant treatment of tongue and floor of the mouth cancers. Recent Results Cancer Res 1978; 68:309–17.

109. Domenge C, Marands P, Douillard JY, et al. Postsurgical adjuvant chemotherapy in extracapsular spread, invaded lymph node (N+ R+) of epidermoid carcinoma of the head and neck. A randomized multicentric trial. Proc Eur Conf Clin Oncol 1987; 4:242.

110. Bitter K. Postoperative chemotherapy versus postoperative cobalt-60 radiation in patients with advanced oral carcinoma: Report on a randomized study (abstr). Head Neck Surg 1981; 3:260.

111. Rossi A, Molinari R, Boracchi P, et al. Adjuvant chemotherapy with vincristine, cyclophosphamide, and doxorubicin after radiotherapy in local–regional nasopharyngeal cancer: Results of a 4-year multicenter randomized study. J Clin Oncol 1988; 6:1401–10.

112. Tejada F, Chandler JR. Combined therapy for stage III and IV Head and Neck cancer (H&N) (abstr # C774). Proc Am Soc Clin Oncol 1982; 1:199.

113. Rentschler RE, Wilbur DW, Petti GH, et al. Adjuvant methotrexate escalated to toxicity for resectable stage III and IV squamous head and neck carcinomas. A prospective, randomized study. J Clin Oncol 1987; 5:278–85.

114. Taylor SG, Applebaum E, Showel JL, et al. A randomized trial of adjuvant chemotherapy in head and neck cancer. J Clin Oncol 1985; 3:672–9.

115. Stell PM, Dalby JE, Strickland P, et al. Sequential chemotherapy and radiotherapy in advanced head and neck cancer. Clin Radiol 1983; 34:463–7.

116. Kun LE, Toohill RJ, Holoye PY, et al. A randomized study of adjuvant chemotherapy for cancer of the upper aerodigestive tract. Int J Radiat Oncol Biol Phys 1986; 12:173–8.

117. Holoye PY, Grossman ThW, Toohill RJ, et al. Randomized study of adjuvant chemotherapy for head and neck cancer. Otolaryngol Head Neck Surg 1985; 93:712–7.

118. Stolwijk C, Wagener DJT, Van den Broek P, et al. Randomized neo-adjuvant chemotherapy trial for advanced head and neck cancer. Neth J Med 1985; 28:347–51.

119. Ervin ThJ, Clark JR, Weichselbaum RR, et al. An analysis of induction and adjuvant chemotherapy in the multidisciplinary treatment of squamous-cell carcinoma of the head and neck. J Clin Oncol 1987; 5:10–20.

120. Head and Neck Contracts Program. Adjuvant chemotherapy for advanced head and neck squamous carcinoma. Final report of the Head and Neck Contracts Program. Cancer 1987; 60:301–11.

121. Jacobs C, Makuch R. Efficacy of adjuvant chemotherapy for patients with resectable head and neck cancer: A subset analysis of the head and neck contracts program. J Clin Oncol 1990; 8:838–47.

122. Stell PM, Rawson NSB. Adjuvant chemotherapy in head and neck cancer. Br J Cancer 1990; 61:779–87.

Concomitant Chemotherapy and Radiotherapy

J. Jassem, L. Dewit, R. Keus, H. Bartelink

Rationale

Concomitant chemoradiotherapy aims at an interaction between the two modalities which results in a greater extra cell killing effect in the tumor than in the surrounding normal tissue. The therapeutic ratio after irradiation, defined as the ratio of incidence of tumor cure to the incidence of complications, should, in principle, always be greater than one. Combination of chemotherapy with radiotherapy should lead to an increase of this ratio. In order to achieve this goal, experimental research needs to provide information on the best choice of cytostatic drugs, the type of interaction involved, and the optimal dose–time sequence in both tumor and normal tissue.

Scientific Considerations

Modification of the Dose–Response Curve for Irradiation

For concomitant chemoradiotherapy to be successful, the net cell killing effect should be larger in the tumor than in the normal tissue. Ideally, a complete dose–response curve is known for both the drug and irradiation. In addition, the extent of modification of the dose–response curve for an agent, given in graded doses, should be obtained. In practice, however, only full dose–response curve for irradiation and the radiation-modifying effects of a drug, given in one or at most a few doses, are usually available.

Radiation dose–response curves for cell survival are characterized on a semilogarithmic scale by a "shoulder" in the low dose region and an almost straight line in the high dose region. Mathematically, they are at best described by a linear–quadratic relationship (36):

$$S/S_0 = e^{-n(\alpha d_n + \beta d_n^2)}$$

where S/S_0 = surviving fraction
n = fraction number
d_n = dose per fraction, expressed in Gy.

α and β are constants of proportionality of the linear term (expressed in Gy^{-1}) and the quadratic term (expressed in Gy^{-2}), respectively. This relationship implies that the dose–response curve for irradiation on a semilogarithmic scale is continuously bending. The linear term is relatively more important at low doses and the quadratic term dominates at high doses. The curvature of the dose−response relationship is dependent on the magnitude of the α and the β components.

The interesting point that has emerged from experimental data in vivo on a large number of tumors and normal tissues is that a fairly clear distinction can be made between early responding normal tissues and tumors on the one hand and late responding tissues on the other (41, 129). In the former, the α-component is considerably larger than the β-component, by a factor of from 7 to >35, whereas in the latter, α is usually only from 1.5 to 5 times larger than β. In general, the α-term is larger for tumors and for early responding normal tissues than for late responding normal tissues, whereas the opposite is true for the β-term (112). The consequence of this phenomenon is that in clinical radiotherapy, where most frequently low radiation doses of from 1.0 to 2.0 Gy are delivered, i.e. cell killing being dominated by the α-term, relatively more cells are killed by irradiation in the tumors and early responding normal tissues than in the late responding tissues. Clearly, this situation is of therapeutic benefit.

An important phenomenon occurring with fractionation is that between two fractions spaced several hours apart, a proportion of the radiation damage in cells is repaired. This process is often referred to as sublethal damage repair. In an in vitro cell survival curve, this is reflected by the reappearance of the initial shoulder of the survival curve after the next fraction. Since in a clinical situation usually from 20 to 35 daily fractions are delivered, the difference in cell killing between tumors/early normal tissues and late normal tissues is magnified to n times the difference at dose d_n. Such a difference is very likely to be

clinically relevant. This will be illustrated with an example below.

When a cytostatic drug is present at the time of irradiation of cells cultured in vitro, in principle, three types of modification of the radiation dose−response curve can occur: either the initial shoulder is reduced or the final slope is increased or both parts of the curve are modified. In modern radiobiological terms, either the α-term or the β-component or both are increased by the drug. Theoretical dose−response curves, using equation (1), with α- and β-values which are typical for a tumor and for an early responding normal tissue, are illustrated in Figure 6.2 A. If a drug enhances the α-term by a factor of 2, while leaving the β-term unaffected, the dose−response relation becomes less curved. The largest relative dose reduction for a given level of cell survival is obtained in the low dose region. If, on the other hand, the drug doubles the β-term without affecting the α-term, the dose−response relation becomes more curved. In this case, the relative dose reduction for a given level of effect becomes larger with higher radiation doses. It is important to notice that in this example the extra cell killing obtained with "β-sensitization" surpasses that achieved by "α-sensitization" only at single doses of radiation beyond 10 Gy.

Figure 6.2 B illustrates radiation dose−response curves that are representative for a late responding normal tissue. Because of a lower α- and a higher β-term, it is more bent than the one for a tumor or an early responding normal tissue. A drug which enhances the α-term by 2 modifies the dose−response curve to a smaller extent than the one for an early responding tissue. In contrast, the change in the dose−response curve when the β-term is increased by 2 is larger than in the previous situation.

Fig. 6.2 **Calculated radiation dose response curves, using the linear quadratic model** [see equation (1)]. A, a typical example of a curve for tumor or an early responding normal tissue (solid line); B, a typical example of a late responding normal tissue (solid line). In both cases, the dashed line represents a dose−response curve when a drug enhances the α-term by a factor of 2, whereas the dotted line illustrates a dose response curve after the β-term was increased by a factor of 2 by the drug

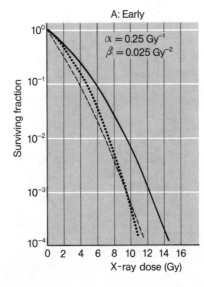

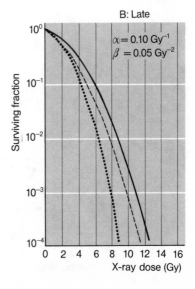

In conclusion, at radiation doses between 2 and 10 Gy, an "α-enhancer" is more effective in enhanced cell killing in a tumor and in an early responding normal tissue than in a late responding tissue, whereas the opposite is true for a "β-sensitizer."

The importance of this observation becomes more clear if we consider the cell killing effect by combination chemoradiotherapy using a commonly used fractionated irradiation regime. Let us assume a patient with a tumor in the head and neck of 150 g, that is approximately 6.5 cm in diameter. Suppose 3% of the cells are clonogenic, this tumor contains 10^{10} clonogenic cells, which need to be eradicated to obtain local tumor control. If the cell survival characteristics of these cells for irradiation are adequately described by equation (1) with α- and β-values as given in Figure 6.2 A and assuming no clonogenic tumor cell proliferation during conventional daily irradiation (2 Gy per fraction), it can be calculated that at least 38 fractions are required to obtain a near 100% tumor cure (Fig. 6.3 A). If a cytostatic drug increases the α-component by a factor of 2 at each fraction, only 21 fractions would be required to obtain the same amount of cell killing. If, on the other hand, the drug would double the β-component, 33 fractions would still be needed for the same effect. In a late responding normal tissue with cell survival parameters as given in Figure 6.2 B and in which we consider, for convenience, 10^{10} clonogenic cells in the irradiated volume, 38 fractions of 2 Gy would kill only approximately 8×10^6 cells (Fig. 6.3 B). A drug which increases the α-term by 2, causes a pronounced increase in cell killing in a late responding tissue, albeit not as much as in the tumor or in the early responding normal tissue. If the drug enhances the β-term by 2, an equally large increase in cell killing is observed, which is larger than that obtained in a tumor.

In conclusion, a cytostatic drug, given in combination with irradiation, is of more therapeutic benefit if it is a strong "α-enhancer" rather than a "β-enhancer." A "β-enhancer" is potentially hazardous, since it increases the cell killing effect of irradiation to a greater extent in a late responding normal tissue than in a tumor or an early responding normal tissue.

This mathemathical approach of modification of a radiation dose response curve by a cytostatic drug, using the linear–quadratic model, is rather new. Consequently, in reviewing the literature data (see below), we will refer to standard terminology as used by the various authors, such as an inhibitor of sublethal damage repair and a radiosensitizer. Using the old concept of an exponential dose–response curve with an initial shoulder for radiation, a repair inhibitor reduces the shoulder, whereas a radiosensitizer increases the final slope of the dose–response curve. In the new concept, the former would be called an "α-enhancer" and the latter a "β-enhancer". It should be realized, however, that both terms—the old one and the new one—are not entirely overlapping, but indicate a slightly different type of modification of a radiation dose–response curve.

Influence on Clonogenic Cell Proliferation

In the previous section, proliferation of the clonogenic cell population occurring during fractionated irradiation has been considered negligible. There is

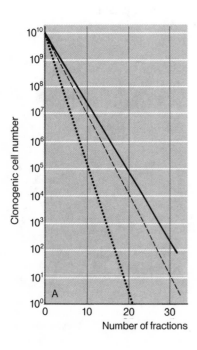

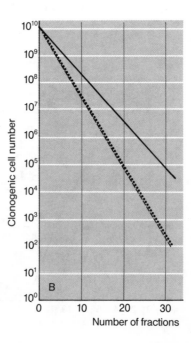

Fig. 6.3 **Calculated clonogenic cell survival as a function of number of radiation fractions of 2 Gy, using the linear quadratic model** [see equation (1)]. A, example of a curve for a tumor or an early responding tissue with the same α- and β-values as in Figure 6.2 (solid line); B, example of a curve for a late responding normal tissue with the same α- and β-values as in Figure 6.2. The same enhancement ratios were used as in Figure 6.2, that is a factor of 2 for the α-term (dashed line) or for the β-term (dotted line). In these calculations, proliferation was considered to be nil during the fractionated irradiation

accumulating evidence, however, emerging from both clinical and experimental studies, that clonogenic cell proliferation is a very important factor determining the net amount of cell killing in tumors as well as in some normal tissues (52, 64, 100, 114, 116). The proliferation factor can be taken into account in the linear−quadratic model as follows:

$$S/S_0 = e^{-n(\alpha d_n + \beta d_n^2) + \lambda t}$$

where t_0 = overall treatment time, and
λ = a constant of proportionality, related to the cell number doubling time.

In contrast to the linear and quadratic term, the proliferation term has a positive sign, which results in an increase in the surviving fraction. Including the proliferation factor into a mathematical formulation is still a subject of much debate (e. g. 42, 100, 112, 130). The above-mentioned equation therefore is not uniformly accepted, but it is a reasonably good approach.

The proliferation rate of clonogenic cells can be readily estimated from labeling tumor cells in vivo with, for instance, halogenated pyrimidines (e. g. iododeoxyuridine) (10). It appears from these analyses that the potential doubling time in head and neck tumors was frequently 5 days or less (12, 34). There is even clinical evidence for accelerated proliferation of clonogenic cells occurring from approximately the third week onwards during conventionally fractionated irradiation (69). Such clonogenic cell proliferation results in a relative increase in cell survival during irradiation. There are now very strong clinical indications that reducing the overall treatment time in radiotherapy results in a higher

cure rate, especially in patients with a short potential tumor doubling time (13a).

Let us consider again the previously mentioned example of a tumor with 10^{10} clonogenic cells for which there is a dose−response relationship for irradiation as illustrated in Figure 6.2, and, which has in addition, a potential doubling time of 5 days. If we assume a constant proliferation rate of the clonogenic cells *during* conventionally fractionated irradiation, that is 5 time 2 Gy per week, cell survival will be gradually higher with increasing fraction number in this situation compared to if no proliferation would occur. Figure 6.4 illustrates that due to such proliferation, the net cell killing effect during irradiation is less than without proliferation: the negative slope of the dose−response curve during the week days when irradiation is delivered is less steep and in the treatment-free weekends the slope becomes even positive. As a result, no tumor cure is obtained after as many as 38 fractions of 2 Gy (i. e. a total dose of 76 Gy in 7.5 weeks). A cytostatic drug which would inhibit such proliferation, when given in combination with irradiation, would increase the tumor cure probability. With complete proliferation inhibition by the drug, cell survival would be as illustrated by curve 1 in Figure 6.4. If the drug is ineffective in blocking proliferation, alternatively the detrimental effect of proliferation during irradiation can be minimized by reducing overall time by giving more than one fraction per day. This is known as "accelerated fractionation."

Dose and Timing Effects of Drugs and Irradiation

In general, the extent of modification by a cytostatic drug of a radiation dose−response curve is drug dose

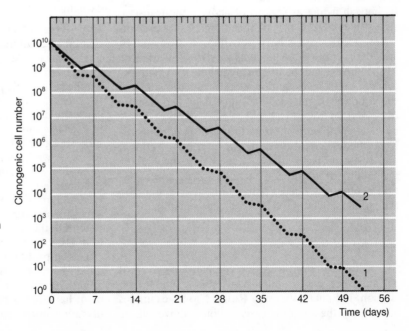

Fig. 6.4 **Calculated clonogenic cell survival as a function of time during a conventionally fractionated irradiation regime of 5 times 2 Gy per week.** Curve (1) represents the situation in which no proliferation occurs whereas curve (2) illustrates cell survival of a clonogenic cell population with a uniform potential doubling time of 5 days

dependent (99). The magnitude of interaction between irradiation and a drug is also time and sequence dependent (99). In most experimental tumors and in early responding normal tissues, radiation enhancement is observed only with time intervals of 1 week or less. This is because at longer time intervals the tissue has recovered from the damage from either agent by repopulation. In late responding, slowly proliferating normal tissues, the radiation enhancement is much less time dependent. Increased radiation damage has been observed in such tissues even at intervals of several months (31). In the past, this phenomenon has been referred to as the "recall-phenomenon." It basically reflects the inability of slowly proliferating normal tissues to recover sufficiently from damage by either a cytostatic drug or irradiation by compensatory proliferation.

In order to maximize the probability of interaction of irradiation and chemotherapy in a tumor, by whatever mechanism, research should focus on investigating the interaction of a drug with important cellular targets, presumed to be also involved in radiation damage. This is a highly complex area of research. First, despite intensive investigations, over many years, the critical lesion from radiation causing cell death is still poorly defined. The critical target for radiation is generally accepted to be DNA, and presumably the unrepaired DNA double strand breaks play an important role (e. g. 17). These DNA lesions are presumed to occur at random over the entire genome. Drugs which also act on DNA have the highest probability of interaction with radiation. The mechanism of action of these drugs in the DNA is usually well known. For certain drugs, the DNA damage is inflicted over the entire genome (i. e. DNA base analogues which are incorporated) whereas for others it occurs in restricted areas (e. g. bleomycin acting in regions of active gene transcription (9), c-DDP acting at specific DNA base sequences (133)). Assays have now become available to study the drug−DNA adducts in vivo. An example of such investigations will be given below. An important topic for investigation therefore is the study of the kinetics of intracellular uptake of a cytostatic drug and of formation and repair of drug−DNA adducts. With such information, a drug administration schedule could be designed on a more rational and scientific basis. It is assumed that the highest probability of interaction between a drug and radiation is obtained when irradiation is delivered at the time of maximal drug−DNA adduct formation.

Preclinical data

We will not attempt to give a complete overview of all published experimental data on concomitant radiation and chemotherapy. Rather, some examples illustrating the scientific basis outlined above will be discussed. Literature data will be selected also on the basis of drugs which were used in combination with irradiation in the clinic.

Modification of the Dose−Response Curve for Irradiation

5-Fluorouracil (5-FU). 5-FU has been extensively investigated in the laboratory. No clear picture has emerged from in vitro and in vivo tumor experiments concerning the mechanism of radiation enhancement by 5-FU. The results varied from a minor radiation-inhibiting effect (65), over noninteractive (65, 103) to enhancement (121, 125). To obtain a maximal effect, it seemed important, however, to expose the tumor cells continuously to 5-FU for a time at least as long as the cell cycle time (18, 121). Moderate radiation enhancement was observed in intestinal crypt cells (53) and in bone marrow (65), whereas no increase in late radiation damage was found in the lung (123). Thus, for clinical application, 5-FU is preferably given in a prolonged continuous infusion during fractionated irradiation. The difference in radiation enhancement between tumors and normal tissues is expected to be small.

Methotrexate (MTX). Experiments on combination irradiation and MTX have yielded similar conclusions as for 5-FU. Variable effects were seen in a number of tumors (65), whereas moderate to severe enhancement ratios were observed in intestinal crypt cells and in skin (76, 91). No effect of the drug was reported on late radiation damage in lung (123) or in spinal cord (117). It is unclear which type of interaction is involved. It is possible that some of the observed effects are attributed to independent cell killing. Cell cycle perturbations by either radiation or the drug are likely to have occurred, which might explain the observed influence of time and sequence.

Hydroxyurea (HU). HU has been extensively investigated in combination with irradiation in head and neck cancer a decade ago. The interest for this drug came from its particular cytotoxic properties. It kills proliferating cells preferentially in S-phase, which is the most radioresistant phase of the cell cycle. It also causes a dose-dependent block in early S, thereby increasing the proportion of cells in the more radiosensitive G1-phase of the cell cycle. In addition, for less well understood reasons, it also causes enhanced cell killing when given some hours after irradiation (93). The "synergistic" effect between HU and irradiation has been well documented in experimental tumors in vitro and in vivo (115). The potential therapeutic benefit comes from the fact that HU is only toxic to and has radiosensitizing effects in proliferating cells, which leaves the slowly dividing, late reacting normal tissues relatively unharmed. Minor to moderate radiation enhancement has been observed experimentally only in proliferating bone marrow cells, intestinal crypt cells, and skin, whereas this effect was absent in resting bone marrow cells and lung (99).

Bleomycin (BLM). Another well investigated drug in the laboratory, which also has been widely used clinically in head and neck cancer patients, is bleomycin. This drug has been shown to inhibit repair of sublethal radiation damage in cultured cells (15, 105). In vivo, modest radiation enhancement after fractionated irradiation was observed in a mouse tumor and in mouse skin (72). More pronounced effects were observed in intestinal crypt cells (77) and in lip mucosa (119). In the latter, the effects were presumably also due to inhibition of sublethal radiation damage repair (119). A significant increase in late radiation damage was found in the mouse lung (73, 123). Hence, this drug does not seem to be a good candidate for improving the therapeutic ratio with combined radiochemotherapy.

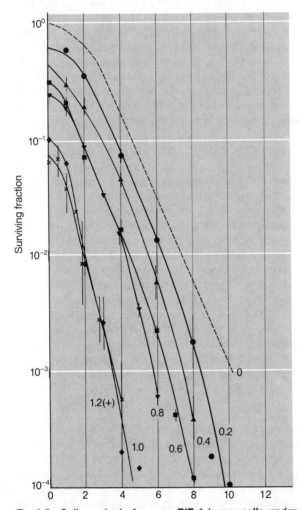

Fig. 6.5 **Cell survival of mouse RIF 1 tumor cells under ambient conditions as a function of radiation dose and graded concentrations of a 1 hour exposure to c-DDP.** [Reproduced from Begg et al. (II) with permission of the authors]

Cisplatin (c-DDP). A good example of a drug dose dependent increase in the slope of a dose–response curve for irradiation in cultured tumor cells comes from studies with c-DDP (Fig. 6.5). The maximum radiation enhancement obtained with c-DDP was a factor of 2.2 at a drug dose causing approximately 90% cell killing as well (11). Inhibition of sublethal damage repair has been found in split-dose experiments in vitro (21, 124) and, to a lesser extent, in vivo (13). The radiation enhancement appears to be cell line dependent and therefore cannot be considered as a general phenomenon (11).

In early responding normal tissues, such as the gut and skin, experimental data have shown a modest increase in radiation effect by c-DDP by a factor of from 1.1 to 1.3 (reviewed by e. g. 32). In some late responding normal tissues such as the kidney and lung, a similar modest radiation enhancement was observed (see review 32 and 57, 75, 104). In the colorectum, no enhancement of late radiation effect was observed (32, 33). A critical analysis of the data on both the early and late responding normal tissues suggests that the enhancement of the radiation effect was mainly due to independent cell killing (32). In the mouse small intestine, however, after correcting for the cell killing effect of the drug, an increase in the β-term of the linear–quadratic relationship by a factor of 2 [see equation (1)] by c-DDP was observed (32). In summary, these experimental studies have demonstrated a larger radioenhancement effect of c-DDP in some tumors than in normal tissues. In clinical application, this combination treatment might therefore lead to an improvement of the therapeutic ratio.

Mitomycin-C (MMC). MMC has been investigated on a limited scale only. In three experimental tumors in vivo, the combination of MMC and irradiation resulted in at most an additive effect (81, 98, 123). A minor increase in late lung damage was seen in mice when the drug was given concurrently with irradiation (123). Hence, based on these experimental data, MMC is unlikely to improve the therapeutic ratio.

Influence on Clonogenic Cell Proliferation

Relatively little attention has been given to the investigation of the effect of a drug on cell proliferation after irradiation. Such effects can be analyzed indirectly from time line experiments. In tumors, highly variable and inconsistent patterns have emerged from this type of experiment (99). In addition, fractionated experiments in vivo under ambient conditions are difficult to interpret because of other processes involved, such as reoxygenation and redistribution. The best way to investigate this issue is in cells cultured in vitro, but its relevance for the clinic is questionable.

In normal tissues, time line experiments are equally difficult to interpret. When cell cycle phase

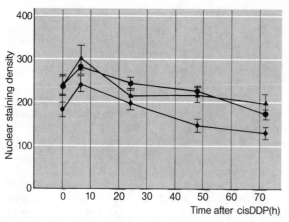

Fig. 6.6 Amount of Pt–DNA adducts, assessed from immunoperoxidase nuclear staining densitometry, as a function of time after 1 hour exposure to c-DDP in approximately equitoxic concentrations. Cell lines investigated were mouse RIF 1 tumor cells (■) and two human ovarian cancer cell lines, A2788 (▼) and A1847 (▲). [Reproduced with permission from Terheggen et al. (110)]

specific drugs are given in combination with irradiation, differences in the amount of cell killing as a function of the time interval might occur due to cell cycle perturbations.

A better approach is to label the proliferating cells in vivo by, for instance, tritiated thymidine. It was shown for c-DDP that, when this drug was given in combination with irradiation, it reduced the proliferation rate of intestinal crypt cells by a factor of 2.3

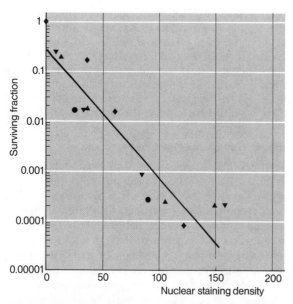

Fig. 6.7 Correlation between cell kill and amount of Pt–DNA adducts measured directly after 1 hour exposure to c-DDP for four cells lines: CHO cells (●), mouse RIF$_1$ tumor cells (■), human ovarian A2788 (▼) and A1847 (▲) cells. [Reproduced with permission from Terheggen et al. (110)]

compared to the repopulation rate after irradiation alone (32). If this effect also occured in patients, it would increase the amount of intestinal crypt cell damage during a daily fractionated irradiation regimen. This type of experiment is therefore required to obtain a better idea of the importance of proliferation inhibition by a drug after irradiation.

Dose and Timing Effects of Drugs and Irradiation

The radioenhancing effect of a drug is mostly drug dose dependent (Fig. 6.5). This drug dose dependence has been demonstrated in tumors as well as in normal tissues (99).

The timing effect has been discussed briefly in the previous section. The optimal time and sequence of administration of a drug is the one which gives the largest increase in cell killing in a tumor relative to that in a normal tissue. Such data are highly dependent on the experimental system used, and are therefore not easily translated into the clinic. Time line studies in patients using increasing drug doses are laborious, not easy to interpret with respect to tumor response, and of some ethical concern as regarding the potential hazardous and unpredictable toxic effects on normal tissues. This problem might be overcome by having a predictive assay for radiation–drug interaction. One way to investigate this issue in the laboratory is to measure the complexes formed between the cytostatic drug and its intracellular target. For c-DDP, for instance, Pt–DNA intrastrand cross links are probably the lesions responsible for the cytostatic effect of the drug. Such adducts can now be measured with a c-DDP–DNA antiserum using an immunoperoxidase staining technique (39, 79, 110). In cells cultured in vitro, the highest number of adducts is obtained at approximately 6 hours after drug exposure (Fig. 6.6). The number of adducts correlates well with the amount of cell killing (Fig. 6.7). This type of investigation can also be performed in experimental tumors and in normal tissues in vivo and even in patients (110, 111). If the number of Pt–DNA adducts would correlate with the radiosensitizing ability of c-DDP, this would provide a suitable predictive assay for designing a combined radiochemotherapy schedule.

Conclusions

In designing a combined radiochemotherapy regimen, some general rules can be deduced from these literature data. The highest tumor cell killing is seen by the concomitant use of radiotherapy and chemotherapy while less damage occurs in normal tissues when there is a long interval between both modalities. In general, a cytostatic drug acts mainly by independent cell killing. Inhibition of sublethal damage repair by a drug is less frequent, whereas "radiosensitization" is rather rare. Each of these

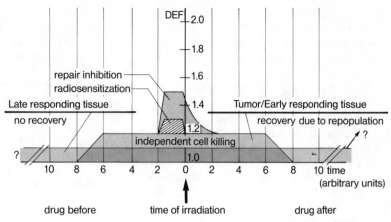

Fig. 6.**8** **Theoretical illustration of expected dose enhancement factor as a function of the time interval between and sequence of administration of a cytostatic drug and irradiation.** Three types of „interaction" are considered. For convenience, the radiation treatment time is concentrated on time point zero, although it usually takes 6–7 weeks. For further explanation, see text

processes might increase the net effect of combined radiochemotherapy. Such increase is quantitatively usually expressed as the dose enhancement factor (DEF), which is the ratio of the radiation dose required for a given level of effect after irradiation alone to the radiation dose after combination radiation and drug treatment. The scientific rationale, which might be taken into account when designing a combined radiochemotherapy regimen, is illustrated in Figure 6.**8**. When a drug causes only an independent cell killing effect, it may lead to a DEF of, for instance, 1.2 in an early responding tissue and 1.1 in a late responding tissue. Recovery in the early responding tissue from such extra damage occurs at an increasing time interval by repopulation. The time for this process to be completed is determined by the stem cell proliferation rate and the transit time of the functional cells. In a late responding tissue, such recovery process after irradiation hardly exists. Due to the continuously progressive nature of expression of late radiation damage at very long times after irradiation, the functional compartment might even be further compromised. This would cause an increase in the DEF, when a drug is administered at such long time intervals *after* irradiation. For the reverse sequence, it is unknown what happens at these long time intervals.

A drug which interacts with instantaneously formed and repaired radiation lesions (e. g. radical formation) causes an increase in radiation damage only when administered at short times *before* irradiation. The time interval between the administration of both agents to obtain an effect is determined by the kinetics of drug uptake in the tumor and the formation of the active complex with critical cellular targets. In this example, it is assumed that the maximal DEF was obtained when the drug was administered in vivo from 0.25 to 3 time units (e. g. hours) before irradiation.

A drug which inhibits repair of sublethal radiation damage obtains its maximal effect depending on the kinetics of interaction with cellular repair processes (e. g. inhibition of certain DNA repair enzymes. In this example, maximal inhibition is assumed when the repair inhibitor was given from 0.25 to 3 time units before irradiation. When given after irradiation, the inhibiting effect of the drug is reduced exponentially with increasing time interval. This is because sublethal damage repair is known to occur at an exponential rate. Half times of this repair process are generally from 0.5 to 1 hour for tumors and early responding tissues, and from 1 to 3 hours for late responding tissues (82).

Irrespective of which process involved, it is obvious that combination chemoradiotherapy is therapeutically beneficial only if the DEF is larger in the tumor than in the early and late responding normal tissue. When designing a treatment schedule, the various processes of interaction, presumed to occur, should be taken into account. The scientific background, mentioned earlier (Fig. 6.**8**), should serve as a guide for designing such treatment schedule.

Phase I and II Clinical Trials

The results of a number of pilot studies evaluating the combination of radiotherapy and chemotherapy given concurrently are now available. Many of these studies were undertaken before the relevant laboratory data on the mechanisms of interaction between radio- and chemo-therapy became available. Usually the most active drugs or drug combinations were simply added to a standard radiotherapy schedule. Only a few studies were designed to take maximum advantage of presumed radiosensitizing properties of the investigated agents. From the point of view of radiobiology, this second approach is more interesting, but strict classification of each individual treatment protocol into one of these two categories is not always possible. Even now, the basic question of whether the observed effect has resulted from true sensitization or mere additivity of radiotherapy and chemotherapy cannot be explicitly answered.

As it has been shown earlier in this chapter, the radiobiological basis for the combination of chemotherapy and irradiation has been a subject of intense investigation that will hopefully lead to more effective use of both modalities. For the time being, however, in view of still unsatisfactory results of surgery and radiotherapy in controlling locally advanced disease, an urgent need exists to define the possible benefit from a combination of irradiation and chemotherapy. For these reasons, this section reviews those studies in which a drug (Tables 6.6 and 6.7) or drug combination (Table 6.8) were given concomitantly with irradiation, irrespective of speculations about whether a real radiosensitization has been achieved.

5-Fluorouracil. The concurrent use of 5-FU and radiotherapy has been explored for almost three decades. Despite its low activity as a single agent in head and neck cancer, 5-FU has been used in a combination with radiotherapy for its "radioenhancing" properties. In early phase I and II studies performed in the 1960s, 5-FU was administered intravenously or intra-arterially (40, 56, 84). These studies demonstrated a rapid tumor regression during radiotherapy and suggested an improvement in local control. Due to excessive early (40, 56, 84) and late (22) local morbidity, the therapeutic ratio of this combination was reduced, however. More recently, Byfield et al. reported a high response rate with 5-FU administered in 5 day (19) and 3 day (20) chemoradiotherapy cycles, the latter employing hyperfractionated radiation. Mucositis was the most common toxicity, but rest periods after each cycle of therapy allowed recovery of normal tissue damage.

These clinical studies are consistent with the experimental data described earlier, in that the therapeutic ratio of combination of 5-FU and irradiation is relatively low because of dose limiting acute local toxicity.

Methotrexate. The number of phase I−II studies with MTX in combination with radiotherapy has

Table 6.6   **Phase I−II studies on concomitant miscellaneous single-agent chemotherapy and irradiation**

Drug Author/date/ref.	No. of patients	Radiotherapy	Chemotherapy	Feasibility
5-Fluorouracil				
Fletcher, 1963 (40)	11	50−60 Gy	iv 12 mg/kg d 1−5, 7.5 mg/kg q × 2/wk	Yes
Jesse, 1969 (56)	25	60−70 Gy	iv 4−8 mg/kg d 1−5, 7−12	Yes
Sato, 1970 (84)	57	70 Gy	ia 250 mg d 10−30	Yes
Byfield, 1984 (19)	18	50−70 Gy, every other week	cii 20−30 mg/kg d 1−5, q 2 wk	Yes
Byfield, 1985 (20)	5	60 Gy, accelerated	cii 40−50 mg/kg d 1−3, q 2 wk	Yes
Methotrexate				
Condit, 1964 (25)	25	50 Gy, conventional or: q × 2/wk or: short intensive	iv 1.3−23 mg/kg q 2 wk	No No Yes
Kramer, 1969 (63)	98	65 Gy	po 7.5 mg/d or: po 25 mg q 3 d or: iv 25 mg q 3 d	No No Yes
Bagshaw, 1969 (6)	25	60 Gy	cia 25 mg/8 h ± FA d 18−44	No
Pointon, 1983 (78)	50	30−55 Gy	iv 100 mg/m^2 ± FA d 0, 14	Yes
Hydroxyurea				
Rominger, 1971 (83)	21	60−70 Gy	po 80 mg q 3 d	Yes
Lerner, 1969 (66)	60	60 Gy	po 80 mg q 3 d	Yes
Bleomycin				
Berdal, 1976 (14)	212	25 Gy, split	im 180 mg over 3 wks	Yes
Kapstad, 1978 (59)	30	45 Gy, split	im 15 mg q × 3/wk	Yes
Tanaka, 1976 (106)	39	25−30 Gy ± surgery	im 7,5 mg q × 2/wk, or iv 10−15 mg q × 2/wk	Yes
Seagren, 1979 (86)	19	50.4 Gy	im 15 U q × 2/wk	Yes
Shah, 1981 (89)	25	40−60 Gy	iv 15 mg q × 3/wk	Yes

Abbreviations: iv, intravenous; po, per os; cii, continuous intravenous infusion; cia, continuous intra-arterial infusion; FA, folinic acid; d, day; wk, week

Table 6.7 **Phase I–II studies on concomitant platinum analogues and irradiation**

Drug Author/date/ref.	No. of patients	Radiotherapy	Chemotherapy	Feasibility
Cisplatin				
Creagan, 1981 (29)	3	60 Gy, split-course	30 mg/m^2 d 2 and 12 of each half of RT	No
Coughlin, 1988 (28)	54	50–70 Gy	100 mg/m^2 q 3 wk × 2 before RT and 20 mg/m^2 q wk × 5 during RT	Yes
Haselow, 1983 (50)	32	68–76 Gy	10–20 mg/m^2 q wk or 30 mg/m^2 q wk	Yes No
Crispino, 1987 (30)	25	70 Gy, split-course	20 mg/m^2 q wk	Yes
Keizer, 1984 (62)	7	30–68 Gy, 1–2 fr/day	6 mg/m^2 q d, or 8 mg/m^2 q d	Yes No
Tobias, 1987 (113)	19	60 Gy	10 mg q d	Yes
Dühmke, 1988 (37)	62	56.7 Gy, accelerated	6 mg/m^2 q d	Yes
Snyderman, 1986 (96)	36	60–66 Gy	15 mg/m^2 d 1–5 q 3 wk × 2	Yes
Chang, 1988 (23)	43	45–65 Gy	20 mg/m^2 d 1–5 q 3 wk × 2	Yes
Bloom, 1985 (16)	34	50 Gy	20 mg/m^2 d 1–5 q 3 wk × 2	Yes
Slotman, 1986 (94)	18	45 Gy + surgery	20 mg/m^2 d 1–5 q 3 wk × 2	Yes
Schmitt, 1983 (85)	22	40–70 Gy + surgery	20 mg/m^2 d 1–5 q 3 wk × 2	Yes
Wheeler, 1988 (128)	17	60–70 Gy	40 mg/m^2 d 1–5 q 4 wk × 3	Yes
Lütgemeier, 1986 (68)	28	60 Gy	60 mg/m^2 d 1–5 q 6 wk × 2	No
Al-Sarraf, 1987 (4)	134	66–73.8 Gy	100 mg/m^2 q 3 wk × 3	Yes
Coughlin, 1988 (28)	17	50 Gy + surgery	100 mg/m^2 q 3 wk × 2	Yes
Miller, 1985 (72)	22	65 Gy	80 mg/m^2 q 3 wk × 3	Yes
Gasparini, 1989 (45)	20	60–70 Gy	80 mg/m^2 q 3 wk × 3	Yes
Carboplatin				
Jacobs, 1989 (55)	26	60–75 Gy	60–100 mg/m^2 q wk, or 400 mg/m^2 q 4 wk	Yes No

Table 6.8 **Phase I–II studies on concomitant multidrug chemotherapy and irradiation**

Author, date/ref.	No. of patients	Radiotherapy	Chemotherapy	Feasibility
Fu, 1979 (43)	15	65–75 Gy, split	CPA 750 mg/m^2 and VCR 1.4 mg/m^2 d 1, BLM 15 U d 3, 4, 5 q wk	No
Glick, 1979 (47)	11	66–74 Gy	VCR 1.4 mg/m^2, BLM 30 mg, MTX 60–200 mg/m^2, ± FA, all q wk	No
Karim, 1983 (60)	22	NR	VCR, BLM, MTX	Yes
Seagren, 1982 (87)	24	54–70 Gy, split	CPA 1000 mg/m^2 d 1, BLM 15 U d 2, 4, 9, 11	Yes
Smith, 1980 (95)	36	55–65 Gy, split	5-Fu 110 mg/m^2 q × 3/wk, ADM 7 mg/m^2 q wk, BLM 4.5 U/m^2 q × 2/wk	Yes
Kaplan, 1985 (58)	42	50–70 Gy, split	MMC 10 mg/m^2 d 1, 5-Fu cii 1000 mg/m^2 d 1–4	Yes
Dobrowsky, 1988 (35)	51	50–75 Gy, split	MMC 15 mg/m^2 d 1, 5-Fu cii 750 mg/m^2 d 1–5	Yes
Souhami, 1988 (97)	30	60–70 Gy	MMC 10 mg/m^2 d 1, MTX 30 mg/m^2 d 1, 5-Fu cii 750 mg/m^2 d 2–4	No
Adelstein, 1988 (2)	54	60 Gy, split	cDDP 75 mg/m^2 d 1, 5-Fu cii 1000 mg/m^2 d 1–4	Yes
Taylor, 1988 (108)	44	70 Gy, every other week	cDDP 60 mg/m^2 d 1, 5-Fu cii 800 mg/m^2 d 2–4 all q 2 wk	Yes
Axelrod, 1987 (5)	10	60 Gy	cDDP 100 mg/m^2 d 0, 20, 5-Fu 200 mg d 8, 9, 15, 16, 35, 36, 42, 43	Yes
Vannetzel, 1987 (118)	41	72 Gy, split	cDDP 25 mg/m^2 d 1–5, 5-Fu cii 500 mg/m^2 d 1–5 all q 3 wk	Yes
Wendt, 1989 (127)	62	70.2 Gy, accel.	cDDP 60 mg/m^2 d 1, 5- Fu 350 mg/m^2 d 1 + FA, 5-Fu cii 350 mg/m^2 d 1–4, all q 3 wk	Yes
Giri, 1987 (46)	18	70 Gy	cDDP 25 mg/m^2 d 1, VCR 1 mg d 2, BLM 15 U d 4 all q wk	Yes
Vokes, 1989 (122)	39	66–80 Gy, every other week	5-Fu cii 800 mg/m^2 d 1–5, HU 500–3000 mg/d all q 2 wk	Yes

Abbreviations: CPA, cyclophosphamide; BLM, bleomycin; VCR, vincristin; MTX, methotrexate; FA, folinic acid; 5-Fu, 5-fluorouracil; MMC, mitomycin C; cDDP, cisplatin; HU, hydroxyurea; cii, continuous intravenous infusion; NR = not reported; accel. = accelerated irradiation.

been relatively small. Condit et al. (25) concluded that MTX added to conventional protracted schedules of radiation therapy resulted in unacceptable drug toxicity, while the combination of MTX and short intensive radiotherapy was considered feasible. Kramer et al. (63) observed a relatively high complete response rate with daily oral MTX and irradiation, but abandoned this schedule for its unacceptable toxicity. Intermittent oral or intravenous administration of MTX resulted in significantly reduced toxicity (63). Intra-arterial infusion of MTX produced a significant increase in severe mucosal reactions, without apparent improvement in local tumor control (6). Pointon et al. (78) administered moderate ($100 \, mg/m^2$) doses of MTX a day prior to commencing radiotherapy and again after 14 days. The application of folinic acid to the patients in whom MTX level was above $0.5 \, \mu mol$ diminished the local and systemic toxicity of combined modality therapy.

Hydroxurea. Concurrent use of HU and radiotherapy was reported in studies conducted in the USA in the 1960s. Lerner et al. (66) and Rominger (83), using HU at a dose of $80 \, mg/kg$ given every third day, found an enhanced radiation response in a majority of the patients without an apparent increase of treatment toxicity.

Bleomycin. BLM alone has only marginal activity in squamous cell head and neck cancer. It has been used together with radiotherapy mainly because of its limited hematologic and immunosuppressive toxicity, ease of administration, and presumed inhibition of sublethal radiation damage repair. The first studies performed in the 1970s suggested the feasibility and relative activity of BLM when combined with radiotherapy (14, 59, 86, 106). This early optimism has been somewhat tempered by the report of Shah et al. (89) who noted that the response rate with BLM was similar to that observed in patients given irradiation alone, whereas the incidence of side effects with combined modality therapy was significantly increased.

In most of the phase II studies with BLM an enhancement of acute radiation effect on normal squamous epithelial tissue, resulting in severe mucositis, was observed. Other toxicities included skin reactions, pulmonary fibrosis, fever, and late soft tissue necrosis. So, as was inferred from experimental investigations, these clinical studies demonstrated no clear therapeutic benefit from combination of BLM and irradiation.

Cisplatin. c-DDP has been the most extensively investigated agent in combination radiochemotherapy of head and neck cancer (Table 6.**7**). The particular interest in c-DDP has been due to its role as both a potential "radiosensitizer" (32) and an active chemotherapeutic agent in cancer of the head and neck (131). Despite extensive experimental investigations on the interaction of c-DDP and radiothera-

py, the optimal time–dose schedule of this combination is still unknown. Consequently, various schedules of c-DDP and radiotherapy, most of them designed on a pure empirical basis have been tested.

Creagan et al. (29) used c-DDP at a dose of $30 \, mg/m^2$ on days 2 and 12 of each half of a split-course radiotherapy regimen. Both systemic and local toxicity were excessive, but this might have been partly due to inadequate hydration ($250 \, mL$ 5% dextrose). c-DDP given at weekly doses of $10–20 \, mg/m^2$ in combination with continuous (27, 50) or split-course (30) radiotherapy was found to be feasible. In contrast, a dose of $20 \, mg/m^2$ given three times a week, or a weekly dose of $30 \, mg/m^2$ caused unacceptable systemic toxicity (27, 50).

Another attractive approach is daily administration of c-DDP since this creates theoretically optimal conditions for radiosensitization. A daily dose of $6 \, mg/m^2$ was found acceptable in a feasibility study (62) yet in a study of Tobias et al. (113) two treatment-related deaths from renal failure were reported with this schedule. Dühmke et al. (37) observed a high complete response rate and acceptable toxicity with a combination of daily c-DDP and accelerated radiotherapy. c-DDP applied in daily doses of $10–20 \, mg/m^2$ over the first and fourth week of conventional irradiation resulted in high response rates (16, 23, 85, 94). The prolonged observation was discouraging, however, in spite of high response rate, disease-free intervals were short and 39% of patients developed renal toxicity (96). In lung cancer this daily concomitant use of c-DDP and irradiation has shown now to be effective. In a randomized phase III trial a significantly improved survival rate has been observed in patients who received daily c-DDP and irradiation compared with irradiation alone, while no improvement has been seen, when weekly c-DDP was added (84a).

Since potentiation of radiation effects by c-DDP in experimental models is dose dependent, the simultaneous application of irradiation and increased doses of c-DDP has been investigated. As expected, the escalation of the drug dose caused increased toxicity of treatment. The c-DDP dose of $40 \, mg/m^2$ given over 5 consecutive days produced considerable systemic and local side effects (128) and a similarly applied dose of $60 \, mg/m^2$ produced unacceptable toxicity and was abandoned (68). Finally, the feasibility and considerable acitivity of c-DDP application in single high doses ($80–100 \, mg/m^2$) repeated every 3 weeks has been investigated (4, 28, 45, 72). This approach, including no fixed temporal relationship between the administration of c-DDP and radiation, exploited the cytotoxic activity of the drug rather than its radiosensitizing properties.

In conclusion, the combination of c-DDP and irradiation has not yet properly been tested in head and neck cancer patients. Few of these studies, if any, however, have utilized earlier mentioned modern techniques, such as measuring Pt−DNA adducts for treatment monitoring. Such studies are urgently needed before embarking on phase III trials.

Carboplatin (CBDCA). This second-generation platinum analogue has been combined with irradiation in a recently reported phase I−II study of Jacobs et al. (55). Twenty-six patients with unresectable stage IV head and neck cancer received CBDCA weekly ($60-100 \, mg/m^2$) or monthly ($400 \, mg/m^2$) with simultaneous conventionally fractionated radiotherapy. Bone marrow depression was dose-limiting toxicity and was severe in patients on monthly schedule.

Multidrug chemotherapy. Multidrug chemotherapy has been combined with irradiation in many recent pilot studies (Table 6.**8**). Drug regimens currently believed to be most active were usually applied, together with standard radiotherapy schedules. The first attempts with this approach were disappointing. Fu et al. (43) administered a combination of cyclophosphamide (CPA), vincristine (VCR), and bleomycin (BLM) in patients with inoperable cancer of the oral cavity, pharynx, and larynx. After completion of radiotherapy, patients were given adjuvant chemotherapy. Treatment toxicity, including enhanced radiation mucositis and infections, was formidable and 20% of patients experienced fatal complications. Similarly, excessive mucositis and bone marrow depression led to discontinuation of the pilot study of RTOG on a combination of VCR, BLM, and MTX (47). Severe toxicity of this regimen when applied concurrently with radiotherapy was also reported by Karim et al. (60), but these authors considered this combination useful, especially in the management of stomal recurrences after laryngectomy (7).

The combination of CPA and BLM failed to result in durable remissions despite impressive early complete response rate in a study by Seagran (87). The toxicity of this regimen in most of the patients approached the limits of tolerance. Smith et al. (95) observed a high response rate but also high mortality with the use of a combination of 5-FU, doxorubicin, and BLM.

Recently a combination of mitomycin C (MMC) and continuous infusion of 5-FU has been found to be feasible and relatively active (35, 58). The combination of MMC, 5-FU, and MTX resulted in unacceptably high morbidity (severe mucositis, xerostomia, and septicemia with two fatal complications) in patients with nasopharyngeal carcinoma (97). Despite a high control rate in this series, the overall survival and disease-free survival were comparable to those reported in the literature with the use of irradiation alone.

Most of the studies performed in the 1980s employed different chemotherapy regimens including

c-DDP. Of these, a combination of c-DDP and 5-FU given in continuous infusion has been the most extensively studied. Recent reports have claimed high response rate with this schedule given with split-course (2, 108, 118) or accelerated (127) radiotherapy. Its limitation is considerable systemic toxicity and the need for patient hospitalization during continuous 5-FU infusion.

A combination of c-DDP, VCR, and BLM produced moderate to severe mucositis in almost all patients and in many cases necessitated an interruption of radiotherapy (46). Most recently a combination of hydroxyurea (HU) and continuous infusion of 5-FU during short cycles of irradiation was reported to be active and menageable (122).

Conclusions. The studies presented here differ considerably in several aspects, of which the most important are: selection of patients, choice of drug, schedule of its administration and dose, and fractionation of radiotherapy. Most of the studies show that local and systemic toxicity make it impossible to use a standard schedules of irradiation when full doses of chemotherapy are applied. For this reason a majority of the attempts included either relatively small doses of drugs combined with conventional doses of irradiation, or only slightly reduced doses of chemotherapy combined with modified schedules of irradiation. Even with these tactics, acute toxicity of combined modality was considerable in most of the trials. This led in many instances to poor compliance with the protocol, the necessity of reduction of the planned radiation dose and, in some instances, to an indefinite interruption of treatment. In some studies an increased number of serious late complications was observed. These data allow us to conclude that in general there is at present little evidence that the addition of chemotherapeutic agents does result in the selective enhancement of sensitivity of the tumor and that at least similar sensitization is observed in normal tissue. Unfortunately, the quantification of enhancement ratios for tumor and normal tissues has only rarely been carried out.

Many studies presented in this section reported a therapeutic advantage when chemotherapy was added to irradiation. These claims, based on historical experience in patients treated with locoregional methods alone, have limited value, however, because of several types of bias. The objective evaluation of treatment effectivity may be achieved only with well designed controlled randomized trials.

Phase III Clinical Trials

In contrast to the extensive literature concerning phase I and II trials, the number of randomized phase III studies on concurrent radiotherapy and chemotherapy in head and neck cancer is relatively small. To the best of our knowledge, the direct comparison of radiotherapy given alone or combined with chemotherapy has been the subject of only eighteen published papers, of which half have enrolled more than 100 patients (Table 6.**9**).

5-Fluorouracil. There have been two phase III controlled studies employing 5-FU to date, both published in the 1970s. In a study of Shigematsu et al. (92) 5-FU infused intra-arterially in patients with cancer of the maxillary sinus produced severe mucosal reactions early in the treatment, which often made it impossible to deliver the planned dose of irradiation. For patients given 5-FU the local recurrence-free rate was superior after 1 year of follow-up, but not after 2 years. Two-year overall survival values were similar in both groups.

In a study from Wisconsin, 5-FU was administered intravenously at a dose of 10 mg/kg/day for the first 3 days, 5 mg/kg on day 4, and 5 mg/kg three times

a week thereafter throughout the course of radiation therapy (60–70 Gy in 6–7 weeks) or until toxicity occurred (48). Patients in the combined treatment group uniformly developed more severe acute mucosal reactions. Many required hospitalization and supportive care, including a nasogastric feeding tube during the treatment course. Major complications, such as soft tissue, bone necrosis, or fistula formation, were seen only in patients given chemotherapy. The report of this study published in 1972 claimed significantly prolonged survival and better local control in the chemotherapy arm (48). This was attributed to an improvement in patients with cancer of the oral cavity and oropharynx. No difference was noted for cancer of the larynx and hypopharynx. The final report, published in 1976 (67), included only patients with oral and oropharyngeal cancer, making

Table 6.**9**   **Phase III randomized studies on concomitant chemotherapy and irradiation**

Drug Author/date/ref.	Tumor site and stage	No. evaluable patients	Impact of chemotherapy		
			Local control	Metastases	Survival
Bleomycin					
Abe, 1978 (1)	Mouth, II–IV	67	NR	NR	NS
Eschwege, 1988 (38)	Oropharynx, II–IV	199	NS	NR	NS
Fu, 1987 (44)	Miscellaneous, III–IV	96	Better	NS	NS
Kapstad, 1978 (59)	Miscellaneous, I–IV	29	NR	NS	NS
Morita, 1980 (74)	Tongue, II–III	45	NS	NR	NR
Shanta, 1980 (90)	Cheek, III–IV	157	Better	NS	NR
Vermund, 1985 (120)	Miscellaneous, II–IV	222	NS	Worse	NS
5-Fluorouracil					
Lo, 1972, 1976 (48, 67)	Miscellaneous, II–IV	185	Better	NS	NS*
Shigematsu, 1971 (92)	Maxill. sinus, II–IV	63	NS	NR	NS
Hydroxyurea					
Hussey, 1975 (54)	Miscellaneous, I–IV	40	NS	NR	NS
Richards, 1969 (80)	Miscellaneous, I–IV	40	NR	NR	NS
Stefani, 1971, 1980 (101, 102)	Miscellaneous, I–IV	150	NS	Worse	Worse
Methotrexate					
Condit, 1968 (26)	Miscellaneous, III–IV	40	NS	NR	NR
Gupta, 1987 (49)	Miscellaneous, I–IV	313	Better	NR	NS+
Mitomycin					
Weissberg, 1989 (126)	Miscellaneous, II–IV	117	Better	NS	NS
Lonidamide					
Magno, 1987 (70)	Miscellaneous	85	Better	NR	NS
Cisplatin					
Haselow, 1990 (51)	Miscellaneous, III–IV	319	NS	NR	NS
Mitomycin + 5-Fu					
Keane, 1988 (61)	Larynx, hypopharynx, III–IV	212	NS	NS	NS

Abbreviations: NR, not reported; NS, not significant.

* mouth better.

+ oropharynx better.

an interpretation of the results for the whole group of patients difficult. The therapeutic benefit obtained with 5-FU was confined to patients with oral cancer.

Methotrexate. Of the two randomized studies with this agent (26, 49) only the latter is large enough for the statistical analysis. This study included 313 patients with head and neck cancer who received radiotheapy with or without two doses of MTX, 100 mg/m^2, on day 0 and 14 of the 3-week course of irradiation. The serum MTX concentration was assayed 24 hours after injection and folinic acid rescue was given when the level of the drug was above 0.4 µmol. This procedure allowed the avoidance of serious complications with combined therapy, and cutaneous and mucosal reactions were only slightly increased. After a median follow-up of 32 months, the local control rate was significantly higher in the MTX group but the incidence of lymph node recurrences was similar. The difference in survival rate just failed the level of statistical significance ($p = 0.075$). A significant improvement both in local control and survival was seen in patients with oropharyngeal cancer while the differences in other locations were insignificant.

Hydroxyurea. This agent was studied in three phase III trials, of which only one included more than 100 patients. The results from this study, performed at the Veterans Administration Hospital, were discouraging (101, 102). A total of 150 patients were given HU, 80 mg/kg, twice weekly, or placebo throughout the period of protracted irradiation (60−100 Gy in 8 to 12 weeks). The preliminary results showed no difference in immediate post-therapy response between the groups and significantly higher incidence of distant metastases in the HU group. For this reason the trial was discontinued. The late report of this study revealed that overall survival was significantly better in placebo group (102).

Bleomycin. BLM has been studied extensively in phase III randomized clinical trials. Seven studies have been reported to date, including four that accrued more than 100 patients. The first paper seemed to be promising. Shanta and Krishnamurthi (90) applied radiotherapy (55−60 Gy in 7 weeks) with placebo or BLM given intravenously, intra-arterially, or intramuscularly in 157 Indian patients with locally advanced buccal cancer. The BLM arm was found to be much more toxic (frequent intense mucositis, four cases of fatal pneumonitis), but showed significantly higher response rate (79% vs. 19% in controls). Moreover, the 5-year disease-free survival was significantly better in patients given BLM (59%) than in control group (23%). The marked difference in treatment results reported in this study might be explained by a specific biological characteristic in this population: in almost all patients the tumor showed features of high differentiation.

Abe et al. (1) compared radiotherapy (30 Gy in 3 weeks) given with or without intravenous BLM, 15 mg twice a week and followed by surgery or further radiotherapy. Mucosal reactions were significantly higher in the BLM arm and so was the complete response rate (44.1% vs. 15.2% in controls). In a study of Morita (74) patients with squamous carcinoma of the tongue were randomized to either radiotherapy alone (40 Gy) or reduced dose radiotherapy (20−24 Gy) combined with daily intramuscular injections of 5 mg BLM. In the second phase of treatment all patients received interstitial irradiation with radium needles. Similar regression rates were found in both groups and the BLM enhancement ratio for tumor response was therefore estimated to be from 1.3 to 1.5. No therapeutic benefit was obtained, however, because the BLM enhancement ratio for the acute reaction of the mucous membrane was estimated to be 1.5. Two-year local control rates were similar for both arms, but no osteonecrosis was seen in patients given radiotherapy alone, as opposed to three cases in BLM arm.

In an NCOG trial performed between 1978 and 1984, patients with stage III and IV inoperable head and neck cancer were randomized to receive BLM (5 U, intravenously, twice a week) during radiotherapy (70 Gy) followed by adjuvant BLM and methotrexate or radiotherapy alone (44). Two-year local control rate was in favour of the combined modality arm, but survival in both groups did not differ significantly. In spite of the low dose of BLM, the acute radiation mucositis was significantly increased.

In a well designed study from Norway (120) employing the method of paired randomization, patients received either daily BLM, 5 mg intramuscularly combined with irradiation, or irradiation alone. The injections had to be discontinued in most of the patients given BLM before the full course of radiotherapy was delivered because of excessive mucositis or other side effects. The results in both arms were similar. No statistically significant differences in locoregional control or 5-year survival were found, except in the number of metastases, which was significantly higher in the BLM group.

These results are in close agreement with those obtained in the EORTC study of oropharyngeal cancer (38). The trial design included administration of radiation therapy (70 Gy in 7−8.5 weeks) with or without BLM (15 mg, intravenously or intramuscularly, twice a week). The rate of local toxic effects (mucositis, epidermitis) was much higher in the BLM arm (72% vs. 21%), while the local control and the 6-year survival rate were almost identical.

Cisplatin. In contrast to the large number of phase I and II c-DDP trials, the data from phase III studies are scarce, although the drug is being presently studied in multicenter phase III trials in the USA

(ECOG, SWOG, and RTOG) and in Europe (EORTC). To date, only early results of the RTOG–ECOG study are available (51). Of 319 evaluable patients, complete response was seen in 30% of patients given radiotherapy alone and in 34% of those treated with both modalities. No difference in survival between two arms have been observed.

Mitomycin-C. This drug has been tested in a recently published phase III study from the Yale University (126). Patients were randomized to receive either radiotherapy alone or radiation with MMC. The limitation of this study was the heterogeneity of the patient population. Of 117 evaluable patients, 48 were treated as an adjuvant to radical surgery, 30 as an adjuvant to nonradical surgery, and only 39 received radiotherapy without surgery. All patients randomized to receive MMC were given the drug intravenously at a dose of 15 mg/m^2 on the fifth day of radiation therapy and patients in the latter two groups received a second course of MMC 6 weeks later. Patients treated with MMC experienced depression of hematologic parameters while the mucosal reactions were similar in both groups. Actuarial local recurrence-free survival was significantly better in the MMC group but overall survival did not differ significantly. There was no difference between the two treatment arms in the incidence of distant metastases.

Lonidamide. This recently developed indazole carboxylic acid derivative has been studied in one phase III trial the results of which have only been reported in abstract form (70). Patients with cancer of the oral cavity were given hyperfractionated radiotherapy (60–66 Gy) with either lonidamide (150 mg three times daily) or placebo. Local control after 2 years was superior in the lonidamide group, but no data on overall survival were presented.

Multidrug chemotherapy. The efficacy of multidrug chemotherapy applied concurrently with radiotherapy was investigated in recently reported study from Canada (61). Patients were randomly allocated to either radiotherapy alone (50 Gy/20 fractions in 4 weeks) or split-course radiotherapy (50 Gy/20 fractions with a 4-week rest period) combined with chemotherapy. The chemotherapy regimen consisted of MMC, 10 mg/m^2, intravenously on day 1 and 42 and 5-FU, 1000 mg/m^2/day, given in continuous infusion on days 1 to 4 and 42 to 45 of the radiation cycle. There was no significant difference in locoregional control and overall survival between the two groups.

The use of alternating chemotherapy and irradiation has recently been tested clinically. This strategy includes temporal separation in the delivery of both modalities allowing for normal tissue recovery. Alternating radiotherapy and multidrug chemotherapy have been compared in a few trials to both modalities given sequentially (3, 24, 71, 88, 109) and none of them have revealed any significant differences in survival between the two procedures.

Treatment schedule dependency. To improve the prognosis for patients with locally advanced head and neck cancer, various treatment strategies for the combination of chemotherapy and radiotherapy have been proposed (100a).

Firstly, induction (neoadjuvant) as well as adjuvant chemotherapy are aimed at improving the prognosis through spatial cooperation by reducing the tumor load locoregionally and eradicating microscopic distant disease. An additive effect of both modalities can also be expected at locoregional tumor sites. Although neoadjuvant chemotherapy can induce an overall response rate of 75% (37a), and those patients achieving a complete response to initial chemotherapy have been repeatedly shown to have the best prognosis, this treatment approach has failed to improve long-term survival (122a, 70a).

Secondly, the concomitant use of chemotherapy and radiotherapy is aimed at both spatial cooperation of the different modalities and the enhancement of radiation effect by the chemotherapy drug or drug combinations. A meta-analysis of the results of twenty-three trials of combined treatment in head and neck cancer was performed by Stell and Rawson in an attempt to detect a change in survival rate since none of the individual studies was large enough to detect a clear benefit in either arm (102a). This meta-analysis of more than 3000 patients randomized to receive whether or not chemotherapy showed no improvement of survival by chemotherapy. In ten trials in which the number of deaths due to toxicity was recorded, the total mortality from chemotherapy was 6.5%. In eight of these ten trials induction chemotherapy was applied. Including toxic deaths, these ten trials showed disappointing results with an overall increase in mortality of 8.9% by adding chemotherapy to standard treatment. Other important findings of this overview were that with respect to the timing of chemotherapy, the synchronous use of radiotherapy and chemotherapy significantly reduced the cancer death rate in contrast to induction or adjuvant chemotherapy. The results of concomitant chemoradiotherapy in head and neck cancer were also reviewed by Vokes and Weichselbaum (122b), in which they found five randomized trials using either 5-FU, bleomycin, or mitomycin, which showed improved survival or disease-free survival. The authors stress the potential for organ preservation when using these regimens, a point which deserves further attention.

Several issues remain to be addressed. It could well be imagined that certain sites of head and neck cancer respond differently to these new approaches. In nasopharyngeal cancer promising findings were observed in two nonrandomized studies with either induction chemotherapy (40a) or concomitant chemoradiotherapy (4a). The best chemotherapy drug or drug combination as well as the optimum radiotherapy fractionation scheme and dose for concomitant, therapy will also have to be established.

The expected small survival benefit in these patients with advanced head and neck cancer, the large number of different sites, and the small numbers of patients in individual departments call for large-scale randomized studies to further clarify the role of combination therapy in the treatment of head an neck cancer. It must be stressed, however, that although the survival gain is small, a reduction in the need for mutilating operations will be important achievements in this field.

Conclusions. Head and neck cancers are a heterogeneous group of malignant tumors that differ considerably in their clinical manifestations and prognosis. They are usually grouped together in clinical studies due to the small number of patients with individual tumor locations. The trials presented here differ greatly in patient selection, including site of the tumor, stage, and operability. In some trials, the investigated methods of treatment were given as adjuncts to surgery. A large spectrum of both radiotherapy and chemotherapy tactics was used, producing a great variety of combination schedules. Most of the trials included small numbers of patients, which did not allow the detection of slight differences in treatment outcome. Duration of follow-up was usually short and extraction of complete data from the individual studies is difficult because of the different methods of reporting the data. All these factors make the interpretation of results difficult.

In general, no marked advantage from the addition of chemotherapy to irradiation has been demonstrated. In spite of the rapid tumor regression observed in most of the studies, significant gain in survival could not be detected. Of eighteen presented trials significantly superior overall survival with chemotherapy was found in two (49, 67) and in both of these studies the gain was confined to only one subset of patients (oral cancer and oropharyngeal cancer, respectively). In one study (102) survival was better with radiotherapy alone and in fourteen studies no significant difference in survival was shown, or the number of patients was inadequate for the statistical analysis of survival.

Based on the available data, it is not possible to indicate the type of drug or drug combination that would potentially be advantageous in combination with radiotherapy. Marginal effects in selected groups of patients have been detected with the use of 5-FU and MTX, while with the other drugs effects were either insignificant (MMC, BLM, combination chemotherapy) or detrimental (HU). The role of daily cisplatin, which has been demonstrated to improve survival in non-small cell lung cancer (84a) is not yet established.

Many studies reported a beneficial effect of chemotherapy resulting in higher response rate and disease-free survival. This conclusion should be treated with caution. The improvement in response rate and disease-free survival demonstrates merely an antitumor activity of the drug. The therapeutic gain from this approach cannot be proved until the prolongation of overall survival and improvement in quality of life has been achieved.

In the majority of head and neck cancer patients, quality of life is highly dependent on local tumor control. Some of the trials analyzed here have shown improved local control rates in patients given chemotherapy. This has usually been achieved at the expense of significantly increased toxicity of treatment. If the drug is to act mainly by independent cell kill, similar results might have been achieved by increasing the total radiation dose (8). Two trials (61, 74) were designed to compare combinations of chemotherapy and irradiation to radiotherapy alone at equal level of normal tissue damage by adjusting the radiation dose or treatment time in the combined modality arm. No significant differences were found for any endpoint in these studies.

None of the analyzed trials have shown any reduction in the incidence of metastatic failure that may have been expected with the addition of systemic therapy. On the contrary, in three large randomized trials an increase in the incidence of distant spread with chemotherapy was observed (44, 102, 120) and in two of them the difference was significant (102, 120).

All the studies consistently reported an increased morbidity with combined modality therapy. Chemotherapy usually enhanced acute local reactions which led to a compromise in the dose of irradiation, interruption of treatment, and an increased number of treatment refusals. An increased number of late local complications was mentioned in some studies. Serious systemic effects of chemotherapy and an increase in the number of treatment-related deaths were frequently observed.

Taken together, the results presented here disappoint the hopes of an improvement in treatment results in head and neck cancer from radiotherapy—chemotherapy combinations. In part, this outcome may be attributed to the factors discussed above (limiting toxicity and increased number of distant failures). The fact that irradiation and chemotherapy in many studies were given as independent agents with a large time interval, significantly, reduced the chance of real radiosensitization. One could also argue that some beneficial effects of this approach might have been overlooked due to inadequate methods of testing (small studies, heterogenous groups of patients, lack of quality control, suboptimal drugs and dosages, etc.). On the other hand, for most other solid tumors studied so far, the strategy of synchronous administration of irradiation and chemotherapy has also shown only marginal, if any, impact on survival (107).

Radiation therapy and chemotherapy are two effective modalities in the management of cancer, but are most active against the same group of cells, i.e. well oxygenated and actively proliferating. It is very probable that there are some subpopulations of tumor cells that are resistant to both treatment modalities. If so, only a subadditive effect from the use of a combined approach could be expected. In addition, the advantage from radiosensitization of the tumor cells by chemotherapy is reduced by the fact that similar effects are usually observed in normal tissues.

Cell killing from chemotherapy shows either an exponential or a biphasic dose dependency and eradication of the tumor is strictly dependent on the number of viable cells. Head and neck tumors can be successfully managed with local treatment modalities at early stages. Yet systemic therapy as an adjuvant to radiotherapy was tested mainly in locally advanced head and neck cancer. At this stage, the chance of detecting an advantageous effect is probably small.

In conclusion, the data presented here do not justify the use of the combination of radiotherapy and chemotherapy in the standard management of head and neck cancer. Marked enhancement of treatment-related morbidity with this approach seems to outweigh the improvement in local tumor control observed in some studies. In 1963 Fletcher et al. (40), in their pioneer clinical studies of concomitant use of chemotherapy and irradiation, noted "unexpectedly rapid regression of the primary tumor." In the final conclusions they stated: "faster regression rates do not necessarily mean an increase in permanency of control," and proposed: "in order to carry out statistically significant studies in a reasonable period of time cooperative studies between institutions . . . are essential. . ." After three decades of clinical investigations there is not much to be added to these statements.

Concluding Remarks and Future Prospects

The lack of therapeutic gain from the use of concomitant chemo- and radio-therapy in most phase III trials may be due to a number of reasons, such as the use of ineffective drugs, inadequate translation of experimental data into the clinic, and, until recently, the nonavailability of predictive assays for individual patient selection. Too many feasibility studies have been carried out in the past aiming to find the "maximal tolerated drug dose" that should be given in combination with irradiation. The time and sequence of administration has been chosen too often on a purely empirical basis. These data were used for designing phase III trials without any knowledge about drug access to the tumor and about the kinetics of formation of interactive complexes with intracellular targets. The large number of phase III trials with

a negative outcome is therefore hardly surprising. It cannot be overstressed that, as long as we remain ignorant of processes such as drug access and drug-target complex formation, patients continued to be exposed to a potentially hazardous treatment, the efficacy of which can only be assessed after a considerable time by standard criteria such as local tumor control and normal tissue toxicity.

In view of the limited sensitivity of head and neck tumors to the currently available cytostatic drugs, more effective agents are sorely needed to improve the efficacy of combined radiochemotherapy. We would strongly advise the following requirements to be met for applying this treatment modality: good evidence for a positive interaction of radiotherapy and the drug under study, intratumoral drug uptake sufficient for a significant radiosensitization, and an acceptable increase in early and late normal tissue radiation damage. In order to maximize differential effects against tumor and late reacting normal tissues, accelerated fractionation schedules counteracting tumor cell repopulation should be investigated. In addition, research should include cytostatic drugs which inhibit proliferation during radiotherapy.

In designing future clinical studies, the methodological pitfalls observed in previous investigations should be avoided. Single-arm studies should be strictly confined to evaluation of feasibility of the new schedule. Their results cannot be accepted as the new standard therapy, but should provide a basis for prospective randomized trials. In phase III trials, the large heterogeneity of head and neck tumors calls for rigid selection and stratification criteria. These studies should be carried out within multi-institutional groups allowing the recruitment of large number of patients in a reasonable time. A standardization of measurements of endpoints and careful quality control are essential. The reporting of treatment results should strictly follow international recommendations (132). Publications should be based on a reasonable duration of observation and should report late effects of treatment.

The need for improvement of currently used methods calls for continuing search for new treatment strategies. The option discussed in this chapter, however, is not yet ready for its incorporation into the standard of care.

References

1. Abe M, Shigematsu Y, Kimura S. Combined use of bleomycin with radiation in the treatment of cancer. Recent Results Cancer Res 1978; 63:169.
2. Adelstein DJ, Sharan VM, Earle AS, et al. Simultaneous radiotherapy and chemotherapy with 5-fluorouracil and cisplatin for locally confined squamous cell head and neck cancer. NCI Monogr 1988; 6:347.
3. Adelstein DJ, Sharan VM, Earle S, et al. A prospective randomized trial of simultaneous (SIM) vs. sequential (SEQ) chemoradiotherapy (CRT) for squamous cell head and neck cancer (SCHNC). Proc. Am Soc Clin Oncol 1989; 8:167.

4. Al-Sarraf M, Pajak TF, Marcial VA, et al. Concurrent radiotherapy and chemotherapy with cisplatin in inoperable squamous cell carcinoma of the head and neck. An RTOG Study. Cancer 1987; 59:259.

4a. Al-Sarraf M, Pajak TF, Cooper JS, et al. Chemoradiotherapy in patients with locally advanced nasopharyngeal carcinoma: a radiation therapy oncology group study. J Clin Oncol 1990; 8:1342.

5. Axelrod RS, Mohr R, Abayomi O, et al. CDDP, 5FU, RT in advanced head and neck cancer. Proc. Am Soc Clin Oncol 1987; 6:133.

6. Bagshaw MA, Doggett RLS. A clinical study of chemical radiosensitization. Front Radiat Ther Oncol 1969; 4:164.

7. Balm AJ, Snow GB, Karim AB, et al. Long-term results of concurrent polychemotherapy and radiotherapy in patients with stomal recurrence after total laryngectomy. Ann Otol Rhinol Laryngol 1986; 95:572.

8. Bartelink H, Breur K, Hart G. Radiotherapy of lymph node metastases in patients with squamous cell carcinoma of the head and neck region. Int J Radiat Oncol Biol Phys 1982; 8:983.

9. Beckman RP, Agostino MJ, McHugh MM, et al. Assessment of preferential cleavage of an actively transcribed retroviral hybrid gene in murine cells by deoxyribonuclease I, bleomycin, neocarcinostatin or ionizing radiation. Biochemistry 1987; 26:5409.

10. Begg AC, McNally NJ, Shrieve DC, et al. A method to measure the duration of DNA synthesis and the potential doubling time from a single sample. Cytometry 1985; 6:620.

11. Begg AC, van der Kolk PJ, Dewit L, et al. Radiosensitization by cisplatin of RIF1 tumour cells in vitro. Int J Radiat Biol 1986; 50:871.

12. Begg AC, Moonen L, Hofland I, et al. Human tumour cell kinetics using a monoclonal antibody against iododeoxyuridine: Intratumour sampling variations. Radiother Oncol 1988; 11:337.

13. Begg AC, Bohlken S, Bartelink H. The effect of cisplatin on the repair of radiation damage in RIF1 mouse tumours in vivo. Radiother Oncol 1989; 15:79.

13a. Begg AC, Hofland I, Moonen L, et al. The predictive value of cell kinetic measurements in a European trial of accelerated fractionation in advanced head and neck tumors: An interim report. Int J Oncol Radiat Biol Phys 1990; 19:1449.

14. Berdal P. Head and neck carcinoma: Treatment with bleomycin and radiation. GANN Monogr Cancer Res 1976; 19:133.

15. Bleehen NM, Gillies NE, Twentyman PR. The effect of bleomycin and radiation in combination on bacteria and mammalian cells in culture. Br J Radiol 1974; 47:346.

16. Bloom EJ, Green MD, Cooper JS, et al. Concomitant use of cisplatinum (CDDP) chemotherapy and radiation therapy (RT) in the treatment of advanced head and neck cancer. Proc. Am Soc Clin Oncol 1985; 4:137.

17. Bryant PE. Use of restriction endonucleases to study relationships between DNA double-strand breaks, chromosomal aberrations and other end-points in mammalian cells. Int J Radiat Biol 1988; 54:869.

18. Byfield JE, Calabro-Jones P, Klisak I, et al. Pharmacologic requirements for obtaining sensitization of human tumor cells in vitro to combined 5-fluorouracil or ftorafur and X-rays. Int J Radiat Oncol Biol Phys 1982; 8:1923.

19. Byfield JE, Sharp TR, Frankel SS, et al. Phase I and II trial of five-day infused 5-fluorouracil and radiation in advanced cancer of the head and neck. J Clin Oncol 1984; 2:406.

20. Byfield JE, Frankel SS, Sharp TR, et al. Phase I and pharmacologic study of 72-hour infused 5-fluorouracil and hyperfractionated cyclical radiation. Int J Radiat Oncol Biol Phys 1985; 11:791.

21. Carde P, Laval F. Effect of cis-dichlorodiammineplatinum II and X-rays on mammalian cell survival. Int J Radiat Oncol Biol Phys 1981; 7:923.

22. Chan RC, Shukovsky LJ. Effects of irradiation on the eye. Radiology 1976; 120:673.

23. Chang H, Leone LA, Trefft M, et al. Advanced head and neck cancer: Response to and toxicity of multimodality therapy. Radiology 1988; 168:863.

24. Cognetti F, Carlini P, Pinnaro P, et al. Preliminary results of a randomized trial of sequential versus simultaneous chemo and radiotherapy (CT-XRT) in patients (PTS) with locally advanced unresectable squamous cell carcinoma of the head and neck (SCCHN), Proc. Am Soc Clin Oncol 1989; 8:170.

25. Condit PT, Ridings GR, Coin JW, et al. Methotrexate and radiation in the treatment of patients with cancer. Cancer Res 1964; 24:1524.

26. Condit PT. Treatment of carcinoma with radiation therapy and methotrexate. Mo Med 1968; 65:832.

27. Coughlin CT, Grace M, O'Donnell JF, et al. Combined modality approach in the management of locally advanced head and neck cancer. Cancer Treat Rep 1984; 68:591.

28. Coughlin CT. Clinical experience with high-dose cisplatin and radiation for treatment of epithelial malignancies. NCI Monogr 1988; 6:365.

29. Creagan ET, Fountain KS, Frytak S, et al. Concomitant radiation therapy and cis-diamminedichloroplatinum (II) in patients with advanced head and neck cancer. Med Pediatr Oncol 1981; 9:119.

30. Crispino S, Tancini S, Barni S, et al. Simultaneous cisplatinum (CDDP) and radiotherapy in patients with locally advanced head and neck cancer. Proc. Am Soc Clin Oncol 1987; 6:123.

31. D'Angio GJ, Evans AE, Breslow N, et al. The treatment of Wilms' tumor; results of the National Wilms' Tumor Study. Cancer 1976; 38:633.

32. Dewit L. Combined treatment of radiation and cis-diamminedichloroplatinum (II): a review of experimental and clinical data. Int J Radiat Oncol Biol Phys 1987; 13:403.

33. Dewit L, Oussoren Y, Bartelink H, et al. The effect of cis-diamminedichloroplatinum (II) on radiation damage in the rectum after fractionated irradiation. Radiother Oncol 1989; 16:121.

34. Dishe S, Saunders MI, Bennett MH, et al. Cell proliferation and differentiation in squamous cancer. Radiother Oncol 1985; 13:19.

35. Dobrowsky W, Dobrowsky E, Strassl H, et al. Radiochemotherapy of head and neck tumors. Strahlentherapie 1988; 164:7.

36. Douglas BG, Fowler JF. The effect of multiple small doses of X-rays on skin reactions in the mouse and a basic interpretation. Radiat Res 1976; 66:401.

37. Dühmke E, Geibel T, Golms R, et al. Combined modality treatment of advanced head and neck cancer using low dose cisplatinum and accelerated fractionation. Strahlentherapie 1988; 164:11.

37a. Ervin TJ, Clark JR, Weichselbaum RR, et al. An analysis of induction and adjuvant chemotherapy in the multidiscipinairy treatment of squamous cell carcinoma of the head and neck. J Clin Oncol 1987; 5:10.

38. Eschwege F, Sancho-Garnier H, Gerard JP, et al. Ten-year results of randomized trial comparing radiotherapy and concomitant bleomycin to radiotherapy alone in epidermoid carcinomas of the oropharynx: experience of the European Organization for Research and Treatment of Cancer. NCI Monogr 1988; 6:275.

39. Fichtinger-Schepman AMJ, van der Veer JL, den Hartog JHJ, et al. Adducts of the antitumor drug cis-diamminedichloroplatinum (II) with DNA: formation, identification and quantitation. Biochemistry 1985; 24:707.

40. Fletcher GH, Suit HD, Howe CD, et al. Clinical method of resting radiation-sensitizing agents in squamous cell carcinoma. Cancer 1963; 16:355.

40a. Fountzilas G, Daniilidis J, Sridhar KS, et al. Induction chemotherapy with a new regimen alternating cisplatin, fluorouracil with mitomycin, hydroxyurea and bleomycin in carcinomas of nasopharynx or other sites of the head and neck region. Cancer 1990; 66:1453.

41. Fowler JF. Kirk Memorial Lecture: What next in fractionated radiotherapy? Br J Cancer 1983; 49(suppl 6):285.

42. Fowler JF. Potential for increasing the differential response between tumors and normal tissues: can proliferation rate be used? Int J Radiat Oncol Biol Phys 1986; 12:641.

43. Fu KK, Silverberg IJ, Phillips TL, et al. Combined radiotherapy and multidrug chemotherapy for advanced head

and neck cancer: Results of a Radiation Therapy Oncology Group pilot study. Cancer Treat Rep 1979; 63:351.

44. Fu KK, Phillips TL, Silverberg IJ, et al. Combined radiotherapy and chemotherapy with bleomycin and methotrexate for advanced inoperable head and neck cancer: Update of a Northern California Oncology Group randomized trial. J Clin Oncol 1987; 5:1410.

45. Gasparini G, Recher G, Favretto S, et al. Simultaneous cis-platinum (CDDP) and radiotherapy (RT) in inoperable or advanced squamous cell carcinoma of the head and neck (H&N). Proc Am Soc Clin Oncol 1989; 8:170.

46. Giri PGS, Taylor SA. Concurrent chemotherapy and radiation therapy in advanced head and neck cancer. Am J Clin Oncol (CCT) 1987; 10(5):417.

47. Glick JH, Fazekas JT, Davis LW, et al. Combination chemotherapy–radiotherapy for advanced, inoperable head and neck cancer. A RTOG pilot study. Cancer Clin Trials 1979; 2:129.

48. Gollin FF, Ansfield FJ, Brandenburg JH, et al. Combined therapy in advanced head and neck cancer: A randomized study. Am J Roentgenol 1972; 114:83.

49. Gupta NK, Pointon RCS, Wilkinson PM. A randomised clinical trial to contrast radiotherapy with radiotherapy and methotrexate given synchronously in head and neck cancer. Clin Radiol 1987; 38:575.

50. Haselow RE, Adams GS, Oken MM, et al. Cis-platinum (DDP) with radiation therapy (RT) for locally advanced unresectable head and neck cancer. Proc Am Soc Clin Oncol 1983; 2:160.

51. Haselow RE, Warshaw MG, Oken MM, et al. Radiation alone versus radiation with weekly low dose cis-platinum in unresectable head and neck. In: Head and Neck Cancer, Vol. II, ed by WE Fee Jr, H Goepfert, ME Johns, EW Strong, PH Ward. BC Decker Inc Toronto 1990, pp 279–281.

52. Hliniak A, Maciejewski B, Trott KR. The influence of the number of fractions, overall treatment time and field size on the local control of cancer of the skin. Br J Radiol 1983; 56:596.

53. Ho E, Coffey C, Maruyama Y. Enhancement of radiation effect on mouse intestinal crypt survival by timing of 5-fluorouracil administration. Radiology 1977; 125:531.

54. Hussey DH, Abrams JP. Combined therapy in advanced head and neck cancer: hydroxyurea and radiotherapy. Prog Clin Cancer 1975; 6:79.

55. Jacobs MC, Eisenberger M, Chu Oh M, et al. Carboplatin (CBDCA) and radiotherapy for stage IV carcinoma of the head and neck: A phase I–II study. Int J Radiat Oncol Biol Phys 1989; 17:361.

56. Jesse RH, Goepfert H, Lindberg RD, et al. Combined intra-arterial infusion and radiotherapy for the treatment of advanced cancer of the head and neck. Am J Roentgenol 1969; 105:20.

57. Jongejan HTM, van der Kogel AJ, Provoost AP, et al. Interaction of cis-diamminedichloroplatinum II and renal irradiation on renal function in the young and adult rat. Radiother Oncol 1987; 10:49.

58. Kaplan MJ, Hahn SS, Johns ME, et al. Mitomycin and fluorouracil with concomitant radiotherapy in head and neck cancer. Arch Otolaryngol 1985; 111:220.

59. Kapstad B, Bang G, Rennaes S, et al. Combined preoperative treatment with cobalt and bleomycin in patients with head and neck carcinoma—a controlled clinical study. Int J Radiat Oncol Biol Phys 1978; 4:85.

60. Karim ABMF, Snow GB, Versluis RJJ, et al. Concurrent radiation therapy with polychemotherapy VBM in advanced or recurrent H&N cancer. Abstract: Second European Conference on Clinical Oncology, Amsterdam, 1983:162.

61. Keane TJ, Harwood AR, Danjoux C, et al. Results of a randomised trial of radiation compared to radiation and chemotherapy for advanced laryngeal, and hypopharyngeal squamous carcinoma. Abstract Second International Conference on Head and Neck Cancer, Boston 1988:89.

62. Keizer HJ, Karim ABMF, Hian Njo K, et al. Feasibility study on daily administration of cis-diamminedichloroplatinum (II) in combination with radiotherapy. Radiother Oncol 1984; 1:227.

63. Kramer S. Use of methotrexate and radiation therapy for advanced cancer of the head and neck. Front Radiat Ther Oncol 1969; 4:116.

64. Kummermehr J, Trott KR. Rate of repopulation in a slow and fast growing tumor. In: Karcher KH, Kogelnik HD, Reinarts G, eds. Progress in radio-oncology, vol II. New York: Raven Press, 1982:299–307.

65. Lelieveld P, Smink T, van Putten L. Experimental studies on the combination of radiation and chemotherapy. Int J Radiat Oncol Biol Phys 1978; 4:37.

66. Lerner HJ, Beckloff GL, Goodwin MC. Concomitant hydroxyurea and radiotherapy in the management of 63 patients with head and neck cancer. Am Surg 1969; 35:525.

67. Lo TCM, Wiley AL, Jr, Ansfield FJ, et al. Combined radiation therapy and 5-fluorouracil for advanced squamous cell carcinoma of the oral cavity and oropharynx: A randomized study. Am J Roentgenol 1976; 126:229.

68. Lütgemeier J, Seifert R, Neumann D. Kombinierte Therapie von hochdosiertem Cis-Platin und Bestrahlung bei fortgeschrittenen HNO-Tumoren (Phase-II-Studie). Strahlentherapie 1986; 162:709.

69. Maciejewski B, Withers HR, Taylor JMG, et al. Dose fractionated and regeneration in radiotherapy for cancer of the oral cavity and oropharynx: Tumor dose–response and repopulation. Int J Radiat Oncol Biol 1989; 16:831.

70. Magno L, Terraneo F, Scandolaro L, et al. Lonidamine and radiotherapy in head and neck cancer: A preliminary report. Proc. Am Soc Clin Oncol 1987; 6:126.

70a. Martin M, Hazan A, Vergnes L, et al. Randomized study of 5-fluorouracil and cisplatin as neoadjuvant therapy in head and neck cancer: a preliminary report. Int J Radiat Oncol Biol Phys 1990; 19:973.

71. Merlano M, Rosso R, Sertoli MR, et al. Sequential versus alternating chemotherapy and radiotherapy in stage III–IV squamous cell carcinoma of the head and neck: A phase III study. J Clin Oncol 1988; 6:627.

72. Miller B, Yu A, Tefft M, et al. Improved response rate in patients with advanced unresectable cancer of the head and neck. Proc Am Soc Clin Oncol 1985; 4:142.

73. Molin J, Søgaard PE, Overgaard J. Experimental studies on the radiation-modifying effect of bleomycin in malignant and normal mouse tissue in vivo. Cancer Treat Rep 1981; 65:583.

74. Morita K. Clinical significance of radiation therapy combined with chemotherapy. Strahlentherapie 1980; 156:228.

75. Moulder JE, Fish BL. Effect of sequencing on the combined toxicity of renal irradiation and cis-platinum. NCI Monogr 1988; 6:35.

76. Phillips TL. Current status, opportunities and problems in clinical combined chemoradiotherapy. In: Okada S, Imamura M, Terashima T, Yamaguchi H, eds. Proceedings of the Sixth International Congress of Radiation Research, Tokyo, 1979:823–9.

77. Phillips TL, Wharam MD, Margolis LW. Modification of radiation injury to normal tissues by chemotherapeutic agents. Cancer 1975; 35:1648.

78. Pointon RCS, Askill C, Hunter RD, et al. Treatment of advanced head and neck cancer using synchronous therapy with methotrexate and irradiation. Clin Radiol 1983; 34:459.

79. Poirier MC, Lippard SJ, Zwelling LA, et al. Antibodies elicited against cis-diamminedichloroplatinum (II)—modified DNA are specific for cis-diamminedichloroplatinum (II)—DNA adducts formed in vivo and in vitro. Proc Natl Acad Sci USA 1982; 79:6443.

80. Richards GJ Jr, Chambers RG. Hydroxyurea: A radiosensitizer in the treatment of neoplasms of the head and neck. Am J Roentgenol 1969; 105:555.

81. Rockwell S, Kennedy KA. Combination therapy with radiation and mitomycin C: Preliminary results with EMT6 tumour cells in vitro and in vivo. Int J Radiat Oncol Biol Phys 1979; 5:1673.

82. Rojas A, Joiner MC. The influence of dose per fraction on repair kinetics. Radiother Oncol 1989; 14:329.

83. Rominger CJ. Hydroxyurea and radiation therapy in advanced neoplasms of the head and neck. Am J Roentgenol 1971; 111:103.

84. Sato Y, Morita M, Takahashi H, et al. Combined surgery, radiotherapy, and regional chemotherapy in carcinoma of the paranasal sinuses. Cancer 1970; 25:571.

84a. Schaake-Koning C, Van den Bogaert W, Dalesio O, et al. Improved survival and the effect of time dose scheduling of radiotherapy and cis-di-amindichloroplatinum (II) in patints with the inoperable non-small cell lung cancer. A randomized phase III trial of the EORTC Radiotherapy and Lung Cancer Cooperative Groups. N Eng J Med (in press).

85. Schmitt G, Higi M, Stupp H, et al. Ein neues interdisziplinäres Behandlungskonzept bei fortgeschrittenen Kopf–Hals-Tumoren. Strahlentherapie 1983; 159:470.

86. Seagren SL, Byfield JE, Nahum AM, et al. Treatment of locally advanced squamous cell carcinoma of the head and neck with concurrent bleomycin and external beam radiation therapy. Int J Radiat Oncol Biol Phys 1979; 5:1531.

87. Seagren SL, Byfield JE, Davidson TM, et al. Bleomycin, cyclophosphamide and radiotherapy in regionally advanced epidermoid carcinoma of the head and neck. Int J Radiat Oncol Biol Phys 1982; 8:127.

88. SECOG, an interim report from the participants: A randomized trial of combined multidrug chemotherapy and radiotherapy in advanced squamous cell carcinoma of the head and neck. Eur J Surg Oncol 1986; 12:289.

89. Shah PM, Shukla SN, Patel KM, et al. Effect of bleomycin–radiotherapy combination in management of head and neck squamous cell carcinoma. Cancer 1981; 48:1106.

90. Shanta V, Krishnamurthi S. Combined bleomycin and radiotherapy in oral cancer. Clin Radiol 1980; 31:617.

91. Shewell J, Davies RW. Combined therapy of the spontaneous mouse mammary tumour: Methotrexate and hyperbaric oxygen irradiation. Eur J Cancer 1977; 13:977.

92. Shigematsu Y, Sakai S, Fuchihata H. Recent trials in the treatment of maxillary sinus carcinoma, with special reference to the chemical potentiation of radiation therapy. Acta Otolaryngol (Stockh) 1971; 71:63.

93. Sinclair WK. Hydroxyurea revisited: A decade of clinical effects studies. Int J Radiat Oncol Biol Phys 1981; 7:631.

94. Slotman GJ, Cummings FJ, Glicksman AR, et al. Preoperative simultaneously administered cis-platinum plus radiation therapy for advanced squamous cell carcinoma of the head and neck. Head Neck Surg 1986; 8:159.

95. Smith BL, Franz JL, Mira JG, et al. Simultaneous combination radiotherapy and multidrug chemotherapy for stage III and stage IV squamous cell carcinoma of the head and neck. J Surg Oncol 1980; 15:91.

96. Snyderman NL, Wetmore SJ, Suen JY. Cisplatin sensitization to radiotherapy in stage IV squamous cell carcinoma of the head and neck. A follow-up report. Arch Otolaryngol Head Neck Surg 1986; 112:1147.

97. Souhami L, Rabinowits M. Combined treatment in carcinoma of the nasopharynx. Laryngoscope 1988; 98:881.

98. Spremulli EN, Leith JT, Bliven SF, et al. Response of a human colony adenocarcinoma (DLD-1) to X-irradiation and mitomycin C in vivo. Int J Radiat Oncol Biol Phys 1983; 9:1209.

99. Steel GG. The search for therapeutic gain in the combination of radiotherapy and chemotherapy. Radiother Oncol 1988; 11:31.

100. Steel GG, Peacock JH. Why are some human tumours more radiosensitive than others? Radiother Oncol 1989; 15:63.

100a. Steel GG, Peckham MJ. Exploitable mechanisms in combined radiotherapy–chemotherapy: The concept of activity. Int J Radiat Oncol Biol Phys 1979; 5:85.

101. Stefani S, Eells RW, Abbate J. Hydroxyurea and radiotherapy in head and neck cancer. Results of a prospective controlled study in 126 patients. Radiology 1971; 101:391.

102. Stefani S, Chung TS. Hydroxyurea and radiotherapy in head and neck cancer—long term results of a double blind randomized prospective study. Int J Radiat Oncol Biol Phys 1980; 6:1398.

102a. Stell PM, Rawson NSB. Adjuvant chemotherapy in head and neck cancer. Br J Cancer 1990; 61:779.

103. Stephens TC, Peacock JH, Steel GG. Cell survival in B16 melanoma after treatment with combinations of cytotoxic agents: Lack of potentiation. Br J Cancer 1977; 36:84.

104. Stewart FA, Luts A, Oussoren Y, et al. Renal damage in mice after combined treatment with cisplatin and X-rays: a comparison of fractionated and single dose studies. NCI Monogr 1988; 6:23.

105. Takabe Y, Miyamoto T, Watanabe M, et al. Synergism of X-rays and bleomycin on Ehrlich ascites tumour cells. Br J Cancer 1977; 36:391.

106. Tanaka Y, Wada T, Fuchihata H, et al. Combined treatment with radiation and bleomycin for intra-oral carcinoma. A preliminary report. Int J Radiat Oncol Biol Phys 1976; 1:1189.

107. Tannock IF. Combined modality treatment with radiotherapy and chemotherapy. Radiother Oncol 1989; 16:83.

108. Taylor SG IV, Murthy AK, Showel J, et al. Concomitant therapy with infusion of cisplatin and 5-fluorouracil plus radiation in head and neck cancer. NCI Monogr 1988; 6:343.

109. Taylor SG IV, Murthy AK, Showel JL, et al. Comparison of toxicity in a randomized trial of sequential vs. simultaneous cisplatin/5-FU infusion and radiation therapy in head and neck cancer. Proc Am Soc Clin Oncol 1989; 8:175.

110. Terheggen PM, Floot BG, Scherer E, et al. Immunocytochemical detection of interaction products on cis-diamminedichloroplatinum (II) and cis-diammine (1.1-cyclobutanedicarboxylato) platinum (II) with DNA in rodent tissue sections. Cancer Res 1987; 47:6719.

111. Terheggen PM, Dijkman R, Begg AC, et al. Monitoring of interaction products of cis-di-aminedichloroplatinum (II) and cis-di-amine (1.1-cyclobutanedicarboxylato) platinum (II) with DNA in cells from platinum-treated cancer patients. Cancer Res 1988; 48:5597.

112. Thames HD Jr, Suit HD. Tumor radioresponsiveness versus fractionation sensitivity. Int J Radiat Oncol Biol Phys 1986; 12:687.

113. Tobias JS, Smith BJ, Blackman G, et al. Concurrent daily cisplatin and radiotherapy in locally advanced squamous carcinoma of the head-and-neck and bronchus. Radioth Oncol 1987; 9:263.

114. Trott KR, Maciejewski B, Preuss-Bayer G, et al. Dose response curve and split-dose recovery in human skin cancer. Radiother Oncol 1984; 2:123.

115. Tubiana M, Frindel E, Vassort F. Critical survey of experimental data on in vivo synchronisation by hydroxyurea. Recent Results Cancer Res 1975; 52:187.

116. Tubiana M, Courdi A. Cell proliferation kinetics in human solid tumors: relation to probability of metastatic dissemination and long-term survival. Radiother Oncol 1989; 15:1.

117. Van der Kogel A, Sissingh HA. Effects of intrathecal methotrexate and cytosine arabinoside on the radiation tolerance of the rat spinal cord. Radiother Oncol 1985; 4:239.

118. Vannetzel JM, Juillard JC, Colbert N, et al. Combined cisplatin, 5-FU infusion and radiation therapy in squamous cell carcinoma of the head and neck. Proc Am Soc Clin Oncol 1987; 6:142.

119. Vanuytsel L, Feng Y, Landuyt W, et al. The combined effect of bleomycin and irradiation on mouse lip mucosa. 2. Influence on the accumulation and repair of sublethal damage during fractionated irradiation. Radiother Oncol 1986; 6:267.

120. Vermund H, Kaalhus O, Winther F, et al. Bleomycin and radiation therapy in squamous cell carcinoma of the upper aero-digestive tract: A phase III clinical trial. Int J Radiat Oncol Biol Phys 1985; 11:1877.

121. Vietti T, Eggerding F, Valeriote F. Combined effect of X-radiation and 5-fluorouracil on survival of transplanted leukemic cells. J Natl Cancer Inst 1971; 47:865.

122. Vokes EE, Panje WR, Schilsky RL, et al. Hydroxyurea, fluorouracil, and concomitant radiotherapy in poor-prognosis head and neck cancer: A phase I–II study. J Clin Oncol 1989; 7:761.

122a. Vokes EE, Panje WR, Mick R, et al. A randomized study comparing two regimens of neoadjuvant and adjuvant chemotherapy in multimodal therapy for locally advanced head and neck cancer. Cancer 1990; 66:206.

122b. Vokes EE, Weichselbaum RR. Concomitant chemotherapy: Rationale and clinical experience in patients with solid tumors. J Clin Oncol 1990; 8:911.

123. Von der Maase H, Overgaard J, Vaeth M. Effects of cancer chemotherapeutic drugs on radiation-induced lung damage in mice. Radiother Oncol 1986; 5:245.

124. Wallner KE, Li GL. Effect of cisplatin resistance on cellular radiation response. Int J Radiat Oncol Biol Phys 1987; 13:587.

125. Weinberg MJ, Lapointe TA, Rauth AM. Growth delay in murine squamous cell tumor after local radiation and concurrent infusional 5-fluorouracil treatment. Int J Radiat Oncol Biol Phys 1986; 12:1449.

126. Weissberg JB, Son YH, Papac RJ, et al. Randomized clinical trial of mitomycin C as an adjunct to radiotherapy in head and neck cancer. Int J Radiat Oncol Biol Phys 1989; 17:3.

127. Wendt TG, Hartenstein RC, Wustrow TPU, et al. Cisplatin, fluorouracil with leucovorin calcium enhancement, and synchronous accelerated radiotherapy in the management of locally advanced head and neck cancer: A phase II study. J Clin Oncol 1989; 7:471.

128. Wheeler R, Salter M, Stephens S, et al. Simultaneous therapy with high-dose cisplatin and radiation for unresectable squamous cell cancer of the head and neck: A phase I–II study. NCI Monogr 1988; 6:339.

129. Williams MV, Denekamp J, Fowler JF. A review of alpha/beta ratios for experimental tumors: Implications for clinical studies of altered fractionation. Int J Radiat Oncol Biol Phys 1985; 11:87.

130. Withers HR, Taylor JMG, Maciejewski B. The hazard of accelerated tumor clonogen repopulation during radiotherapy. Acta Oncol 1988; 27:131.

131. Wittes RE, Cvitkovic E, Shah J, Gerold FP, Strong EW. Cis-dichlorodiammine-platinum (II) in the treatment of epidermoid carcinoma of the head and neck. Cancer Treat Rep 1977; 61:359.

132. Zelen M. Guidelines for publishing papers on cancer clinical trials: responsibilities of editors and authors. J Clin Oncol 1983; 1:164.

133. Zwelling LA. Cisplatin and new platinum analogs. In: Pinedo HM, Longo DL, Chabner BA, eds. Cancer chemotherapy and biological response modifiers, annual 10. Amsterdam: Elsevier, 1988:64–72.

7 Therapies in Development

Immunobiological Therapy for Head and Neck Cancer

D. R. Parkinson, S. P. Schantz

Introduction

Immunotherapeutic approaches to the treatment of head and neck cancer in the 1970s led to disappointing results. The addition of nonspecific immunoadjuvants such as BCG, *Corynebacterium parvum*, and levamisole to chemotherapy added little or nothing to the antitumor effects of chemotherapy alone, and despite initially encouraging results, controlled adjuvant trials with these same agents, were negative. In this chapter we review new evidence concerning the immunobiology of squamous cell carcinoma of the head and neck and the results of recent clinical trials with recombinant cytokines, activated lymphocytes, and plasma therapies.

It would be naive to assume that immune defense mechanisms are the only factors involved in the control of neoplastic diseases and that immunological approaches to therapy will be uniformly successful. Even in experimental animal models purposefully constructed to demonstrate the relevance of host response against tumor, certain cancers are far more immunogenic than others and thus more effectively regulated by cellular and humoral immune defenses. Factors controlling immunogenicity often relate to whether or not an experimental tumor is spontaneous or induced, as the latter tumors are more characteristically associated with easily demonstrable host–tumor interactions. In addition, how a particular cancer was induced may determine antigenicity; the more intensely a tissue is exposed to a carcinogenic agent, the more antigenic will be the neoplasm which develops (59). Furthermore, cancers developing after viral exposure are generally less immunogenic than chemically induced tumors.

Human cancers also undoubtedly possess a wide spectrum of immunogenicity. Head and neck cancer, in relationship to other human solid tumors, likely falls within the category of tumors that are responsive to immune surveillance, since with respect to etiologic factors for head and neck cancer, several potential carcinogens have been implicated. Tobacco has clearly been defined as an important risk factor for development of this disease (94). Other etiologic factors which may convey immunogenicity to head and neck cancers include viral agents, which have been described as both initiators and promoters of this disease (14, 27, 80). Numerous studies have incriminated herpes simplex virus-type 1 as a mutagenic virus responsible for neoplastic transformation. Moreover, evidence suggests that the latter virus can induce cancer more effectively in concert with tobacco extract (80). In addition, papilloma virus, a known tumor promoter, has recently been identified within cancers at multiple sites within the upper areodigestive tract (14).

The patient's immunologic defenses represent the other side of the host–tumor interaction. The more immunogenic a particular cancer, the more clinically important it may be that the patient has a competent immunologic surveillance system. The interaction between head and neck cancers and the immune system may be relatively significant compared to that with other solid tumors, as the cell-mediated immune defect in patients with head and neck cancer is far more profound than in those with carcinomas of the breast, bladder, or bronchus, or those with melanomas or sarcomas (58). Furthermore, cellular immune responses remain depressed after definitive therapy in the majority of individuals with head and neck cancer. Conversely, immune recovery after therapy for cancer has been described in patients with adenocarcinomas, melanomas, and sarcomas (6, 37, 58).

In this chapter we review the immunobiology of head and neck cancer from a historical perspective. We begin with a discussion of studies of immune responsiveness in patients with head and neck cancer, and conclude with a summary of the results of recent clinical trials of immunotherapy in this group of patients.

Immunobiological Studies in Head and Neck Cancer Patients

Lessons from the Studies of Dinitrochlorobenzene (DNCB) Skin Testing

Eilber and Morton reported one of the first studies assessing cell-mediated immunity in head and neck cancer patients using DNCB skin testing (18). This assay begins with the intradermal application of a sensitizing dose of DNCB, and concludes with quantitation of the cutaneous response to a subsequent intradermal injection. DNCB skin testing thus allows determination of an individual's ability to process antigen and mount an immune response. In the study of Eilber and Morton, 100 cancer patients, including 24 with head and neck cancer, were evaluated for skin sensitivity to DNCB. Following sensitization, 95% of normal controls exhibited delayed cutaneous hypersensitivity to DNCB. In contrast, 60% of patients with potentially resectable cancers lacked skin test reactivity to DNCB. In follow-up, 92% of cancer patients who initially reacted to DNCB were free of disease for 6 months, while 92% of cancer patients who failed to exhibit DNCB hypersensitivity either proved to have inoperable cancers or developed early recurrence after surgery. These results were confirmed in a follow-up study by these same investigators (19). In this study, DNCB positive patients again faired well with 36 of 41 patients at 1 year and 16 of 18 followed for 4 years remaining free-of-desease.

Hypersensitivity reactions to other antigens applied intradermally by Eilber and Morton did not yield similar results (18). Patients who reacted to DNCB often lacked reactivity to other recall antigens such as mumps, purified protein derivatives, and dermatophytin. One explanation for this phenomenon is that the generation of response to many of the latter antigens requires adequate prior exposure to that specific antigen as well as an intact host response. The adequacy of previous exposure to the latter antigens often cannot be ascertained. In contrast, DNCB is effective in eliciting a response in more than 95% of normal people when used in a controlled sensitization program.

Following these early studies of DNCB reactivity in patients with head and neck cancer, numerous subsequent studies with both similar and conflicting results were published. Wanebo et al. noted that 30% of patients with T1N0 head and neck cancers were DNCB negative, with a greater degree of immune impairment present in patients with more advanced lesions (87). Furthermore, and distinct from the findings of Eilber et al., a response to PPD was a better predictor for survival at 1 year than response to DNCB (84% survival versus 75% survival, respectively). The predictive value of skin test reactivity was most evident in patients with early stage lesions as compared to those with advanced disease. In patients with stage IV head and neck cancer, DNCB reactivity did not predict for survival.

Bosworth, et al. reported the significance of delayed hypersensitivity on local control in patients treated by radiotherapy for head and neck cancer (3). Patients reactive to DNCB demonstrated a better response to radiotherapy than those anergic to DNCB. Maisel and Ogura noted that 2 years postoperatively 91% of patients who were DNCB reactive were tumor free whereas 55% of those individu-

als who were DNCB nonreactive developed recurrence (39).

On the other hand, two studies have questioned the clinical significance of DNCB skin test reactivity. Gilbert et al. determined the predictive effect of skin test reactivity to DNCB in 85 consecutive patients with squamous cell carcinoma of the upper aerodigestive tract (23). All patients were treated with radiation therapy alone or combined radiation plus surgery. Based on retrospective analysis, the authors concluded that DNCB response was not sufficiently predictive of disease status at 2 years to be useful in making prospective treatment decisions. In review of Gilbert et al.'s data, however, 29 of 35 patients who were successfully treated were DNCB positive. These data suggest some prognostic value for DNCB response.

Chretien et al. also failed to determine a prognostic value for DNCB testing in patients with head and neck cancer (9, 10). Conflicting results have also been noted in studies relating tumor stage to DNCB reactivity. While several studies have demonstrated a relationship between DNCB response and advancing tumor stage, others have not (6, 49, 52, 87).

Our purpose in describing results of DNCB hypersensitivity is to provide a framework for discussion about more recent studies of immunologic monitoring in patients with head and neck cancer. The use of skin test hypersensitivity to DNCB is prototypical of results from subsequent in vitro and in vivo assays of immune status which when negative reflect an impaired immune status and correlate with advanced disease and a poor prognosis. Collectively, the studies of DNCB reactivity as well as many of the subsequent assays of immune status, are flawed by a remarkable lack of consistency in the generation and interpretation of test results.

The heterogeneity of DNCB test results may in part be secondary to differences in methodology. The technique of DNCB sensitization can be described as follows (5). The volar aspect of the arm is cleansed and allowed to dry. The sensitizing dose of DNCB (1000 µg per 3 cm^2) is applied. The injection sites are examined at 24 hours for an initial reaction characterized by erythema and induration, and at 7 and 14 days for a spontaneous flare. The occurrence of the flare indicates sensitization. In the absence of a spontaneous flare by 14 days, a challenge dose is applied, and the injection site is reexamined for a delayed cutaneous reaction at 24 and 48 hours.

Bates et al. have reviewed the various methodologies for skin testing with DNCB (2). Several methods differ in their definition of a positive reaction. Thus, the same test observation may be considered positive in one study and negative in another. Additionally, results may vary based on factors such as the concentration of DNCB used, the time interval between the administration of sensitizing and challenge doses, as well as the length of time between skin dose application and subsequent analysis. The authors concluded that one technique for DNCB sensitization should be utilized in subsequent clinical studies, and they recommended the methodology of Catalona et al. (5).

While standardization is critical, advances in immune monitoring through the acceptance of „the best way" to perform an assay have not been fruitful. It is unlikely that variability in DNCB reactivity can be entirely explained by a lack of test standardization. Other more fundamental biological factors must be considered.

The Heterogeneous Head and Neck Cancer Population

Foremost among factors which may account for variability in immunologic test results is patient heterogeneity. The determinants of disease progression and immunologic status may be extremely diverse. In one individual the lack of DNCB reactivity may be a fundamental observation that reflects a biological parameter critical to the likelihood of disease progression. Undoubtedly, however, the circumstance in which the capacity to generate an immune response (as reflected by the DNCB assay) is the sole and major determinant of disease progression is rare. However, the fact that a test has limited clinical relevance does not imply that it has no biological significance. Rather, the test most likely represents only one determinant of many factors important in the process of disease progression.

The prognostic significance of any factor likely depends on its relative position in the chain of events which lead to disease progression. For instance, the most significant factor leading to disease progression within a given patient with head and neck cancer may be the inherent genetic stability of their individual tumor cells. As a tumor grows, these genetic changes provide an opportunity for selection of the most adaptive viable cancer (48).

Evidence of this phenomenon comes from cytogenetic observations as well as experimental models. Cytogenetic observations generally reveal an association between increasingly more virulent tumors, and an increased number of chromosomal abnormalities. Research with leukemia has been illustrative (65, 81). In chronic myelogenous leukemia, the chromosome 9 to 22 translocation (Philadelphia chromosome) which typifies the less virulent stage of the disease typically becomes associated with additional karyotypic abnormalities as the leukemia progresses (65). Likewise, serial translocations in a low-grade lymphoid tumor involving first one oncogene (bcl-2) and then another (c-myc) will convey a greater malignant potential in that tumor (13). Thus, malignant potential can be considered a sum-

mation of serial genetic events occurring within a particular cancer cell an its offspring.

Numerous factors contribute to the genetic instability of a malignant tumor, and the rate at which genetic changes occur may vary from one patient to the next. Furthermore, one genetic event may predispose to another. For example, Nowell notes that aneuploidy could result from a particular sister chromatid exchange or break, and that once present, it could contribute to the production of further genetic errors through an increased probability of nondisjunctions (48). The degree of cellular heterogeneity within a tumor may contribute to genetic instability through interactions among the preexisting subpopulations of tumor cells (57). Furthermore, a particular oncogenic virus may lead to the initiation of a cancer cell and with the persistence of the viral genome contribute to a cancer cell which is increasingly unstable (68). Finally, the tendency for genetic instability in a particular cancer may be constitutionally inherited and differ from one individual to another. Individuals with chromosome fragility syndromes, such as patients with the Bloom syndrome, ataxia−telangiectasia, and Fanconi anemia may have tumors which likewise have error-prone replication processes that lead to increasing genetic alterations. It may be relevant that head and neck cancer patients express such chromosome fragility when their lymphocytes are exposed in vitro to mutagens (75).

With time, increased genetic instability and associated genetic events result in a tumor that is biologically more aggressive and has an accelerated growth rate. With continued genetic change, tumors may become less antigenic. The tumors may activate certain oncogenes, such as those of the ras oncogene family, which have been shown to convey increased metastatic potential (46). Cancer cells may acquire characteristics which convey to them an increased capacity to progress such as an increased agglutination potential, the production of proteolytic enzymes, or membrane molecules such as laminin and fibronectin (47). The cancer cell should be viewed as a dynamic entity which contains within it a multiplicity of genetic determinants that govern its malignant potential.

When a cancer cell has reached its most progressive state, immune deficiency may play only a minor role in determining disease progression. The cancer cell would be able to survive and grow regardless of the host's capacity to mount a cellular and humoral defense. Conversely, when tumor cells are in a stage of differentiation in which the genetic code is relatively stable, their capacity to adapt to a changing environment may be limited and their proliferative capacity minimal. Under such circumstances the role of immune response would become more dominant. Patients that can maintain a host response in pace with the invasive potential of a particular tumor may not experience disease progression.

Studies of Natural Immunity

Studies of natural immunity exemplify the heterogeneity in the immune status of patients with head and neck cancer. Natural immunity refers principally to a cellular defense mechanism which has the capacity to lyse target cancer cells without need for previous sensitization (85). Unlike the T-cell surveillance system, natural immunity does not require prior exposure to a target in order to exert its effect. The recognition and triggering mechanisms which govern its lytic capacity are inherently determined. The cell responsible for natural immunity, the natural killer (NK) cell, is characterized by its capacity to lyse cancer targets without regard to the target's expression of major histocompatibility class (MHC) cell surface antigens. Target cells do not need to express the latter antigens in order to be efficiently recognized by the NK cell. The natural immune system differs from the adaptive, MHC-restricted cytotoxic T-cell defenses as the latter only recognizes cancer cells that express foreign antigens in concert with MHC antigens. The natural immune system is a primitive system which makes its appearance early in animal phyla long before the appearance of its T-cell counterpart (69). The role of this primitive non-MHC-restricted defense mechanism may be as a defense against non-self rather than altered self as would be the case of T-cell mechanisms (33).

Multiple reports have addressed natural immunity within head and neck cancer patients (43, 70−73, 84, 90, 93), and it is worthwhile noting how the results of studies of natural immune function have paralleled those with DNCB skin testing. Takasugi first described natural immune function in head and neck cancer patients in 1973. He analyzed 64 cancer patients and compared results to 65 concurrently examined age-matched controls (84). It was noted that the cancer-bearing population demonstrated a diminished capacity to lyse a series of allogeneic cancer targets. Furthermore, this deficiency appeared to be most evident in patients with advanced disease. Early stage patients expressed NK cell activity that was two-thirds that of healthy controls. Advanced stage patients expressed levels only one-fourth as effective. Whether or not the defect in natural immune surveillance was a cause or a result of disease progression with these patients could not be determined. These results were subsequently confirmed by Cortesina et al. in a population of untreated patients with laryngeal carcinoma (12).

In the ensuing years Wustron and Zenner reported results of studies of NK cell function in 57 patients with untreated pharyngolaryngeal squamous cell carcinomas (93). Wustrow and Zenner were unable to define any deficit of NK cell function in these individuals as compared to a group of concurrently examined healthy controls. In addition, Wustrow and Zenner were unable to define differences in NK cell function as a factor of disease stage.

Another permutation of possible results was observed by Wolf et al. (90). The latter authors showed that head and neck cancer patients with advanced disease were suppressed in their natural immune status. Interestingly, however, early stage patients actually had an enhanced natural immune status. Finally, Schantz et al. performed a study of natural immunity on 111 previously untreated patients with cancer at multiple primary sites including the oral cavity, pharynx, and larynx (70). Deficient NK cell function was found to exist in the population as a whole, but the degree to which the population was deficient was not marked. Furthermore, a broad overlap in individual values between the cancer population and an age-matched healthy control population was apparent. The authors noted that levels of NK cell function were independent of disease stage. Those individuals with early disease were as likely to have diminished NK cell function as those with more advanced stages.

As was the case for DNCB skin testing, the observed variations in natural immune function in patients with head and cancer may be attributed in part to the lack of a standard methodology for determination of this function. The techniques utilized in studies of NK cell number and activity were less than ideal and differed from one study to another. For example, natural immunity was determined in one study not by functional analyses but through a quantitative assessment of natural killer cells using a monoclonal antibody against the Leu 7 antigen, a surface antigen of NK cells (1, 90). It is known today that the anti-Leu 7 antibody is not specific for the NK cell as the antigen is readily expressed on T-cells. Furthermore, as might be expected, anti-Leu 7 assay results do not correlate with functional assays of natural immune status such as the standard chromium release assay (71). When NK cell function has been evaluated, nonstandard methods have frequently been employed. For example, Wustrow and Zenner estimated NK cell function via quantification of target cell viability by vital staining rather than by the more standard chromium release assay.

Subsequent to reports correlating NK cell function and disease stage, other studies have examined the relationship between NK cell cytotoxicity and disease progression. Schantz et al. concluded that NK cell function has prognostic implications for disease progression, with individuals having deficient NK cell function being at risk for disease progression (71−73). In these studies, decreased NK cell function was also associated with death from metastatic disease. Remarkably, NK cell cytotoxicity did not identify patients at risk for progression of disease at local sites (71).

Schantz et al. also explored the relationship between a tumor's histopathologic differentiation and immune defense (73). In a study of 153 untreated patients with head and neck cancer, NK cell function significantly correlated with treatment outcome only in patients with poorly differentiated cancers, i. e. cancers with < 25% keratinization on histopathologic assessment. For patients with differentiated cancers (> 75% keratinization), quantitation of natural immune mediated cytotoxicity provided no prognostic information.

It is pertinent to note that poorly differentiated head and neck tumors can be distinguished by their lack of expected cell surface antigens. Esteban et al. demonstrated that poorly differentiated tumor cells frequently lack MHC-class I antigen expression (20). The results of Schantz may be explained by recalling the relative importance of NK cell cytotoxicity against cells which lack MHC antigens. As espoused by Karre et al. the primitive NK cell system is highly conserved throughout phylogenetic development and recognizes (non-self) cells which fail to express major histocompatibility antigens. The more adaptive T-cells recognize altered self and constitute a second type of cell-mediated defense (33). In the latter instance, T-cells destroy antigenically altered tumor cells only if those cancer cells express self MHC antigens in concert with the abnormal antigen. Which cell-mediated immune defense is operative against a given tumor therefore may depend in part on the phenotypic characteristics of the patient's cancer.

The impact of tumor cell phenotype on host response has been studied using the murine RMA lymphoma (33). Karre et al. selected subclones of the high MHC-class I RMA lymphoma for their lack of MHC class I antigens. C57BL mice were then injected with both the parent RMA lymphoma and the negative MCH-class I subclones. Upon comparison, the parent line was noted to have a higher metastatic potential than the subclone. In vitro the parent cells were resistant to NK cell function, while subclone cells without MHC-class I antigen were sensitive. Thus, the parent RMA cell possessed an intrinsic capacity to metastasize. However, with changes in specific characteristics of that cell, i. e. the expression of certain cell surface antigens, the NK cell system became functionally relevant and a tumor's metastatic potential declined.

The relationship between tumor biology and NK cell function has also been evaluated by Schantz and Goepfert (72). In their study of patients with and without lymph node metastases at presentation, NK cell function correlated with eventual distant metastatic spread only in patients with regional lyph node metastases. NK cell function was not associated with distant relapse in those without lymph node metastases at presentation. Once again, the functional significance of the immune system appears dependent on biologic properties intrinsic to a tumor, in this case, the tumor's potential for spread to regional lymph nodes. The heterogeneity of determinants for disease progression in patients with head and neck cancer is again emphasized as is limited relevance of any known immune parameter when measured in isolation.

Thus far we have presented only two immune parameters, antigen-recall testing and natural killer cell cytotoxicity, of the many that have biologic significance in patients with head and neck cancer. Others that have been studied in these patients include: lymphocyte blastogenesis in response to mitogens such as phytohemagglutinin (PHA), concanavalin A (ConA), and pokeweed mutagen (PWM); peripheral blood lymphocyte counts; and various measures of humoral immunity including circulating IgA levels and circulating immune complexes.

Other Studies of Cell-mediated Immunity

Lymphocyte reactivity to mitogens, i.e., in vitro stimulated blastogenesis, was one of the initial measures of cell-mediated immune function. In this assay, lymphocytes are incubated with a particular mitogen, such as PHA, PWM, or ConA. After a period of time, incubated cells are exposed to tritiated thymidine. This DNA precursor is incorporated in lymphocytes which have been induced to divide through exposure to the mitogen. The amount of radiolabeled thymidine incorporated into DNA is then quantitated. Low levels of thymidine incorporation have generally been considered to reflect a more deficient immune system, a system less responsive to antigen stimulation. Using this assay, Wanebo et al. noted lymphocyte activity to be deficient in head and neck cancer patients (87). Furthermore, those individuals with advanced disease were more likely to express that deficiency than those with limited disease (87). This correlation between disease stage and a depressed lymphocyte stimulated blastogenesis, however, has not been universally observed. In addition, other studies have failed to report significant correlations between survival and in vitro measured lymphocyte reactivity (78).

Characterization of peripheral blood lymphocyte subsets has also been evaluated as a prognostic factor for patients with head and neck cancer. The general consensus of these studies is that both overall lymphocyte counts and those of specific subsets are decreased in patients with head and neck cancer (8, 17, 50, 53, 78). Furthermore, quantitation of lymphocytes may have prognostic value, as Check et al. noted that absolute lymphocyte counts isolated by Ficoll–hypaque density gradient centrifugation are good predictors of survival (8). Others have failed to confirm a relation between survival and T-lymphocyte counts (17, 87).

Wolf et al. have extensively investigated the prognostic value of lymphocyte subsets quantitated by the use of monoclonal antibodies to lymphocyte surface markers and flow cytometric analysis (92). These authors noted a poor survival in patients with either an absolute decrease in peripheral blood CD8+ (cytotoxic/suppressor) lymphocytes, or a relative decrease in CD8+ lymphocytes with an increased CD4+ (helper T-cell)/CD8+ratio. Results of this study maintained their significance in a multivariate analysis which included standard clinical staging parameters. Strome et al. noted similar results; in their study patients with diminished CD4+/CD8+ ratios were more likely to remain disease free than those with increased ratios (83). These authors also noted high CD4+/CD8+ ratios in patients whose primary disease was located in the pharynx as compared to the oral cavity or larynx. Conflicting results have been published by Schuller et al. who determined that CD4+/CD8+ ratios do not have prognostic value (77).

Lymphokine production has also been evaluated as a prognostic factor for patients with head and neck cancer. Wolf et al. quantitated lymphokine production using a migration inhibition assay (89). In this assay peripheral blood leukocytes are mixed with agarose and placed in the center of flat-bottomed microtiter wells. The cells are then cultured for 18 hours with and without PHA stimulation. After incubation, areas of migration in each well are viewed and measured. The percent migration inhibition in response to PHA is calculated in relationship to inhibition with media alone; and a range of values can be established for the normal population. Wolf and associates noted that certain patients had lymphocytes which did not inhibit migration when stimulated with PHA, a distinctly abnormal result. Furthermore, the patients whose lymphocytes demonstrated impaired migration inhibition were more often those with pharyngeal but not laryngeal cancer and also were those with an elevated C4+/C8+ ratio, a characteristic typically associated with a worse prognosis (92).

Somewhat different conclusions regarding lymphokine production in patients with head and neck cancer were noted in studies of interleukin-2 (IL-2). Hargett et al. measured the IL-2 producing capacity of lymphocytes from head and neck cancer patients (24). In their study, peripheral blood lymphocytes were exposed in vitro for 6 hours to the mitogen, PHA. Supernatant was then harvested and evaluated for its capacity to support the growth of mouse CT6 cells. The growth of this cell line can be converted to units of IL-2, i.e. that dilution of supernatant that produced 50% of the maximum response produced by reference material. A wide range of lymphocyte IL-2 production was noted in 67 evaluated patients, with no relationship apparent between IL-2 produc-

tion and stage of disease. It should be noted however, that the IL-2 bioassay is imprecise.

Huang et al. (28) similarly studied IL-2 production by lymphocytes in 64 patients with head and neck cancer. In this study, a broad range in the expression of IL-2 was also noted, but collated results were not appreciably different than healthy controls. Interestingly, those cancer patients whose lymphocytes produced the highest levels of IL-2 had a shortened disease-free survival compared to others (28). The reason for this anomalous result is unclear. Huang and colleagues proposed that high levels of IL-2 production reflected more intense stimulation of the immune system by abundant tumor associated antigens. In theory, the more extensive a patient's disease is, the higher their level of tumor associated antigens, and the greater the stimulation of their immune response. For studies of lymphokine production as for other measures of immune response such as skin test reactivity and lymphocyte quantitation, the heterogeneity of test results bring to question the biological and clinical significance of the assays used.

Humoral Immunity

Quantitative measures of humoral immunity have also been analyzed for their prognostic value. Perhaps the most studied parameter of this type is a patient's quantitative IgA level (4, 34, 74, 76). Brown et al. first noted that patients with head and neck cancer as well as those with cancers of the skin, intestinal tract, lung, and uterus had elevated IgA levels (4). Results from additional studies of patients with cancer revealed that the hypergammaglobulinemia is not confined to IgA. Lesser degrees of elevation have been noted for IgG, IgM, and IgE (34, 76).

The biological association between mediators of humoral immunity and cancer has not been fully established. However, there is evidence to suggest that elevated levels of immunoglobulins, principally IgA, have a detrimental effect on host−tumor interaction and therefore promote tumor progression. IgA, in contrast to IgG or IgM is incapable of binding tissue-damaging complement or mediating tumor lysis in conjunction with cellular effector mechanisms, and may thus function as a blocking agent (51).

For patients with head and neck cancer, elevated immunoglobulins, principally IgA, portend a worse prognosis (34, 74). Katz studied 243 untreated patients and noted that 13 of 16 with levels of IgA above 600 µg/dl eventually succumbed to their disease (34).

In contrast, only 50% of patients with IgA levels below 600 µg/dL died. This difference in death risk was statistically significant before and after adjustment for standard staging parameters in a multivariate analysis. A subsequent report from Schantz and colleagues confirmed Katz's observations (74). The assay for IgA, in contrast to other immunologic assays, has been standardized and results from different institutions can be readily compared. The principal limitation of IgA quantitation is that it provides prognostic information only for a small subset of patients, since only a markedly elevated IgA level has prognostic value.

Given the growing list of immune assays that correlate with prognosis in head and neck cancer, the relative independence of these assays must be questioned. For example, patients with head and neck cancer and an elevated IgA may have a diminished lymphocyte blastogenesis upon exposure to mitogens, altered skin test reactivity, or impaired natural immune function. Multiparameter studies of immune function are required to determine the relative independence of the various immune assays.

Unfortunately, relatively few such studies have been performed. In one study by Schantz and associates, various measures of cellular and humoral immunity were examined in 73 patients with head and neck cancer (74). Individual test results were correlated with each other as well as with disease extent and patient outcome. As expected, each of the parameters assayed, including the IgA level, NK cell activity, total lymphocyte count, and lymphocyte subsets, individually correlated with prognosis. Upon comparison with one another, however, several important observations were made. For example, no significant relationship was found between a patient's peripheral blood NK cell activity and their IgA level. However, a patient's IgA level was correlated with their lymphocyte blastogenesis response to PHA ($p < 0.005$), ConA ($p = 0.05$) and PWM ($p = 0.10$). As the IgA level increased, so did the lymphocytic response to mitogens. The latter result was not expected given previous results associating an improved survival with an enhanced mitogen response, and a decreased survival with elevated IgA levels.

In the aforementioned study, Schantz and colleagues also found no relationship between the level of IgA and the absolute lymphocyte count. The absolute lymphocyte count and lymphocytic blastogenesis response were, however, inversely related, i. e. as the absolute number of peripheral blood lymphocytes increased, the patient's blastogenesis response increased. The latter results similarly appear contrary to previous studies which individually associated a poor prognosis with decreased peripheral blood lymphocytes and a diminished blastogenesis response.

It is clear that abnormal results from one immune assay do not necessarily imply parallel abnormalities in all immune parameters within that same patient. No two parameters provide the same information regarding how, when, or with what likelihood a patient's disease will recur. The heterogeneity and limitations of the biological determinants of disease progression within the patient with head and neck cancer is again emphasized.

The clinical value of immune monitoring may be greater if the tests are combined with each other than when they are used individually. Schantz et al. addressed this question in their study of IgA and natural immune mediated cytotoxicity (74). As previously mentioned, Schantz and associates found no correlation between IgA levels and NK cell function in patients with head and neck cancer yet both parameters were individually correlated with prognosis. In this study, IgA was predictive of disease recurrence but failed to provide information as to where that disease was likely to recur. In contrast, patients with deficient NK cell function were significantly more likely to die with progressive metastatic disease, both regional and distant. Patients with elevated natural immune function died less frequently. When that death occurred in the latter group, however, it most often occurred due to uncontrolled local disease.

Table 7.**1** demonstrates results from combining IgA levels and NK cell cytotoxicity as published by Schantz et al. (74). This table records the recurrence

Table 7.1 **Patients with elevated IgA: patterns of recurrence defined by natural killer (NK) cell cytotoxicity***[+]

NK cell cytotoxicity	Total patients	Patients with recurrence	Sites of recurrence		
			Local	Regional	Distant
≤ 60 LU[+]	12	7	2	2	6
> 60 LU	7	4	4	2	1

* As previously published (74)

[+] These 19 patients represent a sub-group of 55 untreated patients with head and neck cancer in whom IgA and NK cell activity had been assessed prior to treatment. The 19 patients had IgA levels > 255 mg/dL and represented the population with the highest incidence of death due to disease.

[+] LU, lytic unit.

patterns of patients with high IgA levels. After stratification by NK cell function, the relative risk of developing recurrent disease is noted to be similar, but the pattern of recurrence is different. Within the subgroup of patients with high IgA levels, low NK cytotoxicity was associated local recurrence while high NK cell cytotoxicity was associated with relapse at distant sites. Combining IgA level and NK cell cytotoxicity provided more information regarding failure than either parameter alone. This observation suggests that these immune parameters reflect distinct aspects of the host—tumor interaction.

Studies of Tumor-infiltrating Lymphocytes

Attention has recently been focused on lymphocytes which infiltrate solid tumors as opposed to those which circulate in peripheral blood. In murine studies, tumor-infiltrating lymphocytes (TIL) were found to be more 50 to 100 times more active in eliminating established tumors than lymphokine-activated killer cells isolated from spleen (63). Furthermore, TIL expanded ex vivo demonstrated autologous specific tumor reactivity. These cells were thus able to mediate significant antitumor effects in vivo without concomitantly administered IL-2. They were also effective against relatively large tumor burdens (62).

Studies of TIL from human solid tumors reveal significant heterogeneity in their composition of lymphocytes. Itoh and colleagues demonstrated that the majority of cytotoxic lymphocytes generated from melanoma biopsies after IL-2 activation were CD3+, CD8+ and CD16− autologous specific cytotoxic T-lymphocytes. The latter cells recognized undefined melanoma target antigens by a mechanism which involved the T-cell receptor and classical MHC-restricted cytotoxicity (32). In contrast, similar studies of TIL from renal cell carcinoma biopsy specimens demonstrated that cytotoxicity was mediated by both CD3+ and CD3− cells, and was not MHC-restricted. The majority of TIL found in head and neck squamous carcinomas are CD3+ T-lymphocytes, as demonstrated both by immunohistochemical (91) and cytofluorometric techniques (25). Cultures from different patients yield different proportions of CD4+ and CD8+ (25).

As with TIL from other tumors, lymphocytes isolated de novo from head and neck cancers exhibit little functional activity, respond poorly to mitogens, and exhibit little or no antitumor cytotoxicity (42). Following in vitro culture with high concentrations of IL-2 (1000 units/mL), however, large numbers of TIL exhibiting non-MHC restricted cytotoxicity can be obtained (25, 88). Heo, Whiteside, and colleagues have shown that both CD3+ Leu 19+ and CD3− cells mediate this cytotoxicity (25, 88).

To date there have been no detailed studies confirming the existence of autologous tumor-specific MHC-restricted T cell cytotoxicity in head and neck cancer. Ongoing studies of TIL from patients with head and neck cancer seek to define the lymphocyte populations present, the spectrum of cell surface antigens recognized by these cells, and the extent to which the activity of these cells is influenced by local inhibitory factors such as transforming growth factor beta, or other tumor-secreted immunosuppressive molecules. These studies will be greatly facilitated by the development of permanent cell lines established from individual patients with head and neck cancer (26, 67).

Immunobiological Approaches to Head and Neck Cancer Therapy

Despite the aforementioned data which suggest immunological defects in patients with head and neck cancer, the early trials of immunotherapy for patients with head and neck cancer were disappointing. These studies used nonspecific immunoadjuvants such as BCG (Bacille Calmette—Guérin), Corynebacterium parvum, and levamisole. The negative results observed may be attributed to the poor immunogenicity of these tumors, the immunosuppressed state of many patients, the relatively large tumor burden that was often present, and to the nonspecific and relatively ineffective therapeutic agents used. In addition, clinical benefit may not be apparent in the overall results if that benefit existed only for a limited subset of patients.

Interest in immunotherapy for patients with head and neck cancer has been rekindled by an improved understanding of the immunobiology of these tumors as well as by the availability of new treatment approaches. Recombinant cytokines have recently been evaluated in several clinical trials of patients with head and neck cancer. Some cytokines, like the interferons, have direct antitumor effects as well as immunomodulating properties. Others, like IL-2, have no direct effects on tumors but rather exert their antitumor effects exclusively through by immunomodulation.

The results of initial trials utilizing these agents are summarized as follows. These studies, however, must be reviewed with the knowledge that our understanding of the immunobiology of head and neck cancer and immunotherapy remains limited. Although numerous potential effector cells have been described, the biology of their regulation and cellular interactions is incompletely understood as is their role in the control of tumor progression. The biology of individual cytokines as well as their optimal therapeutic dose and administration schedule need further clarification. These concerns, however, are now evaluable with current technology.

Interferons Alpha and Beta

Interferons alpha and beta belong to a group of proteins that were initially recognized for their antiviral properties, but are now known to possess a spectrum of biological activity. While distinct proteins, they are classified as Type I interferons as they bind to a common receptor and share immunological cross-reactivity as well as biological activity (56). These interferons have direct effects on tumor cell surface antigens including the induction of expression of Class I major histocompatibility antigens. They also have potent antiproliferative effects owing to the inhibition of protein synthesis by the interferon-induced enzyme $2'5'$-oligoadenylate synthetase and to the direct inhibition of the expression of growth-related proteins encoded by oncogenes (66).

A series of interferon-inducible genes has recently been recognized. Understanding the nature and function of these genes will help define the mechanisms of interferon-mediated antitumor activity as well as mechnisms of resistance to interferon (36). The homozygous deletion of Type I interferon genes has recently been described for a number of malignant cell lines. This finding suggests that in the normal cell these genes may functionally behave as tumor suppressor genes, and that the loss of the gene products might be one factor associated with tumor progression (15).

Due to these antiproliferative and immunomodulating activities, interferon alpha has been widely studied in therapeutic trials. The cytokine has single agent activity in a wide range of hematopoietic malignancies and solid tumors including, apparently, some activity in squamous cell carcinomas of the head and neck (82). Ikic and colleagues described the shrinkage of head and neck cancers following direct infiltration of crude leukocyte interferon into the tumor itself, or into the area surrounding tumor (29). These workers subsequently reported similar results utilizing recombinant interferon alpha (30). Medenica and Slack treated patients with 6×10^6 units/m^2 of leukocyte interferon intramuscularly three times a week (41). They reported 3 complete and 4 partial responses in 12 evaluable patients with advanced head and neck squamous carcinomas. Of the 3 patients who achieved a complete response, all had been previously treated with chemotherapy and radiotherapy, 2 had undifferentiated carcinomas, and the third a moderately differentiated squamous cell carcinoma. The durations of the complete responses ranged from 4 to 19 months. Fierro et al. using a regimen similar to that of Medenica and Slack, recorded only 1 partial response and 2 stable diseases in 13 treated patients (21). In addition, Miyake et al. were unable to demonstrate any objective responses in a group of patients with head and neck cancer treated with recombinant interferon alpha-2 (44). Cumulatively, this experience would suggest that single-agent recombinant interferon alpha has only modest activity in advanced squamous cell carcinoma of the head and neck. Similarly, Connors described only 2 partial responses in 13 patients with nasopharyngeal carcinoma treated with leukocyte interferon (11).

That interferon alpha can have significant activity against squamous cell carcinomas is apparent in studies of combination therapy for patients with refractory skin cancer. As reported in later in this chapter by Lippman and Hong (Differentiation Agents), the combination of interferon alpha and 13-cis retinoic acid led to 6 (27%) and 10 (46%) partial responses in 22 patients with this disease (38). Whether or not the activity of this and related combinations with interferon alpha will be reproduced in patients with head and neck cancer remains a question for future study.

Interferon Gamma

Interferon gamma is a protein quite distinct from either of the Type I interferons and is categorized as a Type II interferon (56). It is produced by activated T-lymphocytes, and binds to a specific cell surface receptor. This cytokine has a wider range of immunobiological activity than alpha interferon in addition to its antiviral activity. It activates monocytes and macrophages, upregulates Fc receptors, and increases superoxide production, phagocytosis and killing of intracellular organisms, and in vitro killing of tumor cells (86). Other immunobiological effects include enhancement of NK-cell cytotoxicity, and effects on B-cell immunoglobulin production. In addition, interferon gamma will directly inhibit the growth of some tumor cells in vitro, and causes upregulation of both class I and class II major histocompatibility antigens in tumor cells. The immunomodulatory effects of gamma interferon are dose dependent with very low and very high doses being less immunologically active (40).

Chang et al. demonstrated inhibition of proliferation and differentiation−induction as well es direct cytotoxic effects for interferon gamma in the squamous carcinoma line A431 (7). Richtsmeier studied this cytotoxic effect in detail using a variety of cell lines derived from head and neck carcinomas, and noted optimal results with 24 hours of exposure to interferon gamma at 30 μ/mL or greater (60). Similar direct antitumor effects were not observed with interferon alpha. Moreover, neither additive or synergistic effects were apparent with the combination of alpha and gamma interferons.

The initial attempts to translate these observations to the clinic have been disappointing as no significant antitumor activity was noted in the phase I clinical trials of interferon gamma in patients with squamous cell carcinomas of head and neck (61).

Similarly, interferon gamma was inactive, at doses of $5-10 \times 10^6$ μ/m² administered intramuscularly daily in 14 patients with advanced nasopharyngeal carcinoma (16).

Interleukin-2

IL-2 is a small glycoprotein product of activated lymphocytes which reacts with a specific cell surface receptor on lymphocytes, leading to cellular activation and proliferation. Lymphocyte populations that respond to IL-2 include both T-lymphocytes and natural killer (NK) cells. IL-2 activation of cytotoxic cells leads to the appearance of "lymphokine activated killing" (LAK cell activity), which includes a heterogeneous population of nonantigenic specific cytotoxic effector cells, including activated NK cells and CD3+ non-MHC-restricted cytotoxic lymphocytes. Proliferation of these cells and other antigenic specific activated T-cells can occur. These activated lymphocytes produce a broad range of secondary cytokines including interferon gamma, tumor necrosis factor, and interleukin-6. The wide spectrum of biological consequences of IL-2 action suggest that its antitumor mechanisms are complex, and that toxicity due to IL-2 is largely secondary to induced cytokines (55).

Due to its widespread immunomodulatory effects, IL-2 has been tested extensively in preclinical tumor models as well as in clinical trials in man (55). Principles which have emerged from preclinical models include the fact that IL-2 is active as a single agent in a dose and schedule dependent manner (62), and that the antitumor activity of IL-2 can be enhanced significantly by the addition of other cytokines, such as interferon alpha or tumor necrosis factor, or the coadministration of ex vivo activated and expanded LAK cells or TIL. The effectiveness of therapy with IL-2 is further affected by a variety of factors, including host's immune status, the immunogenicity of the tumor, and the total amount of tumor present at the time of therapy (62).

Based on these principles, IL-2 has been applied to clinical trials of human malignancy (55). Significant antitumor activity has been consistently noted in a minority of patients with melanoma and renal cell cancer. In addition, individual responses have been noted in patients with other solid tumors, including lung and breast carcinoma. The cardiopulmonary toxicity of systemic IL-2 has precluded the treatment of many patients with head and neck carcinoma. Clinical trials using a less toxic IL-2 regimen that includes continuous infusion IL-2 and concomitant interferon alpha have recently been initiated in patients with advanced head and neck cancer.

In an attempt to obtain IL-2 immunostimulatory effects with decreased systemic toxicity, others have administered IL-2 by locoregional injections or delivered IL-2 in association with adoptive cellular therapy. There is abundant rationale for the locoregional administration of interleukin-2 in patients with refractory locoregional disease due to head and neck carcinomas (64). For example in the rat, low doses of IL-2 administered in the region of tumor growth result in local lymphocyte activation and enhanced antitumor activity (45). Cortesina and colleagues have treated head and neck cancer patients with perilymphatic injections of IL-2 in low dose (12). Patients with regional recurrence were injected with 2000 units of IL-2 daily for 10 days at multiple sites around the regional draining lymph nodes. The very low doses of IL-2 used in this approach were not associated with the typical systemic side effects associated with IL-2 therapy. However, local swelling and lymph node pain did occur. Patients later received 10 daily injections of nonrecombinant IL-2 near the insertion of the sternocleidomastoid muscle. Of 10 patients treated in this manner, 3 complete and 3 partial responses lasting several months were observed (22). Remarkably, some responses were noted in involved contralateral lymph nodes. Nonresponding patients included those who had previously undergone radical lymph node dissection or who had a poor performance status at the time of therapy. Confirmatory trials using this approach are now under way.

IL-2 has also been utilized in trials of adoptive immunotherapy in head and neck cancer. Ishikawa and associates have treated 6 patients (5 maxillary and 1 lingual squamous carcinomas) with adoptive immunotherapy (31). In this study, all patients were previously untreated and had T3 or greater primary lesions. Two patients had cervical metastases. From these patients, peripheral blood lymphocytes were isolated, treated with mitomycin-C, and co-cultured ex vivo for 5 to 15 days with autologous or allogeneic tumor cells alone and with recombinant IL-2. These cultured autologous lymphocytes were then administered to patients by direct arterial infusion of 1.5 to 8 $\times 10^8$ cells into the superficial temporal artery at the bifurcation of the maxillary artery, or, in a single case, by direct catheterization of the lingual artery. Patients received from four to fifteen infusions with up to 9.9×10^9 total cells infused. In addition, 500 units of IL-2 (Takeda Pharmaceuticals) were delivered by bolus infusion twice daily throughout the period of administration of cultured autologous lymphocytes. Side effects of this therapy included mild temperature elevation, and in 1 patient, cheek pain at the time of regional infusion. All 6 patients were noted to have a significant reduction in tumor size. In those patients who subsequently underwent surgical resection, tumor necrosis with lymphocyte and macrophage infiltration was apparent on histologic examination. The nature of the lymphocyte cytotoxicity generated ex vivo was not described in this report.

These provocative results suggest that further studies of IL-2 together with adoptive immunotherapy are indicated in patients with head and neck cancer.

Plasmapheresis

A wide range of potentially immunosuppressive factors have been described in the blood of patients with head and neck cancer as well as other solid tumors. These factors include antigen–antibody complexes, acute phase reactants, and less well defined soluble immunosuppressive proteins. Therapeutic strategies employed to remove these factors have included plasma exchange by plasmapheresis and extracorporeal immunoadsorption of immune complexes from plasma with *Staphylococcus* protein A (54).

To date, no studies using extracorporeal immunoadsorption have been reported in patients with head and neck cancer. However, objective tumor regressions in patients with head and neck cancer have been reported following plasma exchange (35, 79). When it occurred, clinical response was associated with pain, pruritus, and erythema at the tumor site, either during or soon after the plasma exchange. In those who responded, pretreatment IgA levels were elevated, and with therapy, IgA levels decreased, serum IgE level increased, and in vitro lymphocyte functions were partially restored. This limited experience suggests that therapeutic removal of immunosuppressive substances may be a useful adjunct to future trials of immunostimulatory therapies.

Conclusion

The studies described in this chapter reveal the biological heterogeneity of patients with head and neck cancer, the limitations of immunologically evaluating patients with this disease, and the difficulty therefore of developing rational immunologic treatments. This biological heterogeneity, when improperly controlled for in the design, conduct, or interpretation of clinical studies frequently contributes to conclusions that are falsely positive or falsely negative. While studies have been performed that are properly controlled and evaluate an adequate number of subjects, the immunobiology literature of head and neck cancer frequently records conclusions which are drawn from the analysis of an insufficient number of patients. In this setting, results from different studies are frequently in conflict and unchallenged generalizations on the immunobiology of head and neck cancer are few in number.

Despite this heterogeneity, various patient subgroups have been associated with a high or low probability of disease control and prolonged survival after conventional treatment. Such correlations, whether positive or negative, are crucial to our understanding of the immunobiology of head and neck cancer, the design of future studies and the eventual selection of specific therapies for specific patients. For example, establishing that deficits in peripheral blood natural immune function are correlated with death from disease in untreated patients is a fundamentally important positive conclusion. That natural immune function does not predict local disease progression, the prognosis of patients with well-differentiated cancers, or disease progression in those whose cancers lack intrinsic metastatic potential is an equally important negative observation.

The studies described in this chapter also provide evidence that objective responses to immunobiologic therapy can be achieved in individual patients with single-agent as well as combination cytokine therapy. While such responses are encouraging, they are relatively infrequent and an improved understanding of the mechanisms of response and resistance to biological therapies is necessary prior to the creation of optimal treatment strategies. Furthermore, given the heterogeneity of head and neck cancer, the use of any single biologic agent or the adoptive transfer of any single type of cellular effector mechanism is unlikely to be successful in all patients. Rather, in those limited circumstances in which an antitumor effect has been identified it will be important to define that individual both immunologically as well as clinically. Defining biological groups with different prognoses to immunologic treatment would lead to more effective clinical trials, and facilitate the rapid development of successful therapies. In addition, patients who are unlikely to respond to biologic agents will be spared the morbidity of an inactive therapy. An increased understanding of the immunobiology of squamous carcinomas, and further definition of the immunologic status of individual patients will provide the necessary background for continued advances in the biological treatment of head and neck cancer.

References

1. Abo T, Balch CM. A differentiation antigen of human NK and K cells identified by a monoclonal antibody (NHK 1). J. Immunol, 1981; 127:1024–29.
2. Bates SE, Suen JY, Tranum BL. Immunologic skin testing and interpretation. A plea for uniformity. Cancer 1979; 43:2306–13.
3. Bosworth JL, Thaler S, Ghossein NA. Delayed hypersensitivity and local control of patients treated by radiotherapy for head and neck cancer. Am J Surg 1976; 132:46–8.
4. Brown AM, Lally ET, Frankel A, Harwick R, Davis LW, Rominger CJ. The association of the IgA levels of serum and whole saliva with the progression of oral cancer. Cancer 1975; 35:1154–62.
5. Catalona WJ, Taylor PT, Rabson AS, Chretien PB. A method for dinitrochlorobenzene contact sensitization–clinicopathologic study. N Engl J Med 1972; 286:399–402.
6. Catalona WJ, Sample WF, Chretien PB. Lymphocyte reactivity in cancer patients: Correlation with tumor histology and clinical stage. Cancer 1973; 31:65–71.

7. Chang EH, Ridge J, Black R. Interferon-gamma induces altered oncogene expression and terminal differentiation in A431 cels. Proc Soc Biol Med 1987; 186:319−26.

8. Check I, Hunter R, Lounsbury B, Rosenberg K, Matz G. Prediction of survival in head and neck cancer based on leukocyte sedimentation in Focoll–hypaque gradients. Laryngoscope 1980; 90:1281−90.

9. Chretien PB, Catalona WJ, Twomey PL, Sample F. Correlation of immune reactivity and clinical status in cancer. Ann Clin Lab Sci 1974; 4:331−39.

10. Chretien PB. Unique immunobiological aspects of head and neck squamous carcinoma. Can J Otolaryngol 1975; 4:222−35.

11. Connors JM, Andiman WA, Howarth CB, et al. Treatment of nasopharyngeal carcinoma with human leucocyte interferon. J Clin Oncol 1985; 3:813−17.

12. Cortesina G, DeStefani A, Giovarelli M, et al. Treatment of recurrent squamous cell carcinoma of the head and neck with low doses of interleukin-2 injected perilymphatically. Cancer 1988; 62:2482−5.

13. Croce LM, Nowell PC. Molecular basis of human B cell neoplasia. Blood 1985; 65:1−7.

14. deVillers EM, Weidauer H, Oho H, zurHausen H. Papillomavirus DNA in human tongue carcinomas. Int J Cancer 1985; 36:575−8.

15. Diaz MO, Ziemin S, LeBeau MM. Homozygous deletion of the alpha- and beta-interferon genes in human leukemia and derived cell lines. Proc Natl Acad Sci USA 1988; 85:5259−63.

16. Dimery IW, Jacobs C, Tseng A Jr, et al. Recombinant interferon-alpha in the treatment of recurrent nasopharyngeal carcinoma. J Biol Response Mod 1989; 8:221−6.

17. Eastham JR, Mason JM, Jennings BR, Belew PW, Maguda TA. T-cell rosette test in squamous cell carcinoma of the head and neck. Arch Otolaryngol 1976; 102:171−5.

18. Eilber FR, Morton DL. Impaired immunologic reactivity and recurrence following cancer surgery. Cancer 1970; 25:362−7.

19. Eilber FR, Morton DL, Ketcham AS. Immunologic abnormalities in head and neck cancer. Am J Surg 1974; 128:534−8.

20. Estaban F, Concha A, Huelin C, et al. Histocompatibility antigens in primary and metastatic squamous carcinoma of the larynx. Int J Cancer 1989; 43:436−42.

21. Fierro R, Johnson J, Myers E, et al. Phase II trial of non-recombinant interferon alpha in recurrent squamous cell carcinoma of the head and neck. Proc. Am Soc Clin Oncol 1988; 29:156.

22. Forni G, Cavallo GP, Giovarelli M, et al. Tumor immunotherapy by local injection of interleukin-2 and non-reactive lymphocytes. Prog Exp Tumor Res 1989; 32:187−212.

23. Gilbert HA, Kagan AR, Miles J, et al. The usefulness of pretreatment DNCB in 85 patients with squamous cell carcinoma of the upper aerodigestive tract. J Surg Oncol 1978; 10:73−7.

24. Hargett S, Wanebo HJ, Pace R. Interleukin-2 production in head and neck cancer patients. Am J Surg 1985; 150:456−60.

25. Heo DS, Whiteside TL, Johnson JT, Chen K, Barnes EL, Herberman RB. Long term interleukin-2 dependent growth and cytotoxic activity of tumor infiltrating lymphocytes from human squamous cell carcinomas of the head and neck. Cancer Res 1987; 47:6353−62.

26. Heo DS, Snyderman C, Gollin SM, et al. Biology, cytogenetics and sensitivity to immunobiological effector cells of new head and neck squamous cell carcinoma lines. Cancer Res 1989; 49:5167−75.

27. Hollingshead AC, Lee O, Chretien PB. Antibodies to herpes virus–nonvirus antigens in squamous carcinoma. Cancer 1976; 37:135−42.

28. Huang HT, Mold NG, Fisher SR, et al. A prospective study of squamous head and neck carcinoma: immunologic aberrations in patients who develop recurrent disease. Cancer 1987; 59:1721−26.

29. Ikic D, Padovan I, Brodarec I, Knezevic M, Soos E. Application of human leucocyte interferon inpatients with tumors of the head and neck. Lancet 1981; 1:1025−7.

30. Ikic D, Padovan I, Knezevic M, Pipic N. Subtumoural and intratumoural application of human leucocyte natural interferon and recombinant HuIFN alpha 2 in patients with cancers of the head and neck. J Interferon Res 1988; 8 (suppl 1):117.

31. Ishikawa T, Ikawa T, Eura M, Fukiage T, Masuyama K. Adoptive, immunotherapy of head and neck cancer with killer cells induced by stimulation with autologous or allogeneic tumor cells and recombinant interleukin-2. Acta Otolaryngol (Stockh) 1989; 107:346−51.

32. Itoh K, Platsoucas CD, Balch CM. Autologous tumor-specific cytotoxic T-lymphocytes in the infiltrate of human metastatic melanomas. J Exp Med 1988; 168:1419−41.

33. Karre K, Ljungren HG, Piontek G, Kiessling R. Selective rejection of H-2 deficient lymphoma variants suggest alternative immune defense strategy. Nature 1986; 319:675−8.

34. Katz AE. Immunobiologic staging of patients with carcinoma of the head and neck. Laryngoscope 1983; 93:445−63.

35. Katz AE, Seder RH, Keggins JJ, et al. Plasmapheresis in patients with advanced carcinoma of the head and neck pp 151−156. In: Head and Neck Oncology Research, Proceedings of the second International Head and Neck. Oncology Research Conference. 1988 Kugler Publication Amsterdam − Berkley/Ghedini Editore − Milano.

36. Kessler DS, Levy DE, Darnell JE Jr. Two intereron-induced nuclear factors bind a single promoter element in interferon-stimulated genes. Proc Natl Acad Aci USA 1988; 85:8521−5.

37. Lichtenstein A, Zighelborim J, Dorey F.Brossman S, Fahey JL. Comparison of immune derangements in patients with different malignancies. Cancer 1980; 45:2090−5.

38. Lippman SM, Parkinson DR, Weber RS, Schantz SP, Gutterman JU, Hong WK. Isotretinoin plus alpha-interferon: effective therapy of advanced squamous cell carcinoma of the skin (abstr #650). Proc Am Soc Clin Oncol 1991; 10:197.

39. Maisel RH, Ogura JH. Abnormal dinitrochlorobenzene skin sensitization in head and neck squamous cell carcinoma. Laryngoscope 1973; 83:2012−19.

40. Maluish AE, Urba WJ, Longo DL, et al. The determination of an immunologically active dose of interferon-gamma in patients with melanoma. J Clin Oncol 1988; 6:434−45.

41. Medenica R, Slack N. Clinical results of leukocyte interferon-induced tumor regression in resistant human metastatic cancer resistant to chemotherapy and/or radiotherapy–pulse therapy schedule. Cancer Drug Deliv 1985; 2:53−75.

42. Miescher S, Whiteside TL, Carrel S, von Fliedner V. Functional properties of tumor infiltrating and blood lymphocytes in patients with solid tumors: effects of tumor cells and their supernatants on proliferative responses of lymphocytes. J Immunol 1986; 13:1899−1907.

43. Mickel RA, Kessler DJ, Taylor JMG, Lichtenstein A. Natural killer cell cytotoxicity in the peripheral blood, cervical lymph nodes, and tumor of head and neck cancer patients. Cancer Res 1988; 48:5017−22.

44. Miyake H, Horiuchi M, Togowa K, et al. Recombinant interferon alpha 2 in patients with head and neck cancer. Gan To Kagaku Ryoho 1985; 12:1651−5.

45. Morikawa K, Okada F, Hosokawa M, Kobayashi H. Enhancement of therapeutic effects of recombinant interleukin-2 on a transplantable rat fibrosarcoma by the use of a sustained release vehicle, pluronic gel. Cancer Res 1987; 47:37.

46. Muschel RJ, Williams JE, Lowry DR, Liotta LA. Harvey ras induction of metastatic potential depends upon oncogene activation and the type of recipient cell. Am J Pathol 1985; 121:1−8.

47. Nicolson G, Milas L, eds. Cancer invasion and metastasis. Biologic and therapeutic aspects. New York: Raven press, 1984.

48. Nowell PC. Mechanisms of tumor progression. Cancer Res 1986; 46:2203−7.

49. Olivari A, Pradier R, Feierstein J, Guardo A, Glait H, Rojas A. Cell-mediated immune response in head and neck cancer patients. J Surg Oncol 1976; 8:287−94.

50. Olkowski ZL, Wilkins SA. T-lymphocyte levels in the peripheral blood of patients with cancer of the head and neck. Am J Surg 1975; 130:440−4.

51. O'Neill PA, Romsdahl MM. IgA as a blocking factor in human malignant melanoma. Immunol Commun 1974; 3:427−38.

52. Papenhausen PR, Kirkwa A, Croft CB, Browiecki B, Silver C. Emerson EE. Cellular immunity in patients with epidermoid cancer of the head and neck. Laryngoscope 1979; 89:538−49.

53. Stefani SS, Kerman RH. Lymphocyte response to phytohaemagglutinin before and after radiation therapy in patients with carcinomas of the head and neck. J Laryngol Otol 1977; 91:605−9.

54. Parkinson DR. The status of plasma therapy as cancer treatment. J Clin Oncol 1988; 6:189-90.

55. Parkinson DR. Interleukin-2 in cancer therapy. Semin Oncol 1988; 15 (suppl 6):10−26.

56. Pestka S, Langer JA, Zoon KC, Samuel CE. Interferons and their actions. Annu Rev Biochem 1987; 56:727−77.

57. Poste G, Doll J, Fidler IJ. Interactions between clonal subpopulations affect the stability of the metastatic phenotype in polyclonal populations of B16 melanoma cells. Proc Natl Acad Sci USA 1981; 78:6226−30.

58. Potvin C, Tarpley JL, Chretien PB. Thymus-dervied lymphocytes in patients with solid malignancies. Clin Immunol Immunopathol 1975; 3:476−82.

59. Prehn RT. Relationship of tumor immunogenicity to concentration of the oncogen. J Natl Cancer Inst 1975; 55:189−90.

60. Richtsmeier WJ. Interferon gamma induced oncolysis: an effect on head and neck squamous carcinoma cultures. Arch Otolaryngol Head Neck Surg 1988; 114:432−7.

61. Richtsmeier WJ, Koch WM, McGuire WP, Poole ME, Chang EH. A phase I/II study of advanced squamous cell carcinoma patients treated with recombinant human interferon gamma. Arch Otolaryngol Head Neck Surg 1990; 116:1271−7.

62. Rosenberg SA. Adoptive immunotherapy of cancer using lymphokine-activated killer cells and recombinant IL-2. In: DeVita VT Jr, Hellman S, Rosenberg SA, eds. Important advances in Oncology. Philadelphia: Lippincott, 1986:55−91.

63. Rosenberg SA, Spiess P, Lafreniere R. A new approach to the adoptive immunotherapy of cancer with tumor-infiltrating lymphocytes. Science 1986; 233:1318−21.

64. Roth AD, Kirkwood JM. New clinical trials with interleukin-2: rationale for regional administration. Nat Immun Cell Growth Regul 1989; 8:153−64.

65. Rowley JD. Ph-positive leukemia, including chronic myelogenous leukemia. Clin Haematol 1980; 9:55−86.

66. Rutherford NM, Marrigan GE, Williams BRG. Interferon-induced binding of nuclear factors to promoter elements of the 2−5 A synthetase gene. EMBO J 1988; 7:751−9.

67. Sacci M, Snyderman CH, Heo DS, et al. Local adoptive immunotherapy of human head and neck cancer xenographs in nude mice with lymphokine-activated killer cells and Interleukin-2. Cancer Res 1990; 50:3113−18.

68. Sager R. Genetic instability, suppression and human cancer. In: Sacks L, ed. Gene regulation in the expression of malignancy. London: Oxford University Press, 1985.

69. Savary CA, Lotzova E. Phylogeny and ontogeny of NK cells. In: Lotzova E, Herberman RB, eds. Immunobiology of natural killer cells, vol 1. Boca Raton: CRC Press, 1986:45−63.

70. Schantz SP, Shillitoe EJ, Brown B, Campbell B. Natural killer cell activity and head and neck cancer: a clinical assessment. J Natl Cancer Inst 1986; 77:869−75.

71. Schantz SP, Brown BW, Lira E, Taylor DL, Beddingfield N. Evidence for the role of natural immunity in the control of metastatic spread of head and neck cancer. Cancer Immunol Immunother 1987; 25:141−5.

72. Schantz SP, Geopfert H. Multimodality therapy and distant metastases: the impact of natural killer cell activity. Arch Otolaryngol Head Neck Surg 1987; 113:1207−13.

73. Schantz SP, Ordonez N. Natural killer cell activity predicts metastases from poorly-differentiated head and neck cancer. Proc Am Assoc Cancer Res 1988; 29:374.

74. Schantz SP, Liu FJ, Taylor DL, Beddingfield N, Weber RS. The relationship of circulating IgA to cellular immunity of head and neck cancer patients. Laryngoscope 1988; 98:671−8.

75. Schantz SP, Hsu TC, Ainslie N, Moser RP. Young adults with head and neck cancer express increased susceptibility to mutagen-induced chromosomal damage. JAMA 1989; 262:3313−15.

76. Schantz SP, Lui FJ. An immunologic profile of young adults with head and neck cancer. Cancer 1989; 64:361−6.

77. Schuller DE, Rack RP, Rinehart JJ, Koolemans-Beynen AR. T-lymphocytes as a prognostic indicator in head and neck cancer. Arch Otolaryngol Head Neck Surg 1986; 112:938−41.

78. Scully C. The immunology of cancer of the head and neck with particular reference to oral cancer. Oral Surg Oral Med Oral Pathol 1982; 53:157−69.

79. Seder RH, Vaughn CW, Oh SK, et al. Tumor repression and temporary restoration of immune response after plasmaphersis in a patient with recurrent oral cancer. Cancer 1987; 60:318−25.

80. Shillitoe EJ, Silverman S. Oral cancer and herpes simplex virus. A review. Oral Surg Oral Med Oral Pathol 1979; 48:216−4.

81. Shtivelman E, Lifshitz B, Gale RP, Cananni E. Fused transcript of abl and bcr genes in chronic myelogenous leukemia. Nature 1985; 315:550−4.

82. Spiegel RJ. The alpha interferons: Clinical overview. Semin Oncol (suppl 2) 1987; 14:1−12.

83. Strome M, Clark JR, Fried MP, Rodliff S, Blazar BA. T-cell subsets and natural killer cell function with squamous cell carcinomas of the head and neck. Arch Otolaryngol 1987; 113:1090−3.

84. Takasugi M, Mickey MR, Terasaki PI. Decline of natural non-selective cell-mediated cytotoxicity in patients with tumor progression. Cancer Res 1973; 33:2898−2902.

85. Trinchieri G, Perussia B. Human natural killer cells: Biologic and pathologic aspects. Lab Invest 1984; 5:489−503.

86. Trinchieri G, Perussia B. Immune interferon: a pleiotropic lymphokine with multiple effects. Immunol Today 1985; 6:131−6.

87. Wanebo HJ, Jun MY, Strong EW, Oettgen H. T-cell deficiency in patients with squamous cell cancer of the head and neck. Am J Surg 1975; 130:445−51.

88. Whiteside TL, Heo DS, Takagi S, Johnson JT, Iwatsuki S, Herberman RB. Cytolytic antitumor effector cells in long term cultures of human tumor infiltrating lymphocytes in recombinant interleukin-2. Cancer Immunol Immunother 1988; 26:1−10.

89. Wolf GT, Peterson KA, Lovett EJ, Beauchamp ML, Baker SR. Lymphokine production and lymphocyte subpopulations in patients with head and neck squamous carcinoma. Arch Otolaryngol 1984; 110:731−5.

90. Wolf GT, Amendola BE, Diaz R, Lovett EJ, Hammerschmidt RM, Peterson KA. Definite vs adjuvant radiotherapy: comparative effects on lymphocyte subpopulations in patients with head and neck squamous carcinoma. Arch Otolaryngol 1985; 111:716−26.

91. Wolf GT, Hudson JL, Peterson KA, Miller HL, McClatchey KD: Lymphocyte subpopulations in infiltration squamous carcinomas of the head and neck: correlations with extent of tumor and prognosis. Otolaryngol Head Neck Surg. 1986; 95:142−51.

92. Wolf GT, Schmaltz S, Hudson J, et al. Alterations in T-lymphocyte subpopulations in patients with head and neck squamous carcinoma: correlations with prognosis. Arch Otolaryngol 1987; 113:1200−6.

93. Wustrow TP, Zenner HP. Natural killer cell activity in patients with carcinoma of the larynx and hypopharynx. Laryngoscope 1985; 95:1391−1400.

94. Wynder EL, Bross IJ, Day E. A study of environmental factors in cancer of the larynx. Cancer 1956; 9:86−110.

Differentiation Agents: A Future Direction for the Management of Upper Aerodigestive Tract Squamous Cell Carcinoma

S. M. Lippman, W. K. Hong

Introduction

Upper aerodigestive tract (UADT, i. e. head and neck) and lung epithelial malignancies are a major and increasing problem worldwide. The magnitude of the problem relates directly to the magnitude of tobacco usage, the etiology in over 80% of cases of premalignant or malignant lesions in these anatomic sites (1).

It has been estimated that worldwide in 1986, 1 billion people smoked 5 trillion cigarettes; approximately 2.5 million deaths and 65 billion dollars in health-care and lost-productivity costs that year were attributable to cigarette smoking. The number of smoking-related deaths is expected to rise to 4 million by the year 2000. Although smoking rates are declining by 1.5% per year in developed nations, they are rising by 2% per year in developing countries. In the United States, 50 million people smoke, and the Surgeon General's 1989 report estimates that nearly 400000 deaths occur annually from this habit (2).

In addition, more than 600 million people worldwide chew tobacco or tobacco-containing mixtures. In Asia, the Philippines, and the South Pacific islands, 450 million people chew betel quids (consisting of areca nut, betel leaf, tobacco, and spice). In India and Africa, 100 million people use a tobacco—lime mixture in the gingival groove, and in the Soviet Union, Iran, and Afghanistan, 20 million people use nass (a mixture of tobacco, lime, ash, and oil) under the tongue (3). Thirty million people in North America and Europe use smokeless tobacco, and the number of users is increasing (1, 4).

The National Cancer Institute's (NCI's) Surveillance, Epidemiology and End Results (SEER) program has projected over 200000 new cases of and 160000 deaths from tobacco-related UADT, esophageal, and lung neoplasms in the United States in 1992 (5). These figures correspond to over one-fifth of all new cancer cases and one-third of all cancer deaths in the United States annually. Furthermore, despite two decades of advances in screening, therapy (surgery, irradiation, and chemotherapy), and supportive care, the 5-year survival rates for head and neck, lung, and esophageal cancers have improved by only 11%, 5%, and 3%, respectively. Clearly, new approaches to the management of these disorders are needed.

This chapter focuses on the in vitro, animal, epidemiologic, and clinical data on the differentiation treatment of epithelial neoplastic processes of the UADT. As we shall discuss, several of the differentiation agents (most notably the retinoids) have been widely investigated as chemopreventive, primary, and adjuvant therapy in preclinical and clinical studies. The differentiation-agent approach assumes that premalignant and malignant lesions are reversible. Premalignant cells are the more easily "differentiated", and so the differentiation agents that have fairly low toxicity are particularly well suited for chemoprevention and adjuvant therapy in relatively healthy individuals.

Differentiation agents comprise a variety of compounds, many unrelated, that can induce neoplastic or preneoplastic cells to revert to a more mature (i. e. more differentiated, or normal) phenotype (6—9). However, this simple definition presents a problem because the complex spectrum of activities of differentiation agents overlaps the actitivity of many other anticancer agents. The dividing lines separating the major classes of anticancer agents—that is, cytotoxic, cytostatic, differentiation, and biologic- or immune-response modification—are becoming increasingly blurred as basic scientific research reveals more about the actions of these agents. Although experimental induction of differentiation has mainly been studied in hematopoietic neoplasms, such as myeloid and erythroid leukemias, work of this nature is expanding into solid-tumor studies, including those of head and neck squamous cell carcinoma (HNSCC) (6—10).

The pleiotropic nature of differentiation agents is best illustrated by several well-studied examples. Retinoids modulate both cell differentiation and immune response (11—14). Even more difficult to classify is β-carotene, which can activate the immune system (15), is cytotoxic in several experimental models, and in vivo is converted to retinol and retinoic acid (RA) and thus can perform the activities, including modulation of differentiation, associated with retinoids. Also, as illustrated by the retinoids, specific agents do not always affect the process of differentiation the same way in different types of tumors. In vitro they induce or enhance differentiation in promyelocytic leukemia, embryonal carcinoma, neuroblastoma, and murine melanoma cells and suppress or reverse the abnormal differentiation of squamous cell carcinomas (SCCs) (6, 12—14).

Thus, the definition of a differentiation agent remains somewhat arbitrary and will doubtless change. A "pure" differentiation agent has not yet been identified. This chapter will focus on retinoids, considered to be prototypical differentiation agents, since the vast majority of preclinical and clinical UADT differentiation studies involve this group of agents.

We began our chapter by discussing cancer incidences not only in the UADT but also in the lungs, and the overlap will occur throughout the chapter. The relevance derives from the concept of "field cancerization", first proposed in Slaughter et al.'s classic 1953 report on oral cancer (16). Slaughter et al. and later investigators argue that oral leukoplakia, HNSCC, and other UADT and lung premalignancies and malignancies result from a process in which the entire epithelium has been exposed to repeated carcinogenic insults (e.g. tobacco and alcohol) (17, 18). This exposure increases the likelihood that multiple, independent premalignant or malignant foci will develop in the exposed epithelium.

Biology of UADT and Lung Squamous Differentiation and Carcinogenesis

Human oral and esophageal epithelium is stratified squamous in type. The oral cavity mucosa is noncornified except for the gingival mucosa and the mucosa on the dorsal surface of the tongue, which undergo keratinization (19). The tracheal epithelium is pseudostratified and comprises columnar ciliated cells, nonciliated secretory cells, and nonsecretory basal cells. Unlike skin epithelium, the UADT and the lung epithelial tissues do not undergo squamous differentiation under normal physiologic conditions. However, they do differentiate along the squamous pathway during carcinogenesis (20). Over 90% of oral cavity tumors are SCCs (21).

The development of cancer is a multistep process, which steps are the focus of intense research and an understanding of which is prerequisite to anticipating how differentiation agents might be useful. The following overview of differentiation marker patterns in UADT and lung tissue will set the stage for our discussion of marker modulations by differentiation agents. Preclinical and clinical studies have focused on the oral cavity; hence, we shall detail the normal and carcinogenic patterns of squamous marker expression at this site.

Cytokeratins, a family of at least nineteen intermediate-size filaments that range from 40 to 68 kDa, serve as a squamous markers since they are expressed in different combinations in various human epithelial tissues, the complex pattern of expression of specific keratins apparently correlating with distinct types of epithelial differentiation (22). Major alterations in patterns of keratin expression have been documented in vitro and in vivo during vitamin A deficiency, cigarette-smoke exposure and carcinogenesis (23−31).

In the oral cavity, the normal gingival epithelium resembles epidermis in that the cells express keratins 1, 2, 5, 6, 10, 11, 13, 14, 16, and 17 (19, 32). In contrast, the alveolar mucosa contains only two major keratins, K4 and K13. The noncornifying stratified epithelium that covers the tongue, oropharynx, palatine tonsil, pharyngeal epiglottis, vocal cord, and esophagus expresses substantial amounts of keratins 4 to 6 and 13 to 15 and minor amounts of K19 (32). The high-molecular-weight (68-kDa) K1 can be a very useful squamous differentiation marker for detecting carcinogenic changes in all oral epithelia except the gingiva (where, as just noted, it occurs normally).

The presence or absence of dysplasia is the major determinant of the pattern of squamous marker expression in human premalignant oral lesions. In normal oral mucosa, high-molecular-weight (62- and 67-kDa) keratins are not detected in the basal layer. In leukoplakia without dysplasia, K1 is also absent in the hyperplastic basal cell layer but may occur in large amounts in the superficial and intermediate epithelial cell layers. In dysplastic lesions, the keratin expression pattern is distinctly different, with irregular staining of the basal cell layer for K1 reflecting the intense staining of dysplastic epithelial cells (33). The expression of keratins in human premalignant oral epithelium has also been analyzed immunohistochemically employing two polyspecific antibodies—AE1, which recognizes keratins 10, 14−16 and 19, and AE2, which recognizes keratins 1 and 10 (characteristic of keratinizing cells) (34). Fixation artifacts prevented an interpretation of results with the AE2 antibody. The results with AE1 demonstrated staining in the basal cells of normal epithelium and a shift to staining in irregular suprabasal cells of dysplastic lesions. Because these antibodies are not monospecific, it is not possible to relate the altered staining patterns to any one keratin. The only other study of keratin (K1) and other squamous marker expression in human premalignant oral lesions is part of an ongoing retinoid chemoprevention trial at our institution, reviewed under Clinical Studies below.

Gimenez-Conti et al.'s (35) preliminary results with a monospecific antibody indicated that the expression of K1 increases during 7,12-dimethylbenza(a)anthracene (DMBA)-induced oral carcinogenesis in the hamster cheek pouch in vivo. The normal hamster cheek pouch epithelium, like human buccal mucosa, does not express K1. K1 expression appears to be limited to the hyperplastic cell population in this model; most of the dysplastic and malignant areas did not express K1. These and other investigators have identified several other biomarkers in this model, including epidermal growth factor-receptor (EGF-R), ornithine decarboxylase, certain polyamines, micronuclei, transglutaminase I, γ-glutamyltranspeptidase (GGT) and filaggrin, which will enhance our basic understanding of the oral carcinogenic process and may be useful to monitor the effects of chemopreventive agents (26, 36-38).

Squamous differentiation in epidermis in vivo and in cultured keratinocytes and tracheal cells results in the synthesis of cholesterol sulfate and involucrin, a protein that undergoes extensive cross-linking by the membrane-associated (particulate) enzyme type I transglutaminase. Hence, cholesterol sulfate, involucrin, and transglutaminase I levels increase during squamous differentiation (39−42). In normal and hyperplastic oral and laryngeal epithelia, immunohistochemical staining detects involucrin and transglutaminase I only in the superficial layer; in dysplasia and SCC, staining occurs throughout the thickness of the epithelium, including the basal and suprabasal layers, although it is irregular and focal (26, 43−45).

A preliminary in vivo survey of human premalignant oral (gingival) lesions revealed an inverse relationship between immunoreactivity for transglutaminase I and the degree of dysplasia, whereas staining for involucrin was consistently strong (45). These findings indicate uncoupling of the keratinocyte programming (i. e. levels of transglutaminase I and involucrin immunoreactivity) in premalignant lesions in vivo and in the cells cultured from these lesions. An analogous uncoupling phenomenon has been reported in cultured SCC treated with RA (retinoic acid), which had a much greater inhibitory effect on transglutaminase I than on involucrin (see In Vitro Data, below). Other biologic markers investigated in human UADT carcinogenesis include DNA content, micronuclei, sister-chromatid exchange, blood group antigens, GGT, filaggrin, lectin receptors, and EGF-R (29, 38, 45−50).

In Vitro Data

Vitamin A, Retinoids and Related Agents

Vitamin A and its natural derivatives and synthetic analogues (retinoids) play a critical role in the differentiation of normal epidermis and other stratified epithelia, both in vitro and in vivo (12−14, 51). Vitamin A deficiency leads to hyperkeratosis and hyperplasia of stratified epithelia (e. g. oral mucosa) and to squamous metaplasia of secretory epithelia (e. g. tracheobronchial epithelium). Retinoid replacement reverses these phenomena (12−14, 52−55). Further, the potential importance of retinoids in UADT and lung carcinogenesis is indicated by the preclinical data showing a synergistic effect of vitamin A deficiency and cigarette-smoke exposure in inducing premalignant lesions and SCC at these sites (28, 52).

Retinoids can modulate the expression of various biochemical markers of squamous differentiation, including cornified envelope formation, keratins, type I transglutaminase, involucrin, and other cross-linked envelope proteins (23, 24, 45, 56−62). Retinoids (e. g. retinyl acetate and RA) were found to inhibit envelope competence and cross-linking in normal keratinocytes, especially when the cells were cultured in vitamin A-deficient medium (63, 64). RA completely blocked cornified envelope production by cultured cells derived from chemically induced mouse skin papillomas (58). This blocking effect was attributed in part to a 50% reduction in transglutaminase I activity and in part to decrease in the synthesis of envelope precursor proteins. Very low RA concentrations can suppress type I transglutaminase activity and inhibit envelope formation in human and rabbit tracheal epithelial cells cultured in a serum-free medium (20, 65).

Epidermal cells cultured in 10−20% serum do not synthesize the K1 keratin. Delipidation removes vitamin A and allows the cells to synthesize K1 while decreasing the synthesis of a 52-kDa keratin (K13) and a 40-kDa keratin (K19) (59, 63, 64). The addition of retinyl acetate to the delipidized serum reverses these keratin synthesis patterns, that is, inhibits K1 synthesis and stimulates K13 and K19 synthesis. Retinoid modulation of keratin synthesis occurs at the gene transcription (mRNA) level (64, 66).

The development of squamous metaplasia in tracheas removed from vitamin A-deficient hamsters and placed in vitamin A-free organ culture is accompanied by the synthesis of keratins of 45, 46.5, 48, 50, 52, 55, 56, 58, and 60 kDa (67). However, unlike in vitamin A-deficient corneal, conjunctival, and esophageal epithelia in the same model, 65- to 67-kDa keratins are not present. Adding retinyl acetate to the organ culture medium suppresses keratin production, prevents squamous metaplasia and maintains a mucociliary phenotype (67).

Studies in a variety of cultured cell lines established from oral and facial SCCs have demonstrated retinoid suppression of transglutaminase I, involucrin, and cornified envelope formation (45, 56, 57, 60, 64, 68, 69). Reiss et al. (56) studied RA modulation of terminal differentiation in a human cell line (Sq CC/Y_1) derived from SCC of the buccal mucosa. They showed that physiologic concentrations of RA strongly inhibited this cell line's stratification, keratinization, and ability to form cornified envelopes (all phenotypic markers of terminal squamous differentiation). Involucrin, although markedly decreased in the presence of RA, was still detectable in suprabasal cells.

Lotan and co-workers at M.D. Anderson Cancer Center found that RA inhibited the proliferation of 6 of 7 human HNSCC cell lines in monolayer culture (60, 69). Sensitivity was heterogeneous between the cell lines; 1 was very sensitive, and 5 were moderately sensitive. The poorly differentiated 183 cell line was resistant to RA. The ability to form colonies in semisolid medium, which was present in 3 of the 7 lines, was suppressed by RA. RA's modulation (at

1 μmol × 6 days) of the expression of differentiation markers also varied between the cell lines. Transglutaminase I activity was decreased by more than 50% in 3 cell lines, and the effect was dose dependent in 1 line. Type II (soluble, tissue type) transglutaminase was expressed in 3 cell lines; its activity was increased by RA in 2 lines and decreased in 1 line. Envelope competence was also variably suppressed by RA. Keratin synthesis was suppressed in several cell lines. The suppression of synthesis of K1 in lines grown in medium supplemented with delipidized serum was most prominent. Cholesterol sulfate levels decreased following RA treatment by ≥ 70% in 4 cell lines. Sacks et al. (70) also observed that the growth and involucrin expression of HNSCC multicellular tumor spheroids in liquid medium were suppressed by RA. These results demonstrate that RA inhibits growth and decreases squamous marker expression in HNSCC cells. As suggested in studies of other cell systems, the antiproliferative and differentiation activity of RA may be greatest in more differentiated malignant cells (14). For example, in the well differentiated 1483 HNSCC cell line, RA inhibited growth and colony-forming ability, reduced transglutaminase I and cholesterol sulfate expression, and suppressed cholesterol sulfotransferase activity. In contrast, RA had no effect on growth or transglutaminase I expression in the poorly differentiated 183 HNSCC cell line (60, 69). Similar studies are beginning in oral leukoplakia cell cultures (71). Findings reported by Lotan, Rice, and others on the patterns of transglutaminase I, involucrin, and cholesterol sulfate expression in keratinocytes suggest separate regulation of specific squamous markers in malignant and premalignant epithelial cells (45, 60, 68, 69).

In addition to squamous marker modulation, Lotan reported that RA enhanced the synthesis of cell surface-membrane glycoproteins ranging from 280 000 kDa to > 400 000 kDa and increased sialyltransferase activity in several HNSCC cell lines (45). Couch et al. (72) observed similar RA-induced alterations of cell-surface carbohydrate antigens in KLN205 murine SCC cells. These alterations were associated with significantly decreased experimental metastatic potential in the lung colony assay.

Specific patterns of oncogene expression have been correlated with epithelial differentiation, carcinogenesis, and neoplastic transformation. These observations led investigators at M. D. Anderson Cancer Center to study the effects of RA on oncogene expression in 2 human HNSCC cell lines, 1483 and 183A. RA produced no changes of c-*myc*, c-*fos*, p53, transforming growth factor-α (TGF-α), c-Ha-*ras* or c-*src* mRNA levels. However, there was a significant decrease in EGF-R gene expression in the well differentiated 1483 cells but not in the poorly differentiated 183A cells (45, 73). This finding is exciting in view of the recent reports on the overexpression of the EGF-R gene (*erb*-B1) in experimental oral carcinogenesis and in human oral leukoplakia and HNSCC (74). Further analyses indicated that the EGF-R protein level was not different between untreated and RA-treated cells. However, the tyrosine kinase activity of the EGF-R was suppressed by RA (75). Since the kinase activity of the EGF-R is essential for signal transduction, its inhibition by RA may be one mechanism by which RA modulates SCC growth and differentiation.

Retinoid Mechanism of Action

Mammalian cells contain two cytoplasmic retinoid-binding proteins—cellular retinol-binding protein (CRBP) and cellular RA-binding protein (CRABP)—which bind the corresponding retinoids with high specificity (76–78). It has been suggested that these proteins translocate retinoids into the cell nucleus and thus play a key role in retinoid modulation of gene expression. Many investigators have identified CRBP and CRABP in HNSCC (79–86). The pattern of cytoplasmic receptor expression varies between HNSCC and adjacent tissue; however, it has not been shown to correlate with clinical outcome or to predict retinoid response in experimental studies.

Three human nuclear RA-receptor (RAR) genes (α, β, γ) that bear strong sequence homology to members of the steroid/thyroid hormone-receptor family have recently been cloned (87–93). These RARs may function like the other members of the steroid-receptor superfamily as ligand-inducible *trans*-acting enhancer factors and thus may regulate gene expression. These receptors and their multiple isoforms, differ in their tissue distribution patterns, biologic properties, and binding affinities to different RA analogues (94, 95). The most recent addition to the nuclear RA receptor family (RXR) is structurally and biologically unique from the RAR series (96). The role of the nuclear receptors in cancer development and RA activity is unclear. What is known, however, suggest that RARs mediate the effects of retinoids on cell differentiation and embryogenesis (97). Elegant studies in acute promyelocytic leukemia strongly suggest that the RAR-α gene plays a key role in the development *and* therapy of this leukemia (98, 99). RAR studies in other neoplastic disorders are just beginning. Current study of the cytoplasmic and nuclear RA receptors may help explain the differential in vitro and in vivo response of oral leukoplakia and HNSCC to RA (100).

Physiologic and Mechanistic Relationships of Carotenoids and Retinoids

Provitamin A, or β-carotene, is the precursor for the in vivo synthesis of retinol (93). All-*trans*-RA is a naturally occurring metabolite of retinol that can replace retinol in vivo in many functions, including regulating epithelial differentiation. RA is synthesized from retinol by various tissues, including cultured tracheobronchial epithelial cells. Recently, Napoli and Race (101) found that RA can also be synthesized directly from β-carotene by various target tissues at a sufficiently high rate to make this a potentially important pathway for RA generation in situ. That β-carotene and retinol are converted at significant levels in situ into RA suggests that RA is their active form and mediates their anticarcinogenic effects, possibly through RARs.

Retinol, however, has some unique effects—that is, they cannot be reproduced by RA. The presence of a specific CRBP (discussed above) that can be translocated into the nucleus and modulate gene expression suggests that retinol acts without being metabolized to RA. Since β-carotene has intrinsic free-radical scavenging properties, its anticarcinogenic activity may be vastly different from that of either retinol or RA (93, 101). In contrast to retinol, which is tightly regulated by homeostasis, dietary β-carotene accumulates in a dose-dependent fashion in the serum and target tissue (e. g. oral epithelia), which has major chemoprevention implications. These nonoverlapping activities of β-carotene and retinol, and the additive in situ generation of the active metabolite RA, further support the combined use of these agents in chemoprevention trials (see Chemoprevention Trals below).

Other Differentiation Agents and Combination Studies

Data with differentiation agents outside the retinoid sphere in HNSCC are limited. Van Dongen et al. (102) recently conducted in vitro tests of three other potential differentiation agents—the polar–planar solvents hexamethylene bis-acetamide (HMBA) and *N,N*-dimethylforamide (DMF), and the antimetabolite 5-azacytidine—for activity against human HNSCCs transplanted in nude mice. HMBA was inactive, but DMF was active in 1 of 4 SCC lines in inhibiting growth and increasing differentiation marker expression. 5-Azacytidine was active in 2 to 5 lines so tested. Similar variable results in cellular morphology, in vitro growth, antigenicity, tumorigenicity, and metastatic activity in nude mice were observed in small cell and SCC lung cancer lines with RA and 5-azacytidine (103).

Vitamin E and β-carotene inhibit growth of HNSCC cell lines derived from the DMBA-induced buccal pouch model (see Animal Models, below). Although the precise mechanisms are unclear, tamoxifen has been reported to inhibit growth of the laryngeal UM-SCC cell line (104). Other hematopoietically active differentiation agents such as vit-

amin D$_3$ have not been well studied in solid-tumor model systems.

In vitro solid-tumor studies evaluating the growth-inhibitory efficacy of retinoids combined with other anticancer agents and modalities (an approach also not yet studied in HNSCC) have given mixed results (14). Japanese investigators observed that RA potentiated 5-fluorouracil (5-FU) activity against transformed fibroblasts (105). On the basis of this and other in vitro findings, they designed the FAR regimen to treat HNSCC (see Primary Therapy below). RA plus interferon (α, γ) have enhanced activity in a number of diverse cell lines (106). In other in vitro systems, RA can antagonize the activity of hydrocortisone and butyrate (57, 62, 107, 108).

Animal Models

Differentiation inducers inhibit tumor growth in several in vivo model systems, including HNSCC. In contrast to in vitro cultured cell line work, it is often difficult to establish that the anticarcinogenic effect of differentiation agents is in fact due to an induction of terminal division with concomitant alteration of differentiation or another anticancer mechanism (e. g. cytotoxicity, immune-response modifications). For many tumor types, the lack of established differentiation markers limits this type of study. In this regard, HNSCC is an excellent model to assess chemically-induced differentiation since in addition to the standard characteristics used to assess differentiation (e. g. histology, clonogenicity in semisolid medium, tumorigenicity), there are other well established differentiation markers, including keratins, involucrin (and other cornified envelope precursors), and transglutaminase I. For example, as in the in vitro work discussed above, vitamin A regulates keratin expression in vivo in experimental animals. Vitamin-A-deficient rabbits develop keratinization of esophageal, conjunctival, and corneal epithelia and the abnormal expression of K1, K2, and K10. The altered keratin expression pattern can be reversed by supplementing the diet with vitamin A (109).

Animal studies by Slaga, Moon, Shklar, and others have clearly established that UADT, lung, and several other epithelial cancers evolve through a multistep process influenced by vitamin A (45, 110–113). It has been known for over 60 years that vitamin A deficiency leads to the development of squamous metaplasia of the tracheobronchial epithelium (53–55). Preclinical studies also indicate that the carcinogenic effects of cigarette smoke and alcohol are enhanced by vitamin A deficiency (28, 52, 114). Natural and synthetic retinoid supplementation in vivo and in vitro can reverse this premalignant process (45, 53–55, 115). Data from Moon's group (116) indicate that β-carotene and retinol, although inactive as single agents, have synergistic activity in combination for inhibiting dimethylnitrosamine-induced lung carcinogenesis in the Syrian golden hamster model. Selenium and vitamin E alone or combined were ineffective chemopreventive agents in this model.

Animal model studies by several groups of investigators have indicated that retinoids, carotenoids, and other differentiation agents have significant chemopreventive and therapeutic activity in buccal, lingual, and palatal HNSCC. The most extensively studied model system is the Syrian golden hamster buccal pouch model, which is an excellent experimental system for studying not only the initiation and promotion phases of oral carcinogenesis, but also tumor regression and tumor prevention. When DMBA in mineral oil is topically applied three times weekly for 28 weeks, SCC develops in a fairly consistent sequence, its occurrence preceded by a hyperkeratotic and dysplastic lesion similar to precancerous human oral leukoplakia (117). Hamster pouch carcinogenesis is similar to human oral carcinomas with respect to histologic appearance, metabolic markers, and oncogene (c-erb-B1) expression (75). Animal models using tobacco-containing mixtures have been difficult to develop (118).

Various potential differentiation agents—including retinoids (e. g. isotretinoin and retinyl acetate), prostaglandin synthesis inhibitors (e. g. indomethacin), crude extracts of onion, soybean-derived Bowman−Birk protease inhibitor, extracts of Spirulina−Dunaliella algae (rich in β-carotene, other carotenoids, and vitamin E), vitamin E (α-tocopherol), and β-carotene—have chemopreventive activity, inhibiting cancer development to varying degrees in the hamster cheek pouch model (45, 119−128). As in most animal models, the degree of inhibition is dose dependent and varies with the carcinogen type (e. g. direct vs. indirect) and concentration. For example, vitamin E partially inhibited the development of SCC induced by DMBA at a 0.5% concentration, whereas complete inhibition was achieved when the DMBA concentration was only 0.1% (123). Oral retinyl acetate effectively reduced tumor number and size even when given after the development of leukoplakia and early cancer.

Local injections of (in order of increasing therapeutic efficacy) isotretinoin, canthaxanthine, β-carotene, vitamin E, and extract of Spirulina−Dunaliella algae produced regression of established carcinogen-induced buccal pouch tumors in a study by Shklar et al. (45, 129, 130). Of major clinical importance, the combination of β-carotene and vitamin E caused regression of established tumors even when given orally. Shklar et al.'s work suggests that the mechanism of in vivo tumor destruction with these agents involves the release of

tumor necrosis factor-α (TNF-α) by tumor-infiltrating macrophages (131). Tsiklakis et al. (132) showed that systemic administration of the retinoid Ro-109 359 caused marked oral tumor regression and produced histologic results of necrosis and excessive keratin loss. Finally, despite its chemopreventive activity in this model (indicated in the paragraph above), the prostaglandin synthesis inhibitor indomethacin was not effective in suppressing established buccal pouch tumors (133).

Data for differentiation agents' effects in other HNSCC model systems are more limited. Huang (134) studied four retinoids in Fisher 344 rats with SCC implanted in the palate. The retinoids were given orally 2 weeks after SCC implantation. Response rates were 60% for isotretinoin, 58% for all-trans-RA, 30% for 13-cis-retinal, and 20% for all-trans-retinol. Isotretinoin was not effective, however, in reversing sunlight-induced premalignant or malignant HNSCC skin lesions of the pinna and nose in white-haired cats (135). Alam and Alam (136) have reported that dietary β-carotene has dose-dependent chemopreventive effects on DMBA-induced salivary gland tumors in rats, including a decrease in tumor incidence and weight and an increase in tumor latency. Despite definite chemopreventive efficacy of β-carotene in the DMBA-induced cheek pouch and salivary gland tumors, Goodwin et al. observed no activity with high-dose oral β-carotene in DMBA-induced hamster lingual carcinogenesis. Dietary retinoids and selenium, however, were effective in the lingual model (45, 137, 138).

In contrast to the extensive work with oral carcinogenesis models reviewed above, animal models for esophageal cancer are much less well studied. In the Sprague−Dawley rat, injecting nitrosomethylbenzylamine (NMBA), an N-nitroso carcinogen found in dietary staples of high-risk areas in China, induces SCC of the esophagus with marked organ specificity (45, 139). The protocol of five weekly injections of NMBA at 3.5 mg/kg for 5 weeks induces neoplasia in more than 80% of animals with a short (8- to 10-week) latency. Esophageal SCC in this model follows a characteristic sequence of development from normal squamous epithelium to transient hyperplasia, pseudoepitheliomatous hyperplasia (similar to the premalignant lesions seen in the cervix), dysplasia, and then in situ carcinoma. Two chemoprevention studies using this model have been reported to date. Wargovich et al. (140) have identified a potent dietary chemopreventive agent, diallyl sulfide. Diallyl sulfide is derived from allium vegetables (e. g. garlic and onion), which were found to have an inverse correlation with gastric cancer in a recent dietary epidemiologic study (141), and is a potent inhibitor of chemically induced skin and colon cancer. Nauss et al. (142) observed no effect of mild vitamin A deficiency or supplementation on the development of preneoplastic esophageal lesions. Future work with this model is focusing on other potential chemopreventive agents and combinations, including the newer, third-generation retinoids (arotinoids) and retinoid/β-carotene combinations, and on intermediate-endpoint studies (45).

Nutritional Epidemiology

A growing number of retrospective and prospective epidemiologic studies suggest that total vitamin A and carotenoid intake in the form of green and leafy vegetables has a significant inverse correlation with risk of UADT and lung cancer (143—146). In a series of case-control studies comparing high vs. low vitamin A intake, investigators from Roswell Park Memorial Institute observed in the high-vitamin A group significant reductions in cancer risk: 73% for lung cancer, 44% for esophageal cancer, 59% for tongue cancer, and 54% for laryngeal cancer (147—151). The dietary and serum epidemiologic studies can accurately study deficiencies of carotenoids (not of preformed vitamin A) as a risk factor (143—166). Generally in these carotenoid studies, the influence of the dietary or serum level factors was significant and persisted when controlling for tobacco and/or alcohol usage. The UADT and lung cancer risks associated with carotenoid deficiency may be increased by the interaction with smoking; which reduces β-carotene serum (and dietary) levels by 15% (167). In certain regions of China and Iran, esophageal cancer appears to be related to the dietary factors of nitrosamine exposure and deficiencies of zinc, riboflavin, β-carotene, and vitamins A, C, and E (139, 149, 153, 155).

Several epidemiologic studies of patients with premalignant and malignant UADT and lung lesions have revealed that low serum levels of β-carotene, vitamin A, retinoid-binding proteins, zinc and other elements, and micronutrients correlate with disease occurrence (80—83, 143, 168, 169). Although some of these studies were in patients with early-stage disease, studies of this type in cancer patients do not establish cause and effect (143, 160, 163). Epidemiologic studies are unable to differentiate between the metabolic effects of cancer on micronutrient serum levels and possible serum level effects on carcinogenesis. Prospective and retrospective nutritional (serum and dietary) epidemiologic studies together with the preclinical in vitro and in vivo work provide important clues to the development of specific cancers. Carefully controlled clinical chemoprevention trials (45, 170—173) however, will be required to definitively establish the role of dietary factors in cancer prevention.

Clinical Studies

Chemoprevention Trials
Summary of Results in Oral, Laryngeal, Lung, and Esophageal Premalignancy

Since the most intensive clinical chemoprevention work involves oral leukoplakia, it is important to detail the diagnosis, etiology, pathogenesis, and natural history of this premalignant lesion to better interpret the intervention trial data (21, 143, 174, 175). Oral leukoplakia is defined as a white patch or plaque on the oral mucosa which cannot be removed by scraping and cannot be classified as any other disease entity. The histologic pattern of oral leukoplakia varies from hyperkeratosis with hyperplasia to severe dysplasia. Tobacco use and alcohol ingestion are important etiologic factors. The increasing use of smokeless tobacco by younger people in the United States has resulted in increasing frequencies of premalignant and malignant oral lesions. There are currently over 12 million users of smokeless tobacco in the United States, and use is increasing, especially among young males (1, 4). A recent survey in the United States found oral lesions in 46% of smokeless-tobacco users.

The categorization of oral leukoplakia as a premalignant lesion is based on the following data: (1) epidemiologic studies from Asia indicate that most new cases of oral cancer arise in geographic regions with an endemically high incidence of leukoplakia; (2) a significant percentage of patients with oral cancers have associated leukoplakia lesions; (3) prospective study of patients with leukoplakia indicates a significant rate of malignant transformation to SCC of the oral cavity, depending primarily on the presence of dysplasia (21, 175). In Silverman et al.'s series of 257 patients with untreated leukoplakia (176), the malignant transformation rate at 8 years was 17.5%—4% in the first year, 5% in the second year, and approximately 1—2% in each year after the second year. When only the subset of patients with epithelial dysplasia upon initial biopsy was considered, however, the transformation rate at 8-year follow-up was 36.4% (176). Similar results have been reported by others (21, 175).

In Asian smokeless-tobacco and betel-nut users, the *annual* spontaneous leukoplakia regression rate is 4—5%. Pindborg et al. (177) studied 214 patients from Denmark with leukoplakia and reported a cumulative spontaneous improvement rate of 37.9% with a maximum follow-up of 10 years, including a 9.8% spontaneous improvement rate within the first 2 years. The limited US data suggests lower spontaneous improvement rates in smokers and dysplastic lesions.

Cigarette smoking is the major causative factor in oral leukoplakia and oral cancer in the United States. A recentus study has suggested that discon-

tinuation of smoking after the development of leukoplakia has only a marginal beneficial effect (176).
Leukoplakia patients who discontinued smoking
after diagnosis had a marginally higher improvement
rate than patients who continued smoking (44% vs.
37%), and a marginally lower rate of malignant
transformation (12% vs. 16%). Although these clinical results were not histologically confirmed [nor was
smoking cessation confirmed biochemically (178)],
they do suggest that an effective chemopreventive
approach is needed as an adjunct to the important
primary preventive measure of smoking cessation.

In India, smokeless tobacco is the major cause of
oral leukoplakia and oral cancer. Gupta et al. (179)
conducted a 5-year educational intervention program
involving over 36 000 tobacco users from three districts of India. They designed their program to
reduce the use of tobacco (betel quid chewing; chutta
and bidi smoking) and evaluate the effect of tobacco
cessation on the natural history of leukoplakia. They
observed that the tobacco cessation rates (combined
reducing and stopping rates) of 37% and 65% in two
districts were associated with decreased leukoplakia
rate ratios, ranging from 0.18 to 0.59, compared with
control data obtained 10 years earlier from the same
areas. However, the third district's rate ratio of
leukoplakia increased to 1.31 despite a tobacco cessation rate of 33%. Histologic confirmation and
laboratory studies to validate tobacco cessation, such
as the cotinine assay, will help evaluate the relative
effects of tobacco and alcohol cessation and chemopreventive agents upon the natural history of leukoplakia.

Although surgical excision is current standard
therapy for oral leukoplakia, it is not feasible when
there is extensive involvement. Further, because of
the multifocal nature of the disorder, local approaches often do not prevent disease recurrence or
de novo lesions. Thus, a significant number of patients with oral leukoplakia could benefit from a
chemopreventive approach.

Nine studies including two placebo-controlled
randomized trials have demonstrated the efficacy of
synthetic retinoids in oral leukoplakia (175). Koch
used approximately 1 mg/kg/day of isotretinoin, tretinoin or etretinate for 2 months in treating 75 evaluable patients with multifocal advanced leukoplakia
(180). Patients received 70 mg/day orally of one of
these retinoids for 8 weeks and were followed for
from 2 to 6 years after the end of therapy. Complete
plus partial response rates (CR + PR rates) were
87% for isotretinoin, 59% for tretinoin, and 92% for
etretinate, with relapse rates of 55%, 57%, and 51%.
On the basis of these results, Koch performed a
second study in which 45 evaluable patients for 6
weeks received either oral etretinate or oral etretinate plus topical etretinate paste (181). Response
rates were high in both groups—71% and 83%,

respectively. Cordero observed 2 PRs and 1 CR in 3
patients treated with oral etretinate (182). Three
small studies, totaling 18 patients, including 2 with
AIDS-related oral "hairy" leukoplakia, reported an
89% response rate to topical retinoids (isotretinoin;
tretinoin) (183–185).

Hong et al. reported the first randomized,
placebo-controlled trial is oral leukoplakia (174, 175,
186–189). This study confirmed the positive results
of the earlier, nonrandomized trials that suggested
the efficacy of retinoids in oral leukoplakia. Hong's
patients received isotretinoin at from 1 to 2 mg/kg/day
for 3 months (186). The clinical response rate was
67% in the treated group, compared with only 10%
in the placebo group (p = 0.0002). This study was the
first to histologically assess all patients before and
after therapy. Dysplasia was present in pretreatment
biopsies from 63% of the retinoid-treated group and
40% of the placebo group. A highly significant finding in this study was the reversal of dysplasia in 54%
of the retinoid-treated group compared with only
10% spontaneous improvement in the placebo group
(p = 0.01). Because of these highly significant differences, the study was prematurely terminated, after
44 patients. The major problems with this short-term
study were the notable isotretinoin side effects and
the over 50% relapse rate within 2 to 3 months of the
end of therapy.

Recent trials with natural retinoid and carotenoid
compounds in leukoplakia also have been reported,
and the preliminary results are promising. Stich et al.
(190–194) have performed a pioneering series of
trials in high-risk groups, such as tobacco–betel nut
chewers in India and the Philippines, and Inuits
(using smokeless tobacco) from the Northwest Territories of Canada. Their recent 6-month, three-arm
(placebo, β-carotene at 180 mg/wk, or combined β-
carotene at 180 mg/wk and vitamin A at 100 000 IU/
wk) clinical trial involving 119 patients indicated that
the combination of β-carotene and vitamin A is twice
as active as β-carotene alone in achieving a CR of
established leukoplakia lesions (28% vs. 15%) and
preventing new lesions (8% vs. 15%) (191). Responses were not confirmed histologically. The
major clinical response with the combination (β-
carotene plus vitamin A) was observed at 6 months,
whereas the data with the synthetic retinoid isotretinoin indicate significant response at 3 months.

Four other β-carotene trials using varying doses
(30 mg/d to 120 mg/d) have reported response rates
ranging from 0–71% with no clear dose–response
relationship (175, 191, 193, 195). None of the
reported β-carotene studies have had histologic confirmation.

Despite the inconclusive epidemiologic data with
performed vitamin A (retinol), Stich recently conducted a clinical study of oral leukoplakia in which
he achieved a 57% CR rate with complete suppres-

sion of new lesions in 21 evaluable patients receiving high-dose (0.14 mg/kg/wk or 200 000 IU/wk) vitamin A therapy administered twice weekly (192). In a placebo control group, the CR rate was 3%, and 21% of patients developed new lesions. Responses in the treatment group were histologically confirmed. The vitamin A-induced CR rate was much higher than that of β-carotene or combined retinol (at lower dose) and β-carotene in Stich's other studies. Also, compliance was excellent, and there were no reported retinoid toxicities (e. g. mucocutaneous dryness). Of course, even this regimen's high dose of vitamin A is far smaller than typical doses (from 1 to 2 mg/kg/day) of synthetic retinoids in clinical trials.

All these natural-agent data make it difficult to determine whether vitamin A or β-carotene is the more active agent or whether (as with Moon's animal data) the combination is synergistic. Only the vitamin A/β-carotene combination and high-dose vitamin A were significantly more active than placebo. Most important, however, since these agents are not antagonistic, not toxic, and apparently effective in humans with oral premalignancy (natural-agent response rates compare favorably with those of synthetic retinoids), it is incumbent now to establish significant activity in a rigorously designed randomized trial. Three major NCI chemoprevention trials (two in lung, one in oral premalignancy) are now testing the vitamin A/β-carotene combination (174).

Primary therapy of laryngeal papillomatosis, a hyperproliferative UADT lesion, has been investigated in two trials. Alberts et al. (196) used isotretinoin at from 1 to 2 mg/kg/day to treat 6 patients with recurrent laryngeal papillomatosis, achieving 3 CRs and 1 PR. Bichler (197) reported similar results (67% CR rate) with etretinate at 1 mg/kg/day in 42 patients. Although these positive results occurred in extensive disease, a recent small randomized study by Bell et al. (198) attempting adjuvant isotretinoin treatment of laryngeal papillomatosis did not prevent recurrence.

Several studies have investigated the effects of differentiation agents on lung premalignant lesions (174). Investigators from Europe have reported three nonrandomized trials using the oral synthetic retinoid etretinate in smokers with bronchial metaplasia (199−201). They observed significant regression of metaplastic lesions in treated individuals (*p* < 0.01). The reversal of metaplasia was even more marked in the small number of patients who stopped smoking while receiving retinoid therapy. Based on these results and the supportive preclinical data, two ongoing randomized, placebo-controlled trials, one in Canada using etretinate and the other at M. D. Anderson Cancer Center using isotretinoin, were designed to evaluate retinoid efficacy in reversing the carcinogenic process in the lung (45, 170, 174, 202−205).

Esophageal carcinoma in the United States is strongly associated with tobacco and alcohol abuse. In China this cancer appears to result primarily from nutritional deficiencies (e. g. of retinol, riboflavin, α- and β-carotene, α-tocopherol, ascorbate, and zinc) and possibly from exposure to specific carcinogens, such as *N*-nitroso compounds (139); it thus appears to be similar to the NMBA esophageal cancer model discussed above (140). Endoscopic surveys in high-risk areas of China and Iran have described a premalignant esophageal lesion that; (1) is similar to 1-methyl-1-nitrosamine-induced experimental esophageal carcinoma; (2) is associated epidemiologically with esophageal carcinoma; (3) has a similar anatomic location to malignant lesions; and (4) in prospective follow-up series has a significant transformation rate to esophageal carcinoma.

In accordance with these data, Muñoz and colleagues designed a prospective, placebo-controlled, randomized esophageal cancer chemoprevention study in Huixian, a high-risk area in the Henan Province of the People's Republic of China (206−208). The study comprised 610 subjects, ages from 35 to 64 years, for 13.5 months given either combined low-dose retinol (15 mg, or 50 000 IU) riboflavin (200 mg), and zinc gluconate (50 mg), or placebo. Standard histologic evaluations (including two endoscopic biopsies) were made of 93% of all entered subjects at the completion of the study (no histologic evaluations were made prior to study entry). In addition, micronuclei from esophageal and buccal mucosa cells were obtained before therapy began and after the 13.5 months. Serum levels of vitamin A, β-carotene, riboflavin, and zinc were obtained at 0, 2, and 13.5 months.

Three recent reports have analyzed various aspects of this study. Regarding the basic efficacy question, these investigators observed no significant difference between the placebo and treatment arms in the percentages of the premalignant lesions (206). After 13.5 months of therapy, a normal-appearing esophagus was observed in 54% of the placebo group and in 50% of the active-treatment group. Furthermore, no significant differences in the prevalence or severity of dysplasia appeared between the two groups at the end of therapy. A second report analyzing micronuclei frequency did indicate a significant reduction (0.19% vs. 0.31%; p = 0.04) in the mean percentage of micronucleated esophageal cells in the vitamin-treated group over the placebo group (207). The prevalence of micronuclei in the buccal mucosal cells did not vary significantly between pre- and posttherapy evaluations, which supports the site-specific value of micronuclei as indicators of cancer risk only in the target, or high-risk, tissues.

The third and most recent report is an analysis correlating the serum levels of various micronutrients (regardless of the study arm) with the histologic findings after therapy. This analysis was important because of the substantial improvement in serum micronutrient levels in approximately 50% of the placebo group. The investigators observed that improvement of blood micronutrient levels, regardless of treatment arm, was associated with a reduced prevalence of esophageal lesions (208). (The most significant and consistent effect was observed with retinol.) This finding emphasizes the concern many investigators in this field have regarding the drop-in (or contamination) adherence issue in a placebo-controlled trial using readily available (via diet or over-the-counter vitamin supplements) micronutrients (45, 171–173). The esophageal trial results do suggest that longer treatment may translate into histologic and clinical benefit, since the potential intermediate-endpoint marker of micronuclei in esophageal mucosa showed improved frequencies. The authors also state that the pattern of cell proliferation, another potential intermediate endpoint marker, also improved.

Preliminary results from a phase II study of isotretinoin (1 mg/kg/d) in the Barrett esophagus, a premalignant lesion in which metaplastic columnar epithelium replaces the normal squamous lining and is associated with an increased risk of multifocal adenocarcinoma of the esophagus (209), have been recently reported. Only 11 of 16 patients completed 6 weeks of therapy with no responses (210). Although this trial was flawed by the small numbers, extremely short intervention and poor adherence, the lack of isotretinoin clinical activity is consistent with the in vitro data, which show growth inhibition of the Barrett esophagus cell cultures only at extremely high isotretinoin concentrations (211). Of note, α-difluoromethylornithine (DFMO) had significant in vitro activity and is now being clinically tested in this disorder. This intermediate endpoint trial is monitoring polyamine levels.

Biologic Markers as Potential Intermediate Endpoints of Chemoprevention Trials

Although not strictly differentiation markers, micronuclei and other genotoxic markers are closely linked to abnormal epithelial differentiation. It is important here to review in some detail the micronuclei data in subjects at high risk of UADT cancers. These data have been used by Stich and others as an adjunct to standard clinical and histologic data as a short-term in vivo marker to screen for active chemopreventive agents in animals and humans. Micronuclei data have been critical to the early development of natural retinoids and carotenoids as potential chemopreventive agents (3, 190, 212–216).

Micronuclei are formed from chromosome and chromatid fragments created by clastogenic events, including carcinogenic damage to DNA, which occurs in proliferating cells (212). When nuclei reform after cell division, micronuclei form to enclose any fragments of DNA that are separated from the centromeres. The presence of micronuclei in a tissue is a quantitative reflection of ongoing genetic damage. The micronuclei assay has been utilized in many human tissues during carcinogenic exposure. Micronuclei correlate with target-tissue cancer risk—elevated micronuclei frequencies are observed in exfoliated epithelial cells from individuals at high risk (e. g. tobacco users) for oral, esophageal, uterine cervical, lung, or bladder cancer (3, 190, 204, 207, 213–220).

In a series of pilot studies, Stich's group (3, 190, 193, 213–216, 219) established that high-risk tobacco/betel nut users had elevated oral mucosal micronuclei frequencies. The highest frequencies corresponded to the sites of greatest carcinogenic exposure whether or not a premalignant lesion was observed clinically. Examples of high-risk groups and corresponding mean micronuclei percentages are a 4.4% mean of micronucleated cells in nass users in Uzbekistan; 8.4% mean in tobacco–betel quid chewers in Orissa, India; 4.8% in tobacco–betel quid chewers of the Philippines; 2.8% in Indian users of khaini tobacco; and 1.9% in Inuits who use snuff (3, 190, 193, 214, 216). One important feature of these data is that they derive from high-risk subjects both without and with premalignant lesions. Stich's early studies focused on high-risk tobacco/betel nut users without clinically apparent lesions.

After establishing site-specific elevated micronuclei frequencies in high-risk individuals, Stich embarked on a novel series of β-carotene and vitamin A chemopreventive intervention studies. Initially, Stich treated members of the high-risk groups mentioned above who had no clinically visible premalignant lesions but had increased micronuclei frequencies in the oral mucosal cells. Stich observed that a 3-month intervention of vitamin A (100 000 IU/wk) and β-carotene (180 mg/wk, or 300 000 IU/week), both given in divided doses twice weekly, significantly suppressed micronuclei frequencies in right and left buccal mucosal scrapings of 40 Filipino betel nut and tobacco chewers (219). Substantial micronuclei suppression occurred in 37 (93%) of the subjects, and the overall mean micronuclei percentage decreased 3-fold, from 4.2% to 1.4%. Because of the dramatic micronuclei suppression observed at 3 months, monthly micronuclei analyses in a subset of 11 subjects revealed a roughly 40% reduction in the micronuclei percentage each month for the first 3 months while on vitamin A and β-carotene therapy.

The striking activity of the combination of vitamin A and β-carotene in suppressing micronuclei led to a study in which Stich et al. treated another group of Filipino tobacco–betel nut chewers (also without premalignant lesions) with either β-carotene alone

(180 mg/wk) or vitamin A alone (150 000 IU/wk) for 9 weeks. These investigators observed a β-carotene-induced micronuclei suppression in 22 (88%) of 25 subjects, with an overall mean micronuclei percentage decrease from 3.4% to 1.2% ($p < 0.001$) (213). Vitamin A alone was also highly effective, with micronuclei suppression in 24 (92%) of 26 subjects and a decrease in the overall mean micronuclei percentage from 4.0% to 1.7% ($p < 0.001$). These investigators also used another carotenoid, canthaxanthine (which has excellent free-radical scavenging activity but no in vivo conversion to retinol), at 180 mg/wk, which was ineffective in suppressing micronuclei. Stich's third intervention was a 10-week course of β-carotene (180 mg/wk) for 23 snuff-using Inuits from the Northwest Territories of Canada and was discussed above as Stich's first study in oral leukoplakia (193). The mean micronuclei percentage decreased from 1.9% to 0.7%. However, the frequencies of nucleated cells and of cells with condensed chromatin (two other markers of genotoxic damage) were not changed in response to β-carotene.

Stich's most recent micronuclei intervention study was conducted in tobacco−betel quid chewers living in Kerala, India (191). All entered individuals had well developed premalignant oral leukoplakia. This three-arm study, as noted above, comprised a placebo group, β-carotene (180 mg/wk) group, and β-carotene (180 mg/wk) plus vitamin A (100 000 IU/wk) group. Micronuclei suppression was impressive in both the lesion and the adjacent clinically normal-appearing tissue at 3 months and was equivalent in the two treatment arms. However, there was a twofold greater lesion CR rate in the β-carotene plus vitamin A arm compared with the β-carotene alone arm (28% vs. 15%).

In contrast to the suppression seen in betel nut, snuff, and other smokeless-tobacco users, Stich observed no micronuclei suppression after 4 months of combined therapy with β-carotene (180 mg/wk) and vitamin A (150 000 IU/wk) in exfoliated epithelial cells from the palate or tongue of Asians practicing the so-called inverted style of smoking (lit end in month) who had premalignant oral leukokeratosis (3, 190, 193, 214, 216).

No marker, including the extensively studied micronuclei, has yet been validated as an intermediate-endpoint marker. Response of micronuclei to chemopreventive agents may differ significantly among patients with oral leukoplakia. Although β-carotene and vitamin A, alone or in combination, are effective in suppressing micronuclei in 80−90% of smokeless-tobacco users after 3 months of therapy, the 6-month CR rate between the agents differ markedly, in that vitamin A has a record of 57% CRs and β-carotene's CR rate is 15%. Furthermore, Stich has found no link between elevated micronuclei frequencies and the presence of oral leukoplakia in nass users (3, 190, 193, 214, 216). Stich consistently found that 10−15% of the lesions and adjacent normal-appearing buccal mucosa of betel, tobacco, and snuff users with elevated micronuclei percentages were resistant (i. e. nonsuppressible micronuclei counts) to the vitamin A and/or β-carotene therapy. The significance of this finding is unclear.

Since micronuclei frequency is raised in epithelial cells of individuals at high risk for aerodigestive tract cancer (oral, esophageal, and lung) and can be lowered by chemopreventive agents, this in vivo quantitative assay should be very useful for monitoring ongoing genetic alterations and their modulation by chemopreventive agents. Another attractive feature of the micronuclei assay is that it is amenable to automated quantification by image-analysis systems, facilitating its widespread use as a screening test for chemopreventive agents). Future work with this assay will be important for screening other potential differentiation and chemopreventive agents in humans, such as vitamin D_3, vitamin E, butylated hydroxyanisole (BHA), butylated hydroxytoluene (BHT), DFMO, and the newer synthetic retinoids (e. g. arotinoids, retinamides) (14, 45, 202, 221).

Oral Premalignancy Intermediate-Endpoint Study

The first chemoprevention trial to analyze a panel of biologic markers, including micronuclei, evolved in part out of the randomized, placebo-controlled trial reported approximately 2 years ago by Hong and coworkers at M.D. Anderson Cancer Center. As detailed above, results of their trial established that isotretinoin has significant clinical and histologic activity in oral lesion leukoplakia (186). Besides the significant 67% response rate, Hong's study made the important finding that over 50% of patients relapsed soon after stopping retinoid therapy. M. D. Anderson investigators are now conducting marker studies as part of a two-phase trial of isotretinoin in oral leukoplakia (217). In phase 1, patients received induction therapy with high-dose isotretinoin (1.5 mg/kg/day) for 3 months. In phase 2, treated patients are randomized to a lower dose of isotretinoin (0.5 mg/kg/day) or to β-carotene (30 mg/day) for 9 months in order to study these agents' abilities to prolong remission.

This study's phase 1 goal involves evaluating the modulation of certain abnormally expressed biologic markers, which may indicate intermediate endpoints (222−224) of the oral carcinogenic process. In phase 2, marker studies will continue during and after maintenance therapy. The biomarkers studied were micronuclei and the squamous differentiation markers detailed earlier−K1 keratin, type I transglutaminase and involucrin. These markers were selected for the following reasons: first, although absent or expressed at low levels in normal oral mucosa, they are expressed at higher levels in many patients with premalignant and malignant oral lesions and so may reflect intermediate endpoints of the multistep carcinogenic process; second, these markers can be analyzed from small tissue biopsies or scrapings, which is essential for studies involving relatively healthy subjects; third, RA (retinoid acid) suppresses squamous marker expression in vitro (see "In Vitro Data" above); fourth, retinol suppresses oral micronuclei expression in smokeless-tobacco users.

The early results indicate the feasibility of serially analyzing a panel of biomarkers from very small tissue specimens obtained in a human chemoprevention trial (223). The results also indicate that isotretinoin suppresses the genotoxic marker micronuclei and may modulate certain squamous differentiation markers. Regarding clinical implications, the data indicate that low-dose isotretinoin is significantly more effective maintenance therapy than β-carotene (225).

Although its chemopreventive efficacy in oral premalignancy has been established, standard-to-high dose isotretinoin is inappropriate for long-term study because of its toxicity. We are now planning a long-term chemoprevention trial testing using vitamin A and β-carotene. This study would be significant if it only established the relatively nontoxic natural agents β-carotene and vitamin A as effective chemopreventive drugs against oral premalignancy. This would imply the high potential of these agents for chemoprevention of tobacco-related UADT and lung epithelial cancers. But at least as important is the opportunity in this study to conduct laboratory studies of an extensive panel of genomic, differentiation, and proliferation markers. Small-sample methods will allow expansion of the limited panel of genotoxic and differentiation markers used in the preliminary study. This expanded study will be the first to evaluate the effects of long-term chemopreventive therapy on an extensive panel of molecular and biochemical markers of proliferation and growth regulation. Biomarker studies may help establish intermediate endpoints for monitoring drug efficacy in chemoprevention trials conducted in oral and other epithelial neoplastic processes (214, 222–224). Valid intermediate-endpoint markers would reduce the cost and time it takes to screen many types of chemopreventive drugs.

Safety Issues in Chemoprevention Trials

Establishing the safety of chemopreventive agents is critical, especially since patients in chemoprevention trials are usually relatively healthy individuals without cancer. To achieve the maximum therapeutic effect, patients must take the agents over a long-term period. Significant side effects, either subjective or objective, must therefore be avoided.

β-Carotene has no clinical side effects except for a dose-dependent yellowing of the skin. Natural vitamin A, or retinol, is generally well tolerated. Doses of 200 000 IU/wk were associated with no clinical toxicities (192). Extremely high doses, of 200 000 IU/m^2/day for a total of from 350 000 to 400 000 IU/day, were associated with side effects in 38% of patients but those side effects were generally mild (226). The spectrum of synthetic retinoids' side effects is comparable to that of vitamin A (14). Most frequently observed are mucocutaneous dryness and musculoskeletal complaints. Chronic toxicity resulting from retinoids includes increased values in liver function tests, vertebral osteophyte formation and abnormalities in reproductive function. Severe teratogenic effects have been documented in infants exposed to synthetic retinoids in utero. Therefore, women of child-bearing potential should be excluded from retinoid chemoprevention trials. Although retinoid side effects clearly are less severe than those of most other antitumor agents, the identification of nontoxic and effective agents would be of major importance to the chemoprevention effort. Currently, there is great interest in the United States and elsewhere in the combination of retinoids and carotenoids for long-term use. This combination is quite active as chemoprevention therapy for skin and lung neoplasia in animals and for oral leukoplakia in man.

Two large US studies (> 15 000 subjects), one conducted by McLarty at the University of Texas at Tyler and the other by Goodman in Seattle, Washington, documented the safety of long-term retinol and β-carotene administration as regards cumulative toxicities (45, 170, 174, 202, 227, 228). The Seattle study used β-carotene (30 mg/day) and retinol (25 000 IU/day) and the Texas study used β-carotene (50 mg/day) and retinol (25 000 IU every other day). Toxicities from both studies were minimal, other than the yellowing of skin. These two studies demonstrate that well tolerated doses of β-carotene and retinol are capable of substantially increasing the serum β-carotene and serum retinyl palmitate concentrations without producing liver toxicity or significant increases in serum triglycerides (229).

Differentiation Therapy in HNSCC

Primary Therapy

The extensive preclinical and growing clinical data in UADT preneoplasia have led to retinoid trials in advanced HNSCC (14, 175). Retinoids have major *single-agent* activity in acute promyelocytic leukemia (trans-RA) (99) and modest activity in a limited number of other established malignancies (14), including cutaneous T-cell lymphoma and advanced SCC of the skin. Although high-dose retinol did not produce clinical response in only 4 treated HNSCC patients in a broad phase II study in advanced cancer (226), isotretinoin has produced responses in refractory head and neck cancers. A nonrandomized broad phase II trial at the University of Arizona administered isotretinoin to a subgroup of 29 patients with advanced disease and achieved 3 responses, all PRs of short duration, in the 19 evaluable patients (230).

These and other data led to a prospective, multiinstitutional, randomized phase II trial of isotretinoin in advanced HNSCC (231). Forty patients were randomized to receive very high-dose isotretinoin (3 mg/kg/day) or methotrexate (15 mg/m^2 intramuscularly for 3 consecutive days, each for 3 weeks), the best studied and current standard active single agent for reccurrent disease (21, 232). Three objective responses (16%), including 1 CR, occurred in the 19 evaluable isotretinoin-treated patients. Only 1 minor response (5%) occurred in the methotrexate-treated group. This very low response rate to methotrexate (reported to be in the range of 8−63% for advanced HNSCC) reflects the poor-risk patients with refractory disease included in the trial. These 19 isotretinoin-treated patients, along with an equal number from the earlier Arizona broad phase II trial (230), bring the total up to 38 evaluable patients, for a response rate of 16%. This compares to established single-agent cytotoxic response rates of 15−30% (21, 232).

Advanced SCC skin lesions in the head and neck region can behave clinically similar to the more classic advanced SCC of internal (mucosal) head and neck sites (233). In one chemotherapy series of 68 consecutive patients with advanced *head and neck* SCC, 16 (23%) actually had primary tumors of the *skin* of the head and neck (234). Retinoids in high doses have definite chemopreventive activity in SCC of the skin in high-risk patients and are active against in situ SCC of the skin; however, their clinical use in invasive cutaneous SCC has been limited (235−237). One recent report comprised 4 patients with moderately-to-well differentiated locally advanced cancers that were refractory to local treatment (surgery and/ or irradiation) (237). All 4 patients had marked disease regression beginning within 3 to 4 weeks of starting isotretinoin therapy. This series has now been extended to comprise 11 evaluable patients and has achieved 2 complete, 2 partial, 2 mixed, and 2 minor responses (233). The current study combining isotretinoin with α-interferon in advanced cutaneous SCC has produced promising results with a 68% (95% CI, 49−87%) overall response rate— > 90% response rate in locally advanced disease and < 30% in distant-metastatic and chemotherapy-refractory disease (238). The regimen was reasonably well tolerated—the dose-limiting toxicity in this elderly patient population (median age 67 years) was chronic fatigue. These response data are roughly 2-fold higher than the limited single-agent systemic data using higher drug doses in locally advanced patients. In vivo cell line data suggest additive to synergistic antiproliferative and/or differentiative activity in a number of malignant cell types. Other (platinum-based chemotherapy) regimens with similar reported activity have been more acutely toxic than this regimen, and their ultimate utility in terms of response or survival prolongation either alone or in combination with surgery or radiotherapy, has been elusive. Investigators are interested in this retinoid−interferon regimen as a possible building block for improved combinations. Future work will focus on mechanisms of action and possible dose modifications—both of which are issues of major importance which will be addressed in follow-up studies using this approach. This promising clinical activity in the pilot skin cancer trial provided the rationale for the study of this novel biologic regimen in other advanced cancers (106). Major activity of this regimen has recently been observed in locally advanced SCC of the cervix (239). Studies of other sites including advanced SCC of the UADT and lung are ongoing.

A series of innovative nonrandomized clinical trials developed in the early 1970s by several groups from Japan have investigated the use of the so-called FAR regimen, which incorporates vitamin A, 5-FU, and radiation (105, 240). The FAR regimen has been used either alone or with surgical resection since 1972 in the management of head and neck cancers. This combination is based on in vitro work in cultured transformed fibroblasts indicating that cobalt-60 radiation is potentiated by 5-FU and vitamin A, and that 5-FU's anticancer activity is potentiated by vitamin A. The basic regimen as reported by Komiyama and colleagues (240) is 5-FU at 250 mg intravenously and vitamin A (retinyl palmitate) at 50 000 IU intramuscularly given 1 and 6 hours before each 200-rad fraction of cobalt-60 radiation, the radiation given five times per week for a total planned dose of from 6000 to 7000 rad.

The Japanese investigators reported their FAR results in 191 patients with laryngeal carcinoma, 60 with hypopharyngeal and cervical esophageal cancer, and 23 with epipharyngeal cancer, all treated from 1972 to 1977 (105, 240). The 5-year survivals of radiotherapy-treated laryngeal cancer patients treated with (n = 53) and without (n = 138) FAR therapy were 83% and 65%. Similar results were achieved in hypopharyngeal cancer: 5-year survivals of 38% with FAR and 24% without. The 5-year survivals in laryngeal cancer by tumor size were 80% for T1 lesions, 78% for T2, 65% for T3 and 50% for T4. The 5-year survivals by site were 59% for supraglottic, 76% for glottic, and 100% (9 of 9) for subglottic laryngeal cancer. Another Japanese group substituted etretinate for vitamin A in the FAR regimen and achieved promising pilot-study results in 16 patients (241).

Of interest, two other pilot studies of vitamin A and β-carotene in advanced HNSCC suggest that these agents may ameliorate treatment-related oral mucositis (242, 243).

Based on supportive preclinical data (see Animal Models above), there is growing interest in the use of prostaglandin synthesis inhibitors (e. g. indomethacin) in HNSCC patients (244–247). The mechanism of anticarcinogenic action of these agents is unclear but appears to relate to their immune modulatory effects. Although drugs of this class have not yet been studied as chemopreventive agents in human UADT or lung trials, they have produced promising preliminary results as primary therapy in HNSCC.

Adjuvant Therapy

Standard treatment for advanced (stage III or IV) HNSCC is surgery and/or radiotherapy; neoadjuvant chemotherapy has not improved the survival of these patients (21). Standard treatment for early-stage disease is either surgical excision or radiotherapy. The major causes of failure in patients with advanced disease are local–regional recurrence and distant metastasis. In contrast, the major cause of failure in early-stage disease is the development of second malignant (second primary) tumors (SMTs) (18).

Since adjuvant therapy will most benefit patients with early-stage disease and the major cause of death in these patients is SMTs, we shall define and detail the magnitude of the SMT problem in HNSCC. The definition of SMT in HNSCC, established by Warren and Gates in 1932 (248), is the existence of any biopsy-proved noncontiguous cancers, regardless of histology. Survivors after successful treatment for HNSCC are at a 3%–6% risk per year for developing a second or third primary tumor in the UADT or lung. As diagnostic and therapeutic techniques continue to improve, the expectation is that relative survival rates are likely to increase, with the consequent concern that more patients will live long enough to develop SMTs.

The incidence of SMTs varies little by primary tumor site. A characteristic site distribution pattern has been described, however. SMTs associated with oral cavity primary tumors are most likely to occur in the head and neck area (approximately one-half); approximately one-third of the SMTs are in the lung, and one-fifth are in the esophagus (18, 249). Although primary tumor sites of the oral cavity and pharynx overlap in their distribution of SMTs, laryngeal cancer has a distinctly different pattern, with a relatively high incidence of SMTs (over 40%) in the lung, which is associated with a grave prognosis (median survival, from 5 to 10 months) (250). Since the cure rate for early-stage laryngeal cancer is excellent after radiation therapy or surgery (reported 5-year survival rates of 60–90%), this patient group is at a particularly high cumulative risk to develop SMTs.

To better define the current magnitude of the SMT problem and factors that might influence the development of SMTs, the Radiation Therapy Oncology Group (RTOG) prospectively collected a registry of all its HNSCC patients, including 928 patients treated by radiotherapy (251). A total of 114 SMTs occurred in these 928 patients. Overall estimated risks of developing an SMT were about 10% within 3 years of radiation therapy, 15% within 5 years of radiation therapy, and 24% within 8 years of radiation therapy. Therefore, HNSCC presents a unique opportunity to investigate chemopreventive strategies. SMTs in HNSCC patients are not treatment related (18, 252). It appears that the common etiologic risk factors for the initial tumors are important in the pathogenesis of the SMTs. As stated above in the Biology section, the development of SMTs in the aerodigestive tract may be due to the process of diffuse field cancerization, where the entire epithelium at risk has been exposed to continued carcinogenic insult and has a relatively high probability of developing multiple foci of premalignant or malignant lesions (16–18).

The subject of reducing SMTs by cessation of smoking is controversial. A 1971 study by Moore (253) suggested that stopping smoking reduced the incidence of a SMT developing after successful treatment of an initial tumor. Studies from Castigliano (254) and Wynder et al. (255), however, did not substantiate the predicted reduction of SMT development after stopping smoking. Recent further evidence from Hellquist et al. (256) and Gillis et al. (257) also suggests that smoking cessation may not be as critical to the development of SMTs as once thought. These data are similar to the leukoplakia data discussed earlier (174–176) and suggest that smoking cessation as a primary preventive measure after field cancerization has occurred may be most effective in earlier carcinogenic stages. Pharmacologic intervention with chemopreventive agents as an adjunct to smoking cessation measures could markedly suppress the development of SMTs.

Investigators at M.D. Anderson recently completed a prospective double-blind, randomized study of isotretinoin versus placebo in HNSCC (258). Patient eligibility features were a histologically confirmed diagnosis of HNSCC, stage I to IV (M0) disease and clinically disease-free status after surgery and/or radiotherapy. Each eligible patient was randomly assigned to either high-dose isotretinoin (from 50 to 100 mg/m²/day) or to placebo capsules for a duration of up to 12 months and follow-up for up to 5 years. A total of 103 patients were entered into the study. There were no statistically significant differences between the groups with regard to factors considered to influence prognosis. Site of primary tumor, prior treatment, stage of disease, tumor cell differentiation and history of smoking and alcohol were similar in both groups.

The patterns of failure after isotretinoin or placebo in these 103 patients were initially reported at a median follow-up of 32 months. Differences between local, regional, and distant relapse rates in the isotretinoin group and those in the placebo group were not statistically significant. The data indicate a significant difference, however, between the development of SMTs in the isotretinoin group and in the placebo group, (4 vs. 24%, p = 0.005). With extended follow-up (median 42 months) (175), the overall failure (recurrence plus SMT) difference has reached significance and the SMT difference remains highly significant (6 vs. 28%, $p = 0.005$). Over 80% of SMTs developed in the UADT, esophagus, or lung. In the retinoid arm no SMTs developed during the 1-year therapy and no lung SMTs occurred. Multiple SMTs developed only in patients in the placebo arm. The SMT incidence or patterns were unrelated to smoking in this trial. The major problem with high-dose isotretinoin was the frequent toxicity.

Based on preliminary evidence from this study, these investigators have recently activated a trial with low-dose isotretinoin (30 mg/d) that is designed for long-term intervention to prevent SMTs. Head and neck cancer patients with advanced disease have competing risks of local, regional, or distant relapse and are not suitable candidates for chemoprevention studies because they do not survive long enough to develop SMTs. This NCI-sponsored trial will enroll over 1000 patients from selected RTOG and CCOP (Community Clinical Oncology Program) centers with stage I or II HNSCC in order to determine whether low-dose isotretinoin is efficacious in reducing SMTs and improving survival.

Conclusion

Tobacco-related head and neck, other UADT, and lung neoplasms clearly are a major and increasing worldwide problem. Despite treatment advances, mortality rates from these malignancies have decreased only marginally in the past 20 years. Differentiation therapy provides a new and promising approach which has already demonstrated major activity in certain human hematologic (99) solid tumor (238, 239) systems. The preclinical in vitro and animal studies are generating a wealth of information on the potential clinical applicability of differentiation agents. The key to understanding the general modulation of squamous differentiation may be found in the way these agents modulate differentiation biomarkers such as the pattern of keratin expression.

Retinoids are considered to be the prototype class of differentiation agents. The recent identification of specific nuclear receptors should provide an important insight into molecular mechanisms of retinoid action. Clinical data with differentiation agents are primarily limited to the RA, β-carotene (chemoprevention only) and interferon-α.

As single agents, isotretinoin and interferon-α exhibit modest activity in patients with advanced HNSCC (21). The limited data from clinical studies incorporating these agents with other anticancer agents for treating HNSCC are difficult to interpret because of the lack of randomized trial designs (21).

Current and future differentiation work in established cancers should focus on the development and conduct of controlled, randomized trials to evaluate differentiation agents in combination and with other anticancer agent classes and modalities in advanced disease (6–11, 14, 106, 238, 239, 259–262). These clinical trials should be based on the new data arising from in vitro and animal studies, such as the recent work indicating enhanced activity of retinoid–interferon and other cytokine combinations, cytotoxics, and irradiation. Although differentiation agents may have only limited value as primary single-agent treatment of HNSCC, they still may prove to have a role in combination therapies.

A randomized, placebo-controlled chemoprevention trial in China using riboflavin, zinc, and retinol illustrates the difficulties in conducting nutritional intervention chemopreventive studies in general. Despite the rigorous study design, the ready availability of these nutrients led to significant contamination (e. g. increasing serum retinol levels) in the placebo group. This observation is of great concern for many chemoprevention studies, especially those using natural agents such as β-carotene, which are readily available in many foods and over-the-counter vitamin supplements (222).

The most promising potential use of differentiation agents in the UADT lies in the realm of clinical chemoprevention with established activity of isotretinoin in reversing oral premalignancy and suppressing head and neck SMTs. The requirement for long-term therapy in chemoprevention studies highlights the importance of searching for nontoxic effective agents. One such nontoxic regimen that is receiving extensive clinical study in the United States and elsewhere is the combination of vitamin A and β-carotene. Preliminary data with this combination suggest that it; (1) is nontoxic, even with prolonged (> 5 years) use in humans; (2) synergistic in animal lung and skin carcinogenesis models; (3) may be effective as primary therapy for oral leukoplakia; and (4) can prolong remission in leukoplakia patients. In addition to the β-carotene and vitamin A combination, preclinical studies suggest several promising single agents (e. g. BHT, retinamides, arotenoids, and allium compounds) and combinations (e. g. vitamin E plus β-carotene, and DFMO plus selenium) as candidates for rigorous clinical evaluation in UADT and lung carcinogenesis (14, 131, 140, 221, 262).

A rapidly growing aspect of chemoprevention trials is the parallel and complementary evaluation of biologic markers as potential intermediate endpoints of the carcinogenic process. Intermediate-endpoint studies increase our basic understanding of the expression and modulation of certain abnormal biomarkers associated with specific stages of the multistep carcinogenic process in HNSCC and other epithelial cancers. Historically, the primary problem faced in measuring biologic markers during clinical trials in humans was the large tissue samples needed for analyses. In the past, measurement of these markers required gram amounts of tissue. However, rapid advances in the development of microassay (immunohistochemical, in situ hybridization and PCR) techniques make such measurements possible on serial sections of small (e. g. 1−2 mm biopsies) amounts of tissue. The goal now is to apply these techniques to the study of the multistep process of carcinogenesis in vivo and to use these assays to determine intermediate-endpoint markers for the cellular effects of chemopreventive agents (223).

To date, the most extensively studied marker is micronuclei, which has been studied in lung, oral, and esophageal lesion tissues of high-risk individuals. Evaluation of this short-term marker was critical to the early study of the differentiation agents natural vitamin A and β-carotene as chemopreventive agents in leukoplakia. Early data from studies evaluating micronuclei in oral leukoplakia already indicate the feasibility and utility of serially analyzing a panel of biomarkers in very small tissue specimens, which make laboratory studies in human chemoprevention trials feasible. Given these established small-tissue techniques, M.D. Anderson is now planning to study the modulation of an expanded panel of genomic, growth regulatory and phenotypic (differentiation and proliferation) markers in a long-term oral leukoplakia chemoprevention trial employing low-dose isotretinoin vs. vitamin A and β-carotene.

Positive data from the recently completed high-dose retinoid adjuvant study in HNSCC (258) and low-dose study in oral premalignancy (225) promoted investigators at M.D. Anderson to develop a multicenter large-scale study using low-dose isotretinoin to treat patients with stage I or II HNSCC who have been rendered disease free by primary therapy. A similar trial is in development in the U.S. for stage-I non-small cell lung cancer (174). These studies are aimed at preventing SMTs, which occur in the UADT and lung and are the major cause of mortality in patients who present with early-stage cancer. The important concept of tobacco-related field cancerization, which is still undergoing rigorous basic science study, holds that the entire UADT and the lungs are at risk. The theory links the carcinogenic processes and development of SMTs of the UADT and lung to a basic etiology and pathogenesis.

This work was supported in part by Public Health Service Grant CA 46303 from the National Cancer Institute, National Institutes of Health, Department of Health and Human Services. Dr. Lippman is a recipient of an American Cancer Society Career Development Award.

References

1. Advisory Committee to the Surgeon General. The health consequences of using smokeless tobacco. USDHHS NIH publication no. 86−2874. Bethesda: National Institutes of Health, 1986.
2. Blakeman EM ed. Tobacco use in America conference: final report. Report of a conference held January 27−28, 1989, at the University of Texas M.D. Anderson Cancer Center. Available from The American Medical Association. Public Affairs Group, 1101 Vermont, NW, Washington DC 20 005.
3. Stich HF, Rosin MP. Towards a more comprehensive evaluation of a genotoxic hazard in man. Mutat Res 1985; 150:43−50.
4. Squier CA. Smokeless tobacco and oral cancer. A cause for concern? CA 1984; 34:242−7.
5. Boring CL, Squires TS, Tong T. Cancer statistics, 1992. CA 1992; 42:19−38.
6. Gallagher RE. Control of differentiation. In: Moosa AR and Schimpff SA eds. Comprehensive textbook of oncology. Baltimore: Williams & Wilkins, 1990: 14.
7. Reiss M, Gamba-Vitalo C, Sartorelli AC. Induction of tumor cell differentiation as a therapeutic approach: Preclinical models for hematopoietic and solid neoplasms. Cancer Treat Rep. 1986; 70:201−18.
8. Waxman S, et al. The status of differentiation therapy. New York: Raven Press, 1988.
9. Cheson BD, Jasperse DM, Chun HG, Friedman MA. Differentiating agents in the treatment of human malignancies. Cancer Treat Rev 1986; 13:129−45.
10. Pierce GB, Speera WC. Tumors as caricatures of the process of tissue renewal: prospects for therapy by directing differentiation. Cancer Res 1988; 48:1996.
11. Muto Y, Moriwaki H. Antitumor activity of vitamin A and its derivatives. JNCI 1984; 73:1389−93.
12. Lotan R. Effects of vitamin A and its analogs (retinoids) on normal and neoplastic cells. Biochim Biophys Acta 1980; 605:33−91.
13. Roberts AB, Sporn MB. Cellular biology and biochemistry of the retinoids. In: Sporn MB, Roberts AB, Goodman DS (eds.). The Retinoids II. Orlando: Academic Press, 1984:209−86.
14. Lippman SM, Kessler JF, Meyskens FL. Retinoids as preventive and therapeutic anticancer agents. Cancer Treat Rep 1987; 71:391−405, 493−515.
15. Tomita Y, Himeno K, Nomoto K, Endo H, Hirohata T. Augmentation of tumor immunity against syngeneic tumors in mice by beta-carotene. JNCI 1987; 78:679−81.
16. Slaughter DP, Southwick HW, Smejkal W. "Field cancerization" in oral stratified squamous epithelium: Clinical implications of multicentric origin. Cancer 1953; 6:963−8.
17. Strong MS, Incze J, Vaughan CW. Field cancerization in the aerodigestive tract—Its etiology, manifestation, and significance. J Otolaryngol 1984; 13:1−6.
18. Lippman SM, Hong WK. Second malignant tumors in head and neck squamous cell carinoma: The overshadowing threat for early stage patients (editorial). Int J Radiat Oncol Biol Phys 1989; 17:691−4.

19. Ouhayoun JP, Gosselin F, Forest N, Winter S, Franke WW. Cytokeratin patterns of human oral epithelia: Differences in cytokeratin synthesis in gingival epithelium and the adjacent alveolar mucosa. Differentiation 1985; 30:123−9.

20. Jetten AM. Multistep process of squamous differentiation of tracheobronchial epithelial cells. Role of retinoids. Dermatologica 1987; 175:37−44.

21. Wolf G, Lippman SM, Laramore G, Hong WK. Head and neck cancer. In: Holland JF, Frei E, Bast RC Jr, Kufe DW, Morton DL, Weischelbaum R, eds. Cancer medicine. 3rd ed. Philadelphia: Lea & Febieger, 1992. [In press].

22. Moll R, Franke WW, Schiller DL. The catalog of human cytokeratins: Patterns of expression in normal epithelia, tumors and cultured cells. Cell 1982; 31:11−24.

23. Kim KH, Scwartz F, Fuchs E. Differences in keratin synthesis between normal epithelial cells and squamous cell carcinomas are mediated by vitamin A. Proc Natl Acad Sci USA 1984; 81:4280−4.

24. Kopan R, Traska G, Fuchs E. Retinoids as important regulators of terminal differentiation: Examining keratin expression in individual epidermal cells at various stages of keratinization. J Cell Biol 1987; 105:247−40.

25. Loning T, Staquet MJ, Thivolet J, Seifert G. Keratin polypeptides distribution in normal and diseased human epidermis and oral mucosa. Virchows Arch [A] 1980; 388:273−88.

26. Conti CJ. Markers of keratinocyte differentiation in preneoplastic and neoplastic lesions. In: Russo J, ed. Immunocytochemistry in tumor diagnosis. Proceedings of the Workshop on Immunocytochemistry in Tumor Diagnosis, Detroit, Michigan, 1984. Boston: Martinus Nijhoff, 1984:59−71.

27. Nischt R, Roop DR, Mehrel T, et al. Aberrant expression during two-stage mouse skin carcinogenesis of a type 1 47-kDa keratin, K13, normally associated with terminal differentiation of internal stratified epithelia. Mol Carcinog 1988; 1:96−108.

28. Rutten AAJJL, Bruyntjes JP, Ramaekers FCS. Effect of cigarette smoke condensate and vitamin A depletion on keratin expression patterns in cultured hamster tracheal epithelium: An immunohistomorphological study using monoclonal antibodies to keratins. Virchows Arch [B] 1989; 56:111−17.

29. Seifert G, Caselitz J. Markers of oral and salivary gland tumors: Immunocytochemical investigations. Cancer Detect Prev 1985; 8−23−34.

30. Myoken Y, Moroyama T, Miyauchi S, Takada K, Namba M. Monoclonal antibodies against human oral squamous cell carcinoma reacting with keratin proteins. Cancer 1987; 60:2927−37.

31. Kim KH, Stellmach V, Javors J, Fuchs E. Regulation of human mesothelial cell differentiation: Opposing roles of retinoids and epidermal growth factor in the expression of intermediate filament proteins. J Cell Biol 1987; 105:3039−51.

32. Nagle RB, Moll R, Weidauer H. Nemetschek H, Franke WW. Different patterns of cytokeratin expression in the normal epithelia of the upper respiratory tract. Differentiation 1985; 30:130−40.

33. Itoiz ME, Lanfranchi HE, Gimenez-Conti IB, Conti CJ. Immunohistochemical demonstration of keratins in oral mucosa lesions. Acta Odont Scand 1984; 1:47−9.

34. Reibel J, Clausen H, Dabelsteen E. Staining patterns of human premalignant oral epithelium and squamous cell carcinomas by monoclonal antikeratin antibodies. Acta Pathol Microbiol Immunol Scand [A] 1985; 93:323−30.

35. Gimenez-Conti IB, Shin D, Larcher F, et al. Markers of premalignant progression in hamster cheek pouch chemical carcinogenesis (abstr). Proc Am Assoc Cancer Res 1989; 30:169.

36. Shin DM, Gimenez IB, Slaga TJ, et al. Expression of epidermal growth factor receptor, polyamines, ornithine decarboxylase, micronuclei, and transglutaminase I in DMBA-induction hamster buccal pouch tumor model. Cancer Res. 1990; 50:2505−10.

37. Solt DB, Shklar G. Rapid induction of gamma glutamyltranspeptidase-rich intraepithelial clones in 7,12-dimethylbenz(a)anthracene treated hamster buccal pouch. Cancer Res 1982; 42:285−91.

38. Itoiz ME, Conti CJ, Lanfranchi HE, Mamrack M, Klein-Szanto AJP. Immunohistochemical detection of filaggrin in preneoplastic and neoplastic lesions of the human oral mucosa. Am J Pathol 1985; 119:456−61.

39. Rearick JI, Stoner GD, George MA, Jetten AM. Cholesterol sulfate accumulation in tumorigenic and nontumorigenic rat esophageal epithelial cells: Evidence for defective differentiation control in tumorigenic cells. Cancer Res. 1988; 48:5289−95.

40. Jetten AM, George MA, Nervi C, Boone LR, Rearick JI. Increased cholesterol sulfate and cholesterol sulfotransferase activity in relation to the multistep process of differentiation in human epidermal keratinocytes. J Invest Dermatol 1989; 92:203−9.

41. Thacher SM. Purification of keratinocyte transglutaminase and its expression during squamous differentiation. J Invest Dermatol 1989; 92:578−84.

42. Said JW, Nash G, Sassoon AF, Shintaku IP, Banks-Schlegel S. Involucrin in lung tumors. A specific marker for squamous differentiation. Lab Invest 1983; 49:563−8.

43. Itoiz ME, Conti CJ, Gimenez-Conti IB, Lanfranchi HE, Fernandez-Alonso GI, Klein-Szanto AJP. Immunodetection of involucrin in lesions of the oral mucosa. J Oral Pathol 1986; 15:205−8.

44. Kaplan MJ, Mills SE, Rice RH, Johns ME. Involucrin in laryngeal dysplasia. Arch Otolaryngol 1984; 110:713−16.

45. Lippman SM, Lee JS, Lotan R, Hong WK. Chemoprevention of upper aerodigestive tract cancers: A report of the Upper Aerodigestive Cancer Task Force workshop. Head Neck Surg. 1990; 12:5−20.

46. Ghosh, R, Sharma JK, Ghosh PK. Sister chromatid exchange in the lymphocytes of patients with oral leukoplakia. Cancer Genet Cytogene 1988; 36:177−82.

47. Doseva D, Christov K, Kristeva K. DNA content in reactive hyperplasia, precancerosis, and carcinomas of the oral cavity. Acta Histochem (Jena) 1984; 75:113−19.

48. Fontham E, Correa P, Rodriguez E, Lin Y. Validation of smoking history with the micronuclei test. In: Hoffman D, Harris C, eds. Mechanisms in tobacco carcinogenesis. Cold Spring Harbor: Cold Spring Harbor Laboratory, 1986:113−19.

49. Spitz MR, Fueger JJ, Beddingfield NA, et al. Chromosome sensitivity to bleomycin-induced mutagenesis: An independent risk factor for upper aerodigestive tract cancers. Cancer Res 1989; 49:4626−8.

50. Morgan PR, Shirlaw PJ, Johnson NW, Leigh IM, Lane EB. Potential application of anti-keratin antibodies in oral diagnosis. J Oral Pathol 1987; 16:212−22.

51. Lichti U, Yuspa SH. Inhibition of epidermal terminal differentiation and tumor promotion by retinoids. In: Nugent J, Clars S, eds. Retinoids, differentiation and disease. London: Pitman, 1985: 77−89.

52. Jeffery PK, Brain AP, Shields PA, Quinn BP, Betts T. Response of laryngeal and tracheobronchial surface lining to inhaled cigarette smoke in normal and vitamin A deficient rats: A scanning electron microscopic study. Scanning Microsc 1988; 2:545−52.

53. Wolbach SB, Howe PR. Tissue changes following deprivation of fat soluble A vitamin. J Exp Med 1925; 42:753−77.

54. Saffiotti V, Montesano R, Sellakumar A, Borg S. Experimental cancer of the lung. Inhibition by vitamin A of the induction of tracheobronchial squamous metaplasia and squamous cell tumors. Cancer 1967; 20:857−64.

55. Mossman BT, Craighead JE, MacPherson BV. Asbestos-induced epithelial changes in organ cultures of hamster trachea: Inhibition by retinyl methyl ether. Science 1980; 207:311−13.

56. Reiss M, Pitman SW, Sartorelli AC. Modulation of the terminal differentiation of human squamous carcinoma cells in vitro by all-trans-retinoic acid. JNCI 1985; 74:1015−23.

57. Cline PR, Rice RH. Modulation of involucrin and envelope competence in human keratinocytes by hydrocortisone, retinyl acetate and growth arrest. Cancer Res. 1983; 43:3203−7.

58. Nagae S, Lichti U, De Luca LM, Yuspa SH. Effect of retinoic acid on cornified envelope formation: Difference between

spontaneous envelope formation in vivo or in vitro and expression of envelope competence. J Invest Dermatol 1987; 89:51−8.

59. Glifix BM, Eckert RL. Coordinate control by vitamin A of keratin gene expression in human keratinocytes. J Biol Chem 1985; 260:14026−9.

60. Jetten AM, Kim JS, Sacks PG, et al. Suppression of growth and squamous cell differentiation markers in cultured human head and neck squamous carcinoma cells by β-all-trans retinoic acid. Int J. Cancer 1990; 45:195−202.

61. Wu R, Wu MMJ. Effects of retinoids on human bronchial epithelial cells: Differential regulation of hyaluronate synthesis and keratin protein synthesis. J Cell Physiol 1986; 127:73−82.

62. Thacher SSM, Coe El, Rice RH. Retinoid suppression of transglutaminase activity and envelope competence in cultured human epidermal carcinoma cells: Hydrocortisone is a potent antagonist of retinyl acetate but not retinoic acid. Differentiation 1985; 29:82−7.

63. Fuchs E, Green H. Regulation of terminal differentiation of cultured human conjunctival keratinocytes. Cell 1981; 25:617−25.

64. Green H, Watt FM. Regulation by vitamin A of envelope cross-linking in cultured keratinocytes derived from different human epithelia. Mol Cell Biol 1982; 2:1115−7.

65. Floyd EE, Jetten AM. Retinoids, growth factors and the tracheobronchial epithelium (editorial). Lab Invest 1988; 59:1−4.

66. Eckert RL, Green H. Cloning of cDNAs specifying vitamin A-responsive human keratins. Proc Natl Acad Sci USA 1984; 81:4321−5.

67. Huang FL, Roop DR, DeLuca LM. Vitamin A deficiency and keratin biosynthesis in cultured hamster trachea. In Vitro Cell Dev Biol 1986; 22:223−30.

68. Rice RH, Thacher SM. In: Breiter-Hahn J. Matoltsky AG, Richards KS eds. Biology of the integument. vol. 2. Heidelberg: Springer, 1986:752−61.

69. Lotan R, Sacks PG, Lotan D, Hong WK. Differential effects of retinoic acid on the in vitro growth and cell surface glycoconjugates of two human head and neck squamous cell carcinomas. Int J Cancer 1987; 40:224−9.

70. Sacks PG, Oke V, Vasey T. Lotan R. Retinoic acid inhibition of a head and neck multicellular tumor spheroid model. Head Neck Surg 1989; 11:219−25.

71. Sacks PG, Hong WK, Hittelman WN. In vitro studies of the premalignant process: initial culture of oral premalignant lesions. Cancer Bull 1991; 43:485−9.

72. Couch WJ, Pauli BU, Weinstein RS, Coon JS. Modulation of the metastatic phenotype by 13-cis-retinoic acid. JNCI 1987; 78:971−7.

73. Lee JS, Kim JS, Blick M, Hong WK, Lotan R. Effects of retinoic acid on oncogene expression in a human head and neck squamous carcinoma cell line. In: Wolf GT, Carey TE, eds. Head and neck oncology research. Berkeley: Kugler & Ghedini, 1987:43−8.

74. Wong DTW. Amplification of the C-erb B1 oncogene in chemically induced oral carcinomas. Carcinogenesis 1987; 8:1963−5.

75. Kim JS, Lee JS, Blick M, et al. Effects of retinoic acid (RA) on the gene expression, autophosphorylation, and EGF binding properties of the EGF-receptor in human head and neck squamous carcinoma cells (HNSCC) (abstr). Proc Am Assoc Cancer Res 1988; 29:42.

76. Chytil F, Ong DE. Cellular retinol and retinoic acid binding proteins in vitamin A action. Fed Proc 1979; 38: 2510−14.

77. Chytil F, Ong DE. Cellular retinoid-binding proteins. In: Sporn MB, Roberts AB, Goodman DS, eds. The retinoids II. Orlando: Academic Press, 1984:89−123.

78. Chytil F, Sherman DR. How do retinoids work? Dermatologica 1987; 175:8−12.

79. Ong DE, Goodwin WJ, Jesse RH, Griffin AC. Presence of cellular retinol and retinoic acid-binding proteins in epidermoid carcinoma of the oral cavity and oropharynx. Cancer 1982; 49:1409−12.

80. Bichler, E, Daxenbichler G. Retinoid acid-binding protein in human squamous cell carcinomas of the ORL region. Cancer 1982; 49:619−21.

81. Bichler, E, Daxenbichler G, Marth CH. Vitamin A status and retinoid-binding proteins in carcinomas of the head and neck region. Oncology 1982; 40:336−9.

82. Gates RE, Rees RS. Altered vitamin A-binding proteins in carcinoma of the head and neck. Cancer 1985; 56:2598−604.

83. Fex G, Wahlberg P, Biorklund A, Wennerberg J, Willen R. Studies of cellular retinol-binding protein (CRBP) in squamous-cell carcinomas of the head and neck region. Int J Cancer 1986; 37:217−21.

84. Rallet A, Jardillier JC. Cellular binding proteins for retinol and retinoic acid in head and neck carcinomas and in human breast cancer cell lines. Steroids 1988; 52:397−8.

85. Yanagita T, Komiyama S, Kuwano M. Cellular retinol-binding proteins in head and neck tumors and their adjacent tissues. Cancer 1986; 58:2251−5.

86. Wahlberg P, Biorklund A, Wennerberg J, Willen R. Studies of cellular retinol-binding protein in squamous cell carcinomas of the cervix uteri and of the oral cavity. Int J Cancer 1988; 41:771−6.

87. Gudas LJ. Molecular mechanisms of retinoid action. Am J Respir Cell Mol Biol 1990; 2:319−20.

88. Petkovich M, Brand NJ, Krust A, Chambon P. A human retinoic acid receptor which belongs to the family of nuclear receptors. Nature 1987; 330:444−50.

89. Giguere V, Ong ES, Segui P, Evans RM. Identification of a receptor for the morphogen retinoic acid. Nature 1987; 330:624−9.

90. Brand N, Petkovich M, Krust A, et al. Identification of a second human retinoic acid receptor. Nature 1988; 332:850−3.

91. Krust A, Kastner P, Petkovich M, Zelent A, Chambon P. A third human retinoic acid receptor, hRAR-gama. Proc Natl Acad Sci USA 1989; 886:5310−14.

92. Evans RM. The steroid and thyroid hormone receptor superfamily. Science 1988; 240:889−95.

93. Blomhoff R, Green MH, Berg T, Norum KR. Transport and storage of vitamin A. Science 1990; 250:399−404.

94. Smith S, Eichele G. Temporal and regional differences in the expression pattern of distinct retinoic acid receptor-β transcripts in the chick embryo. Development 1991; 111:245−52.

95. Lehmann JM, Dawson MI, Hobbs PD, Husman M, Pfahl M. Identification of retinoids with nuclear receptor subtype-selective activities. Cancer Res 1991; 51:4804−9.

96. Mangelsdorf D, Ong E, Dyck J, Evans R. Nuclear receptor that identifies a novel retinoic acid response pathway. Nature 1990; 345:224−9.

97. Tabin C. Retinoids, homeoboxes, and growth factors:Toward molecular models for limb development. Cell 1991; 66:199−277.

98. de The Lavau C, Marchio A, Chomienne C, Degos L, Dejean A. The PML-RARα fusion mRNA generated by the t (15:17) translocation in acute promyelocytic leukemia encodes a functionally altered RAR. Cell 1991; 66:675−84.

99. Warrell P, Frankel S, Miller W, et al. Differentiation therapy of acute promyelocytic leukemia with tretinoin (all-trans-retinoic acid). N Engl J Med 1991; 324:1385−93.

100. Hu L, Crowe DL, Rheinwald JG, Chambon P, Gudas LJ. Abnormal expression of retinoic acid receptors and keratin 19 by human oral and epidermal squamous cell carcinoma cell lines. Cancer Res 1991; 51:3972−81.

101. Napoli, JL, Race Kr. Biogenesis of retinoic acid from β-carotene: Differences between the metabolism of β-carotene and retinal. J Biol Chem 1988; 263:17372−7.

102. van Dongen G, Braakhuis BJM, Bagnay M, Leyva A, Snow GB. Activity of differentiation-inducing agents and conventional drugs in head and neck cancer xenografts. Acta Otolaryngol (Stockh) 1988; 105:488−93.

103. Olsson L, Behnke O, Sorensen HR. Modulatory effects of 5-azacytidine, phorbol ester, and retinoic acid on the malignant phenotype of human lung cancer cells. Int J Cancer 1985; 35:189−98.

104. Shapira A, Virolainen E, Jameson JJ, Ossakow SJ, Carey TE. Growth inhibition of laryngeal UM-SCC cell lines by tamoxifen: Comparison with effects on the MCF-7 breast cancer cell line. Otolaryngol Head Neck Surg 1986; 112:1151−8.

105. Takaku F. Clinical trials and cancer risk in Japan. JNCI 1984; 73:1483–5.

106. Dmitrovsky E, Bosl GJ. Active cancer therapy combining 13-*cis*-retinoic acid with interferon-α. JNCI 1992; 84:218–9.

107. Reiss M, Maniglia CA, Sartorelli AC. Modulation of cell shedding and glycosaminoglycan synthesis of human malignant keratinocytes by all-trans-retinoic acid and hydrocortisone in vitro. J Invest Dermatol 1986; 86:683.

108. Bijman J Th, Wagener DJ, van Rennes H, Wessels JMC, Ramaekers FCS, van den Broek P. Modulation of placental alkaline phosphatase activity and cytokeratins in human HN-1 cells by butyrate, retinoic acid catecholamines and histamine. Br J Cancer 1987; 56:127–32.

109. Tseng SCG, Hatchell D, Tierney N, Huang A J-W, Sun T-T. Expression of specific keratin markers by rabbit corneal, conjunctival, and esophageal epithelia during vitamin A deficiency. J Cell Biol 1984; 99:2279–86.

110. Slaga TJ. Cancer: Etiology, mechanisms and prevention—A summary. In: Slaga TJ, ed. Modifiers of chemical carcinogenesis. New York: Raven Press, 1980: 243–62.

111. Sporn MB. Carcinogenesis and cancer: Different perspectives on the same disease. Cancer Res. 1991; 51:6215–8.

112. Moon RC, Mehta RG. Retinoid inhibition of experimental carcinogenesis. In: Boca Rotan FL, Dawson MI, Okamuia WH, eds. Chemistry and biology of synthetic retinoids. Boca Raton: CRC Press, 1990: 501–18.

113. Aldaz CM, Conti CJ, Larcher F, et al. Sequential development of aneuploidy, keratin modifications, and gamma-glutamyltransferase expression in mouse skin papillomas. Cancer Res 1988; 48:3253–7.

114. Mak KM, Leo MA, Lieber CS. Differentiation by ethanol consumption of tracheal squamous metaplasia caused by vitamin A deficiency in rats. JNCI 1987; 79:1001–10.

115. Lasnitzki I, Bollag W. Prevention and reversal by a non-polar arotinoid (Ro 15-0778) of 3,4-benzpyrene- and cigarette smoke condensate-induced hyperplasia and metaplasia of rodent respiratory epithelia grown in vitro. Eur J Cancer Clin Oncol 1987; 23:861–5.

116. Mehta RG, Rao KVN, Detrisac CJ, Kelloff GJ, Moon RC. Inhibition of dimethylnitrosamine-induced lung carcinogenesis by retinoids (abstr). Proc Am Assoc Cancer Res 1988; 29:129.

117. Salley JJ. Experimental carcinogenesis in the cheek pouch of the Syrian hamster. J Dent Res 1954; 33:253–62.

118. Kandarkar SV, Hasgekar NN, Sirsat SM. Optical and ultrastructural pathology of vitamin A pretreated hamster cheek pouch—pouch-exposed to lime (Ca(OH)$_2$) and tobacco over total life span. Neoplasma 1981; 28:729–37.

119. Burge-Bottenbley A, Shklar G. Retardation of experimental oral cancer development by retinyl acetate. Nutr Cancer 1983; 5:121–29.

120. Shklar G, Schwartz J, Grau D, Trickler D, Wallace H. Inhibition of hamster buccal pouch carcinogenesis by 13-*cis*-retinoic acid. Oral Surg Oral Med Oral Pathol 1980; 50:45–52.

121. Suda D, Schwartz J, Shklar G. Inhibition of experimental oral carcinogenesis by topical beta carotene. Carcinogenesis 1986; 7:711–15.

122. Suda D, Schwartz J, Shklar G. GGT reduction in beta carotene-inhibition of hamster buccal pouch carcinogenesis. Eur J Cancer Clin Oncol 1987; 23:43–6.

123. Trickler D, Shklar G. Prevention by vitamin E of experimental oral carcinogenesis. JNCI 1987; 78:165–9.

124. Perkins TM, Shklar G. Delay in hamster buccal pouch carcinogenesis by aspirin and indomethacin. Oral Surg Oral Med Oral Pathol 1982; 53:170–8.

125. Messadi V, Billings P, Shklar G, Kennedy AR. Inhibition of oral carcinogenesis by a protease inhibitor. JNCI 1986; 76:447–52.

126. Schwartz J, Shklar G, Reid S, Trickler D. Prevention of experimental oral cancer by extracts of Spirulina–Dunaliella algae. Nutr Cancer 1988; 11:127–34.

127. Kandarkar SV, Potdar PD, Sirsat SM. Dose response effect of retinyl acetate on DMBA induced carcinogenesis in the hamster cheek pouch. Neoplasma 1984; 31:415–21.

128. Niukian K, Schwartz J, Shklar G. Effects of onion extract on the development of hamster buccal pouch carcinomas as expressed in tumor burden. Nutr Cancer 1987; 9:171–6.

129. Schwartz J, Shklar G. Regression of experimental hamster cancer by beta-carotene and algae extracts. J Oral Maxillofac Surg. 1987; 45:510–15.

130. Shklar G, Schwartz J, Trickler DP, Niukian K. Regression by vitamin E of experimental oral cancer JNCI 1987; 78:987–92.

131. Shklar G, Schwartz J. Tumor necrosis factor in experimental cancer regression with alpha-tocopherol, beta-carotene, canthaxanthin and algae extract. Eur J Cancer Clin Oncol 1988; 24:839–50.

132. Tsiklakis K, Papadakou A, Angelopoulos AP. The therapeutic effect of an aromatic retinoid (RO-109359) on hamster buccal pouch carcinomas. Oral Surg Oral Med Oral Pathol 1987; 64:327–32.

133. Franklin CD, Craig GT. The effect of indomethacin on tumor regression in DMBA-induced epithelial neoplasia of hamster cheek pouch mucosa. Oral Med Oral Pathol Surg 1987; 63:335–9.

134. Huang CC. Effect of retinoids on the growth of squamous cell carcinoma of the palate in rats. Am J Otolaryngol 1986; 7:55–7.

135. Evans AG, Madewell BR, Stannard AA. A trial of 13-*cis*-retinoic acid for treatment of squamous cell carcinoma and preneoplastic lesions of the head in cats. Am J Res 1985; 46:2553–6.

136. Alam BS, Alam SQ. The effect of different levels of dietary β-carotene on DMBA-induced salivary gland tumors. Nutr Cancer 1987; 9:93–101.

137. Goodwin WJ, Bordash GD, Huijing F, Altman N. Inhibition of hamster tongue carcinogenesis by selenium and retinoic acid. Ann Otol Rhinol Laryngol 1986; 95:162–6.

138. Shklar G, Marefat P, Korhauser A, Trickler D, Wallace H. Retinoid inhibition of lingual carcinogenesis. Oral Surg Oral Med Oral Pathol 1980; 49:325–32.

139. Barch DH. Esophageal cancer and microelements. J Am Coll Nutr 1989; 8:99–107.

140. Wargovich MJ, Woods C, Stephens LC, Gray KN. Chemoprevention of *N*-nitrosomethylbenzylamine-induced esophageal cancer in rats by the naturally occurring thioether diallyl sulfide. Cancer Res. 1988; 48:6872–5.

141. You WC, Blot WJ, Chang YS, et al. Allium vegetables and reduced risk of stomach cancer. JNCI 1989; 81:162–4.

142. Nauss KM, Bueche D, Newberne PM. Effect of vitamin A nutriture on experimental esophageal carcinogenesis. JNCI 1987; 79:145–7.

143. Lippman SM, Meyskens FL. Retinoids for the prevention of cancer. In: Moon TE, Micozzi M, eds. Nutrition and cancer prevention: The role of micronutrients. New York: Marcel Dekker, 1989: 243–72.

144. Byers T. Diet and cancer: Any progress in the interim? Cancer 1988; 62:1713–24.

145. Colditz GA, Stampfer MJ, Willett WC. Diet and lung cancer: A review of the epidemiologic evidence in humans. Arch Intern Med 1987; 147:157–60.

146. Bertram JS, Kolonel LN, Meyskens FL. Rationale and strategies for chemoprevention of cancer in humans. Cancer Res. 1987; 47:3012–31.

147. Marshall J, Graham S, Mettlin C, Shedd D, Swanson M. Diet in the epidemiology of oral cancer. Nutr Cancer 1982; 3:145–9.

148. Mettlin C, Graham S, Swanson M. Vitamin A and lung cancer. JNCI 1979; 62:1435–8.

149. Mettlin C, Graham S, Priore R, Marshall J, Swanson M. Diet and cancer of the esophagus. Nutr Cancer 1981; 2:143–7.

150. Graham S, Mettlin C, Marshall J. Priore R, Rzepka T, Shedd D. Dietary factors in the epidemiology of cancer of the larynx. Am J. Epidemiol 1981; 113:675–80.

151. Graham S. Epidemiology of retinoids and cancer. JNCI 1984; 73:1423–8.

152. Winn DM, Ziegler RG, Pickle LW, Gridley G, Blot WJ, Hoover RN. Diet in the etiology of oral and pharyngeal cancer among women from the southern United States. Cancer Res 1984; 44:1216–22.

153. Yang CS, Sun Y, Yang Q, et al. Vitamin A and other deficiencies in Linxian, a high esophageal cancer incidence area in northern China. JNCI 1984; 73:1449–53.

154. Wahi PN, Kehar U, Lahiri B. Factors influencing oral and oropharyngeal cancers in India. Br J Cancer 1965; 19:642–60.

155. Zaride DG, Blettner M, Trapeznikov NN, et al. Survey of a population with a high incidence of oral and oesophageal cancer. Int J Cancer 1985; 36:153–8.

156. Meyskens FL. Thinking about cancer causality and chemoprevention. JNCI 1988; 80:1278–81.

157. DeCosse JJ. Potential for chemoprevention. Cancer 1982; 50:2550–3.

158. Menkes MS, Comstock GW, Vuilleumier JP, Helsing KJ, Rider AA, Brookmeyer R. Serum beta-carotene, vitamins A and E, selenium, and the risk of lung cancer. N Engl J Med 1986; 315:1250–4.

159. Greenwald P, Sondik E, Lynch BS. Diet and chemoprevention in NCI research strategy to achieve national cancer control objectives. Annu Rev Public Health 1986; 7:267–91.

160. Chaudhy NA, Jafarey NA, Ibrahim K. Plasma vitamin A and carotene levels in relation to the clinical stages of carcinoma of the oral cavity and oropharynx. JPMA 1980; 30:221–3.

161. Mellow MH, Layne EA, Lippman TO, Kaushik M, Hostetler C, Smith JC. Plasma zinc and vitamin A in human squamous carcinoma of the esophagus. Cancer 1983; 51:1615–20.

162. Ibrahim K, Jafarey N, Zuberi S. Plasma vitamin A and carotene levels in squamous cell carcinoma of the oral cavity and oropharynx. Clin Oncol 1977; 3:203–7.

163. Mugliston T, Coe A. Serum vitamin A levels in patients with untreated T1 or T2 squamous carcinoma of the larynx: A pilot study. J Otorhinolaryngol Relat Spec 1986; 48:261–4.

164. Bichler E. Plasma levels of retinol and retinol-binding protein in patients with squamous cell carcinomas of the head and neck region. Arch Otorhinolaryngol 1982; 236:115–21.

165. Osler M. Vitamin A and lung cancer: Should smokers eat more vegetables? Lung Cancer 1986; 2:238–46.

166. Kromhout D. Essential micronutrients in relation to carcinogenesis. Am J Clin Nutr 1987; 45:1361–7.

167. Gerster H. Beta-carotene and smoking. J Nutr Growth Cancer 1987; 4:45–9.

168. Friedman GD, Blaner WS, Goodman DS, et al. Serum retinol and retinol-binding protein levels do not predict subsequent lung cancer. Am J Epidemiol 1986; 123:781–9.

169. La Via MF, Weathers DR, Kreitzman SN, Waldron CE, Teti G. Relationship of vitamin A intake and E rosette inhibition to oral dysplasia and neoplasia. Cancer Detect Prev 1981; 4:121–8.

170. Cullen JW. The National Cancer Institute's intervention trials. Cancer 1988; 62:1851–64.

171. Meyskens FL Jr. Coming of Age—the chemoprevention of cancer. N Engl J Med 1990; 323:825–7.

172. Hennekens CH. Issues in the design and conduct of clinical trials. JNCI 1984; 73:1473–6.

173. Greenberg E, Baron J, Stukel T, et al. A clinical trial of beta carotene to prevent basal-cell and squamous-cell cancers of the skin. N Engl J Med 1990; 323:789–95.

174. Lippman SM, Hong WK. Chemoprevention of aerodigestive tract carcinogenesis. Cancer Bull 1991; 43:525–33.

175. Lippman SM, Hong WK. Retinoid chemoprevention of upper aerodigestive tract carcinogenesis. In: DeVita VT, Hellman S, Rosenberg SA, eds. Important advances in oncology. Philadelphia: Lippincott, 1992: 93–109.

176. Silverman S, Gorsky M, Lozada F. Oral leukoplakia and malignant transformation: A follow-up study of 257 patients. Cancer 1984; 53:563–8.

177. Pindborg JJ, Jolst O, Renstrup G, Roed-Petersen B. Studies in oral leukoplakia: A preliminary report on the period prevalence of malignant transformation in leukoplakia based on a follow-up study of 248 patients. J Am Dent Assoc 1968; 76:767–71.

178. Stookey GK, Katz BP, Olson BL, Drook CA, Cohen SJ. Evaluation of biochemical validation measures in determination of smoking status. J Dent Res 1987; 66:1597–601.

179. Gupta PC, Pindborg J, Bhonsle RB, et al. Intervention study for primary prevention of oral cancer among 36 000 Indian tobacco users. Lancet 1986; 1:1235–8.

180. Koch HF. Biochemical treatment of precancerous oral lesions: The effectiveness of various analogues of retinoic acid. J Maxillofac Surg 1978; 6:59–63.

181. Koch HF. Effect of retinoids on precancerous lesions of oral mucosa. In: Orfanos CE, Braun-Falco O, Farber EM, et al., eds. Retinoids: Advances in basic research and therapy. Berlin: Springer, 1981: 307–12.

182. Cordero AA, Allevato MAJ, Barclay CA, Traballi CA, Donatti LB. Treatment of lichen planus and leukoplakia with the oral retinoid Ro 10-9359. In: Orfanos CE, Braun-Falco O, Farber EM, et al., eds. Retinoids: Advances in basic research and therapy. Berlin: Springer, 1981: 273–8.

183. Raque CJ, Biondo RV, Keeran MG, Honeycutt WM, Jansen GT. Snuff dippers' keratosis (snuff-induced leukoplakia). South Med J 1975; 68:565–8.

184. Shah JP, Strong EW, DeCosse JJ, Itri L, Sellers P. Effect of retinoids on oral leukoplakia. Am J. Surg 1983; 146: 466–70.

185. Schofer H, Ochsendorf FR, Helm EB, Milbradt R. Treatment of oral 'hairy' leukoplakia in AIDS patients with vitamin A acid (topically) or acyclovir (systemically) (letter). Dermatologica 1987; 174:150–1.

186. Hong WK, Endicott J, Itri LM, et al. 13-cis-retinoic acid in the treatment of oral leukoplakia. N Engl J Med. 1986; 315:1501–5.

187. Hong WK, Doos WG. Chemoprevention of head and neck cancer. Otolaryngol Clin North Am 1985; 18:543–9.

188. Lotan R, Kim JS, Maaroui M, Schantz SP, Hong WK. Vitamin A, retinoids and the prevention and treatment of head and neck cancer. Cancer Bull 1987; 39:93–7.

189. Lotan R, Schantz SP, Hong WK. The use of retinoids in head and neck cancer. In: Jacobs C, Cancers of the head and neck. The Hague: Martinus Hijhoff, 1987: 177–91.

190. Stich HF, Dunn BP. DNA adducts, micronuclei and leukoplakias as intermediate endpoints in intervention trials. In: Bartsch H, Hemminki, eds. Methods for detecting DNA damaging agents in humans: Applications in cancer epidemiology and prevention. New York: Oxford University Press, 1988: 137–45.

191. Stich HF, Rosin MP, Hornby AP, Matthew B, Sankaranarayanan R, Nair MK. Remission of oral leukoplakias and micronuclei in tobacco-betel quid chewers treated with beta-carotene and with beta-carotene plus vitamin A. Int J Cancer 1988; 42:195–9.

192. Stich HF, Hornby AP, Mathew B, Sankaranarayanan R, Nair MK. Response of oral leukoplakias to the administration of vitamin A. Cancer Lett 1988; 40:93.

193. Stich HF, Hornby AP, Dunn BP. A pilot beta-carotene intervention trial with Inuits using smokeless tobacco. Int J Cancer 1985; 36:321–7.

194. Rosin MP. Genetic and proliferation markers in clinical studies of the premalignant process. Cancer Bull 1991; 43:507–14.

195. Garewal HS, Meyskens FL, Killen, D, et al. Response of oral leukoplakia to beta-carotene. J Clin Oncol 1990; 8:1715–20.

196. Alberts DS, Coulthard SW, Meyskens FL Jr. Regression of aggressive laryngeal papillomatosis with 13-cis-retinoic acid (Accutane). J Biol Response Mod 1986; 5:124–8.

197. Bichler E. The role of aromatic retinoid in treatment of laryngeal keratinizing disorders and dysplasias. In: Spitzy KH, Karrer K, eds. Proceedings of the Thirteenth International Congress of Chemotherapy. Vienna: VH Egermann, 1983: 201–29.

198. Bell R, Hong WK, Itri L, McDonald G, Strong S. The use of 13-cis-retinoic acid in recurrent respiratory papillomatosis of the larynx. Am J Otolaryngol 1988; 9:161–4.

199. Gouveia J, Hercend T, Lemaigre G, et al. Degree of bronchial metaplasia in heavy smokers and its regression after treatment with a retinoid. Lancet 1982; 1:710–12.

200. Mathe G, Gouveia J, Hercend T, et al. Correlation between precancerous bronchial metaplasia and cigarette consumption, the preliminary results of retinoid treatment. Cancer Detect Prev 1982; 5:461–6.

201. Misset JL, Mathe G, Santelli G, et al. Regression of bronchial epidermoid metaplasia in heavy smokers with etretinate treatment. Cancer Detect Prev 1986; 9:167–70.

202. Lippman SM, Hittelman WN, Lotan R, Pastorino U, Hong WK. Recent advances in cancer chemoprevention—A meeting report. Cancer Cells 1991; 3:59−65.

203. Port C, Sporn M, Kaufman D. Prevention of lung cancers in hamsters by 13-cis-retinoic-acid (abstr). Proc Am Assoc Cancer Res 1975; 16:24.

204. Lippman SM, Peters EJ, Wargovich MJ, et al. The evaluation of micronuclei as an intermediate endpoint of bronchial carcinogenesis. In: Engstrom PF, ed. Advances in cancer control VII. New York: Alan R Liss, 1990; 339:165−77.

205. Browman GP, Arnold A, Booker L, Johnstone B, Skingley P, Levine MN. Etretinate blood levels in monitoring of compliance and contamination in a chemoprevention trial. JNCI 1989; 81:795−8.

206. Muñoz N, Bang LJ, Day NE, et al. No effect of riboflavine, retinol, and zinc on prevalence of precancerous lesions of oesophagus: Randomized double-blind intervention study in high-risk population of China. Lancet 1985; 2:111−14.

207. Muñoz N, Hayashi M, Bang LJ, Wahrendorf J, Crespi M, Bosch FX. Effect of riboflavin, retinol and zinc on micronuclei of buccal mucosa and of esophagus: A randomized double-blind intervention study in China. JNCI 1987; 79:687−91.

208. Wahrendorf J, Muñoz N, Jian-Bang L, Thurnham DI, Crespi M, Bosch FX. Blood, retinol and zinc riboflavin status in relation to precancerous lesions of the esophagus: Findings from a vitamin intervention trial in the People's Republic of China. Cancer Res 1988; 48:2280−3.

209. Rabinovitch PS, Reid BJ, Haggitt RC, Norwood TH, Rubin CE. Progression to cancer in Barrett's esophagus is associated with genomic instability. Lab Invest 1988; 60:65−71.

210. Sampliner RE, Garewal HS. Phase II trial of 13-cis retinoic acid (isotretinoin) in Barrett's esophagus. Gastroenterology 1988; 94:A396.

211. Garewal H, Sampliner R. Barrett's esophagus: A unique premalignant lesion for adenocarcinoma. Prev Med 1989; 18:749−56.

212. Heddle JA. A rapid in vivo test for chromosomal damage. Mutat Res 1973; 18:187−90.

213. Stich HF, Stich W, Rosin MP, Vallejera MO. Use of the micronucleus test to minotor the effect of vitamin A, beta-carotene and canthaxanthin on the buccal mucosa of betel nut/tobacco chewers. Int J Cancer 1984; 34:745−50.

214. Rosin MP, Dunn BP, Stich HF. Use of intermediate endpoints in quantitating the response of precancerous lesions to chemopreventive agents. Can J Physiol Pharmacol 1987; 65:483−7.

215. Stich HF, Dunn BP. Relationship between cellular levels of beta-carotene and sensitivity to genotoxic agents. Int J Cancer 1986; 38:713−17.

216. Stich HF, Rosin MP. Micronuclei in exfoliated human cells as a tool for studies in cancer risk and cancer intervention. Cancer Lett 1984; 22:241−53.

217. Lippman S, Toth B, Batsakis J, et al. The evaluation of biologic markers as intermediate endpoints in a chemoprevention trial of 13-cis-retinoic acid (13cRA) in human premalignant oral lesions (abstr). Proc Am Soc Clin Oncol 1989; 8:168.

218. Reali D, Di Marino F, Bahramandpour S, Carducci A, Barale R, Loprieno N. Micronuclei in exfoliated urothelial cells and urine mutagenicity in smokers. Mutat Res 1987; 192:145−9.

219. Stich HF, Rosin MP, Vallejera MO. Reduction with vitamin A and beta-carotene administration of proportion of micronucleated buccal mucosal cells in Asian betel nut and tobacco chewers. Lancet 1984; 1:1204−6.

220. Lippman SM, Peters E, Wargovich M, et al. Bronchial micronuclei as a marker of an "early" intermediate endpoint of carcinogenesis in the tracheobronchial epithelium. Int J Cancer 1990; 45:811−15.

221. Modiano MR, Dalton WS, Lippman SM, Joffe L, Booth AR, Meyskens FL. Phase II study of fenretinide (N-[4-hydroxyphenyl]retinamide) in advanced breast cancer and melanoma. Invest New Drugs 1990; 8:317−9.

222. Lippman SM, Spitz MR. Intervention in the premalignant process. Cancer Bull 1991; 43:473−4.

223. Lippman SM, Lee JS, Lotan R, Hittelman W, Wargovich MJ,

Hong WK. Biomarkers as intermediate endpoints in chemoprevention trials. JNCI 1990; 82:555−60.

224. Lipkin M. Biomarkers of increased susceptibility to gastrointestinal cancer: New application to studies of cancer prevention in human subjects. Cancer Res. 1988; 48:235−45.

225. Lippman SM, Toth BB, Batsakis JG, et al. Low-dose 13-cis-retinoic acid (13cRA) maintains remission in oral premalignancy: More effective than β-carotene in randomized trial. Slide pres. Proc Amer Soc Clin Oncol. 1990; 9:59. Washington: ASCO, 1990.

226. Goodman GE. Phase II trial of retinol in patients with advanced cancers. Cancer Treat Rep 1986; 70:1023−4.

227. Omenn GS, Goodman GE, Kleinman GD, et al. The role of intervention studies in ascertaining the contribution of dietary factors in lung cancer: The Seattle chemoprevention trial of retinoids in asbestos-exposed workers. Ann NY Acad Sci 1988; 534:575−83.

228. Prentice RL, Omenn GS, Goodman GE, et al. Rationale and design of cancer chemoprevention studies in Seattle, NCI Monogr 1985; 69:249−58.

229. Kalman DA, Goodman GE, Omenn GS, Bellamy G, Rollins B. Micronutrient assay for cancer prevention clinical trials: Serum retinol, retinyl palmitate, alpha-carotene, and beta-carotene with the use of high-performance liquid chromatography. JNCI 1987; 79:975−82.

230. Meyskens FL Jr, Gilmartin E, Alberts DS, et al. Activity of isotretinoin against squamous cell cancers and preneoplastic lesions. Cancer Treat Rep 1982; 66:1315−19.

231. Lippman SM, Kessler JF, Al-Sarraf M, et al. Treatment of advanced squamous cell carcinoma of the head and neck with isotretinoin: A phase II randomized trial. Invest New Drugs 1988; 6:13−17.

232. Hong WK, Bromer R. Chemotherapy in head and neck cancer. N Engl J Med. 1983; 308:75−9.

233. Weber RS, Lippman SM, McNeese MD. Advanced basal and squamous cell carcinoma of the head and neck. In: Jacobs C, ed. Head and neck oncology. Norwell: Kluwer Academic Publishers, 1990: 61−81.

234. Holoye PY, Byers RM, Gard DA, Goepfert H, Guillamondegui OM, Jesse RH. Combination chemotherapy of head and neck cancer. Cancer 1978; 42:1661−9.

235. Kraemer KH, DiGiovanna JJ, Moshell AN, Tarone RE, Peck GL. Prevention of skin cancer in xeroderma pigmentosum with the use of oral isotretinoin. N Engl J Med 1988; 318:1633−7.

236. Lippman SM, Meyskens FL. Results of the use of vitamin A and retinoids in cutaneous malignancies. Pharmacol Ther 1989; 40:107−22.

237. Lippman SM, Meyskens FL. Treatment of advanced squamous cell carcinoma of the skin with isotretinoin. Ann Intern Med 1987; 107:499−501.

238. Lippman SM, Parkinson DR, Itri LM, et al. 13-cis-retinoic acid and interferon α-2a: effective combination therapy of advanced squamous cell carcinoma of the skin. JNCI 1992; 84:235−41.

239. Lippman SM, Kavanagh JJ, Paredes-Espinoza M, et al. 13-cis-retinoic acid plus interferon α-2a: highly active systemic therapy for squamous cell carcinoma of the cervix. JNCI 1992; 84:241−5.

240. Komiyama S, Kudoh S, Yanagita T, Kuwano M. Synergistic combination therapy of 5-fluorouracil, vitamin A, and cobalt-60 radiation for head and neck tumors: Antitumor combination therapy with vitamin A. Auris Nasus Larynx 1985; 12:S239−43.

241. Edamatsu, H, Chikuda K, Hasegawa M. Vitamin A: Disorder of otorhinolaryngology. Otorhinolaryngology 1982; 54:941.

242. Thatcher N, Blackledge G, Crowther D. Advanced recurrent squamous cell carcinoma of the head and neck: Results of a chemotherapeutic regimen with adriamycin, bleomycin, 5-fluorouracil, methotrexate, and vitamin A. Cancer 1980; 46:1324−8.

243. Mills EED. The modifying effect of beta-carotene on radiation and chemotherapy induced oral mucositis. Br J Cancer 1988; 57:416−17.

244. Pange WR. Regression of head and neck carcinoma with a

prostaglandin-synthesis inhibitor. Arch Otolaryngol 1981; 107:658−63.

245. McCormick KJ, Panje WR. Indomethacin-induced augmentation of lymphoproliferative responses in patients with head and neck cancer. Cancer Immunol Immunother 1986; 21:226−32.

246. Jung TTK, Berlinger NT, Juhn SK. Prostaglandins in squamous cell carcinoma of the head and neck: A preliminary study. Laryngoscope 1985; 95:307−12.

247. Wanebo HJ, Riley T, Katz D, Pace RC, Johns ME, Cantrell RW. Indomethacin sensitive suppressor-cell activity in head and neck cancer patients: The role of the adherent mononuclear cell. Cancer 1988; 61:462−74.

248. Warren S, Gates O. Multiple primary malignant tumors: A survey of the literature and statistical study. Am J Cancer 1932; 51:1358−403.

249. Licciardello JTW, Spitz MR, Hong WK. Multiple primary cancer in patients with cancer of the head and neck: Second cancer of the head and neck, esophagus, and lung. Int J Radiat Oncol Biol Phys 1989; 17:467−76.

250. McDonald S, Haie C, Rubin P, Nelson D, Divers LD. Second malignant tumors of laryngeal carcinoma: Diagnosis, treatment, and prevention. Int J. Radiat Oncol Biol Phys 1989; 17:457−65.

251. Cooper JS, Pajak TF, Rubin P, et al. Second malignancies in patients who have head and neck cancers: Incidence, effect on survival and implications for chemoprevention based on the RTOG experience. Int J Radiat Oncol Biol Phys 1989; 17:449−56.

252. Parker RG, Enstrom JE. Second primary cancers of the head and neck following treatment of initial primary head and neck cancers. Int J Radiat Oncol Biol Phys 1988; 14:561−4.

253. Moore C. Cigarette smoking in cancer of the mouth, pharynx, and larynx—A continuing study. JAMA 1971; 218:553−8.

254. Castigliano SC. Influence of continuous smoking on the incidence of second primary cancers involving mouth, pharynx and larynx. J Am Dent Assoc 1968; 77:580−5.

255. Wynder EL, Dodo H, Bloch DA, Gantt RC, Moore OS. Epidemiologic investigation of multiple cancer in the upper alimentary and respiratory tracts. Cancer 1969; 24:730−9.

256. Hellquist H, Lundgren J, Olofosson J. Hyperplasia, keratosis, dysplasia, and carcinoma in situ of the vocal cords. Clin Otolaryngol 1982; 7:11−27.

257. Gillis TM, Incze J, Strong MS, Vaughan CW, Simpson GT. Natural history and management of keratosis, atypia, carcinoma in situ and microinvasive cancer of the larynx. Am J Surg 1983; 146:512−19.

258. Hong WK, Lippman SM, Itri LM, et al. Prevention of second primary tumors with isotretinoin in squamous-cell carcinoma of the head and neck. N Eng J Med 1990; 323:795−801.

259. Braakhuis BJ, van Dongen GA, van Walsum M, Leyva A, Snow GB. Preclinical antitumor activity of 5-aza-2′-deoxycytidine against human head and neck cancer xenografts. Invest New Drugs 1988; 6:299−304.

260. Waxman S, Scher W, Scher BM. Basic principles for utilizing combination differentiation agents. Cancer Detect Prev 1986; 9:395−407.

261. Lotan R, Nicolson GL. Can anticancer therapy be improved by sequential use of cytotoxic and cytostatic (differentiating or immunomodulating) agents to suppress tumor cell phenotypic diversification? Biochem Pharmacol 1988; 37:149−54.

262. Malone WF, Kelloff GJ. Chemoprevention strategies utilizing combinations of inhibitors of carcinogenesis. JNCI 1989; 81:824.

Index

NB: Page numbers in *italics* refer to figures and tables.